PRINCIPLES OF PATHOBIOLOGY

PRINCIPLES OF

SECOND EDITION

Edited by Mariano F. La Via

New York · OXFORD UNIVERSITY PRESS

PATHOBIOLOGY

and Rolla B. Hill, Jr.

London · 1975 · Toronto

Library of Congress Catalogue Card Number: 74-83989
Printed in the United States of America

FOREWORD

Classically, the pathologist has contributed to the study of human disease by describing advanced changes in cells and tissues, and it has often appeared that disease states differed fundamentally from the normal condition. More recently, because of tremendous advances in our knowledge of biochemistry, physiology, and microbiology as applied to medicine, we have been able to trace the pathogenesis of many disorders from their early onset. This new book presents the concept of disease as an abnormal biological process that differs quantitatively, rather than qualitatively, from normal biological mechanisms. This approach will illuminate for medical, dental, and biology students the study of disease and will fill a significant deficit in the textual material presently available.

The book consists of seven chapters covering the basic areas of pathology. The chapters on cellular changes, inflammation, and host-parasite relations discuss several states in the reaction to injury, progressing from the molecular to the organismal level. These sections are written by active experimental pathologists who recognize that the compartmentalization of knowledge, a laudable and necessary goal in the research laboratory, cannot be the objective of students. Rather, students must integrate an infinite number of changes in ultrastructural organization and intermediary metabolism caused by multiple insults at the cellular level, and superimpose an awareness of the interactions and control processes of cells and tissue at the organ and organismal level.

Although growth is a response to injury as well as a normal phase of development, uncontrolled growth or neoplasia has assumed a unique role in pathology. Recent progress in understanding the implications of viruses, hormones, and immunological factors in carcinogenesis is of intense current interest to all biologists; in addition, the older work on physical and chemical carcinogens has taken on new relevance. The chapter on neoplasia is one of the few available in the literature which makes a careful review of the entire field.

Immunological mechanisms play a dual role in injury and defense reactions. Antibody response to foreign moieties, such as bacteria and viruses, may protect an individual against clinical disease. Acute and delayed hypersensitivity, formerly associated with anaphylaxis, serum sickness, and tuberculosis, have now proven to be a serious problem in organ transplantation. "Self-injury" or autoimmunization has become of great importance in diseases affecting all organs, but particularly the kidney, thyroid, bowel, heart, and central nervous system.

In the final chapter we are reminded that, in addition to well-documented biochemical inborn errors of metabolism, cytogenetic abnormalities, and teratologic defects in development, all disease states have a genetic basis that eventually determines the fate of the organism.

The editors have done a splendid job of identifying six basic areas of pathobiology or general pathology. They have presented their information in a succinct, integrated manner in a beautifully illustrated text, small enough to be used in core curricula, and large enough to provide an excellent review of the current state of the field.

DONALD WEST KING
Delafield Professor of Pathology
College of Physicians and Surgeons
Columbia University

PREFACE

It is a truism that several conflicting forces are making the design of curricula in the biological and medical sciences very difficult. The much-touted information explosion of recent years must somehow be dealt with in these curricula. Disciplines are losing their discrete identities, and it is not always clear what is medical and what is biological. Disciplinary teaching time in required courses in medical schools is rapidly diminishing to allow for more electives and "integrated" interdisciplinary courses.

In its own field this textbook is an attempt to reconcile these conflicts and to fill a void that has existed for several years. The subject matter is that which has been known as General Pathology—the interface between biology and pathology, encompassing growth, metabolism, and biologic interaction as well as the effects of external and internal injuries on these general processes. It will be useful in those medical and dental schools where pressures have forced the adoption of a limited "core" curriculum in general pathology; it will be equally appropriate for biology or zoology departments that feel the need to expose their students to the principles governing some of the extremes of biological activity known as disease. The book is designed for easy use by busy students; it deals with current knowledge directly and intelligibly, avoiding the reconditeness and jargon of research papers.

In organizing this book it has been necessary to make some hard decisions. Some areas in general pathology that might be considered important have been either omitted or dealt with very briefly because of space limitations. Other relatively rare entities have been stressed because of fundamental concepts that they illuminate. We make no apologies for these decisions, which have been made consciously but which will obviously differ from the decisions that might have been made by others. Similar thought has gone into the bibliographies, which are thorough but in no sense exhaustive. It has been our abiding rule to consider the needs and capabilities of the student in the modern curriculum.

ROLLA B. HILL, JR.
MARIANO F. LA VIA

February 1971

Note to the Second Edition

This second edition is coming out earlier than originally planned—thanks to the enthusiastic reception accorded the first edition and the understanding of our publisher, who concurred in our wish to keep this book as up-to-date as possible for maximum usefulness to the readers. Thus, our thanks go to all who made this second effort possible. Each chapter has been revised and updated extensively; the second chapter has been rewritten entirely, with the purpose of presenting the material in a context that more closely relates it to human pathology. It is our sincere hope that this small contribution to the literature of pathology will be, as we intend it to be, an aid to all who need it.

M. F. L.
R. B. H.

September 1974

ACKNOWLEDGMENTS

Chapter 2	Supported by NIH grants SAM15440 and GM00431 to B.F.T. and by grants from Sigrid Juselius Foundation and the Finnish National Research Council for Natural Sciences to A.U.A. The authors wish to express their appreciation to the following colleagues who reviewed the manuscript and made many helpful suggestions: Peter J. Goldblatt, Hal K. Hawkins, David T. Janigan, Susan R. Panny, Elizabeth M. McDowell, John D. Shelburne, and Robert E. Stowell. Dr. Raymond T. Jones provided valuable assistance in the editorial work.
Chapter 4	The author wishes to express his appreciation to Mrs. Ala Jo Koonts for secretarial work.
Chapter 6	Supported by NIH grants CA–08856, CA–06927, CA–05255, CA–13456, RR–05539, and by an appropriation from the Commonwealth of Pennsylvania.

CONTRIBUTORS

ANTTI U. ARSTILA, M.D.

Professor and Chairman
Department of Cell Biology
University of Jyvaskyla, Finland
Assistant Professor of Pathology
University of Maryland
Baltimore, Maryland 21201

ROLLA B. HILL, JR., M.D.

Professor and Chairman
Department of Pathology
State University of New York
Upstate Medical Center
Syracuse, New York 13210

MARIANO F. LA VIA, M.D.

Professor
Department of Pathology
and Laboratory Medicine
Emory University School of Medicine
Atlanta, Georgia 30322

CHARLES E. MCCALL, M.D.

Associate Professor of Medicine
Associate in Pharmacology
The Bowman Gray School of Medicine
Winston-Salem, North Carolina 27103

RICHMOND T. PREHN, M.D.

Senior Member
The Institute for Cancer Research
Fox Chase
Philadelphia, Pennsylvania 19111

ROBERT H. SHIKES, M.D.

Assistant Professor
Department of Pathology
University of Colorado
Medical Center
Denver, Colorado 80220

BENJAMIN F. TRUMP, M.D.

Professor and Chairman
Department of Pathology
University of Maryland
Baltimore, Maryland 21201

PETER A. WARD, M.D.

Professor and Chairman
Department of Pathology
University of Connecticut Health Center
Farmington, Connecticut 06032

CONTENTS

PRINCIPLES OF PATHOBIOLOGY

1

PATHOBIOLOGY AND THE MEDICAL SCIENCES

Rolla B. Hill, Jr., M.D.

> Contemplations of nature and of bodies in their simple form break up and distract the understanding, while contemplations of nature and bodies in their composition and configuration overpower and dissolve the understanding . . . for that school is so busy with the particles that it hardly attends to the structure, while the others are so lost in admiration of the structure that they do not penetrate to the simplicity of nature.
>
> *Francis Bacon*

During its short life the discipline of cellular biology has grown with astonishing rapidity. Enormous and unenvisioned knowledge has been gained. The mechanism of transfer of genetic information is being steadily clarified; the mysteries of the control and expression of that genetic information are gradually yielding to experimentation; tools are being applied which allow the forbidding problems of morphogenesis, differentiation, and maturation to be approached.

Progress toward general understanding of disease at the molecular or cellular level has not kept pace with advances in normal biology, yet there are many isolated examples of brilliant work illuminating aspects of abnormal biology. For instance, our understanding of the nature of viral parasitism, of the specific enzymatic defects in the inborn errors of metabolism, of aspects of immunological deficiencies and diseases, and of the causes of hemoglobinopathies, has been greatly enriched by knowledge gained in the study of normal biology.

These new contributions to the study of disease have been achieved by close cooperation among scientists from disciplines previously devoted separately to normal or abnormal biology. From this fruitful union came pathobiology, a science integrating cell biology and classical pathology, encompassing normal processes of growth, metabolism, and biologic interaction, and the effects of external and internal injuries on these processes.

This science has not been with us long enough to have generated a strong philosophical basis, and we still grope at times to find applicability and meaning. Nevertheless, we must attempt a modern approach to what, in the heyday of descriptive morphologic pathology, was the unity of structure and function, when disease (dysfunction) was to be understood as a reflection of altered anatomy. Dyspnea and cyanosis in pneumonia were caused by the presence of inflammatory debris in the alveoli. Jaundice occurred because blockage of ducts prevented the excretion of bilirubin. Even this approach, which may seem grossly mechanistic to us, is little more than two hundred years old. For the long centuries prior to Morgagni, Bernard, Pasteur, and Virchow, the concept of a direct pathogenetic relation between altered structure and disease was foreign to medical thinking. The concept still has considerable utility, but the time is ripe for a refinement of thought not possible previously.

In 1943 W. D. Forbus, in his book *Reaction to Injury,* attempted to crystallize what was then a relatively new viewpoint in pathology: that disease did not exist except as a reaction to injury. A monumental two-volume work classifying diseases according to types of injurious agents instead of topology set forth this view. Although the format was not widely adopted in teaching programs, the vision insinuated itself into pathology. A dialectical outgrowth of Forbus's contribution has been the concept that disease is *not the imposition of new, different structure and function, but simply the quantitative alteration–increase or decrease–of existing pathways.* The synthesis of these views is that to understand pathology we must understand the changes in structures and functions which occur in response to various injuries. The injurious agents themselves may determine the direction that a reaction will take, but they are bystanders to the disease itself. Once an injury has occurred, forces within the cell, tissue, or organism are brought into action; the interaction of these forces is what produces disease. Responses to injury can be isolated, dissected, and classified, and eventually the individual factors making up the total response can be identified. Although these individual responses are not infinite, they can occur in a bewildering number of combinations and strengths.

This is the subject of pathobiology–the alterations in normal biological mechanisms that occur in response to injury. Alterations in ribosome structure are as important as alterations in cardiac structure, and interference with oxidative phosphorylation is as crippling as interference with blood flow. Neoplasia and immunity are two parts of a general problem of control of cell division, cell growth, and cell differentiation. The proteins important in blood coagulation are synthesized by the same mechanisms and under the same general controls as intracellular enzymes.

The long list of etiological agents of disease does not reflect an equally long list of pathogenetic mechanisms. The dictum that all life processes depend on the cell leads inevitably to questions about these mechanisms. Which category of cellular processes determines the integrity of the cell in response to injury? Although gene action may be a primary directing force, the manifestations of disease must reflect disturbances of enzymatic activity.[1]

This is not to suggest that each injurious agent has a specific enzymatic target. Enzymatic anactivity, hypoactivity, and hyperactivity may result from a direct change in the number of enzyme molecules (through interference with genetic control or any of the steps leading to its expression), or from changes in the physical state of the molecule, or from effects on cofactors, pH, substrates, and other things. Study of the purified enzyme *in vitro* may often not reveal these effects; since this highly artificial situation introduces vast changes in availability of cofactors and substrates, ionic strength and physical state, factors of architectural or spatial relations (for example, enzyme complexes and membrane-bound enzymes) may be totally shattered. Evaluation of enzymes under these conditions may thus indicate an enzyme deficiency which is not in fact present, or it may fail to reveal the presence of an actual functional deficiency. In addition, injuries usually have more than a single target and produce much wider effects than a single enzymatic defect. The enormous discoveries of molecular biology have focused attention on the isolated cell and on isolated injury. The multicellular and the multi-organ organism have so many interlocking, mutually dependent, often mutually corrective mechanisms, that such isolation *in vivo* is indeed rare.

In analyzing injury one can distinguish injuries immediately affecting enzymatic activity from injuries which directly affect a mediating process that then deranges enzymatic activity. These mediators of injury may be chemical structures—e.g., DNA—from which activity of the enzymes originally springs, or physical structures such as a membrane or a polysome, or aggregations of cells whose functions interdependently rely on architectural relations among them.

Variations in enzymatic activity occur frequently in tissue under normal physiological conditions; in fact, such variations are completely essential to survival. Hormones, differentiation and biological rhythms control enzymatic activities, and it may be difficult to distinguish between normal variation and variation due to injury, which can be identical quantitatively and qualitatively. Indeed,

1. I am indebted to Dr. Renzo Rendi for making clear to me the central importance of this.

small, virtually undetectable injuries are constantly occurring and the slight corrective responses which approximate servo-mechanisms constitute homeostasis—the means by which an organism maintains its precarious identity in spite of the myriad internal and external injuries which beset living things.

It is the reaction to injury, not the injury itself, that produces the manifestations of disease. In the hereditary condition known as glucose-6-phosphate dehydrogenase deficiency, *in vitro* tests reveal a decrease in assayed enzyme activity of erythrocytes. This certainly reflects a genetic injury, but there are no symptoms, no overt responses, unless a second circumstance (the ingestion of fava beans, for instance, or doses of the drug primaquin) supervenes. The disease, characterized by hemolysis, does not occur without a secondary agent, but the genetic injury is demonstrably present throughout life.

It must be emphasized that pathology and pathobiology are not separate disciplines but simply subdisciplines of the over-all science of biology. There are no new metabolic pathways occurring in an injured cell; there is simply accentuation, diminution, or loss of existing pathways.[2] There are no new structures; there is simply an increase or decrease in structures that occur in so-called normal cells. Paul Weiss has said: "Even the grossest deformity is produced by the same rigorously lawful molecular and cellular interactions that govern normal development" (1960). Minor injuries occur constantly and cause small perturbations in homeostasis which are corrected as servo-mechanisms are thrown into play. All organisms float restlessly between the states of health and disease.

By now the reader is becoming aware of the difficulties surrounding the use of the word *injury*. It is almost axiomatic that traumatic damage—e.g., a knife wound in the skin—causes injury to tissues which elicits certain predictable homeostatic responses in the injured tissues. It is clear that sustained anoxia causes predictable damage and death to cells; a mild degree of hypoxia, however, causes qualitatively similar changes that result not in death but in a reversibly altered, viable cell. Is this injury? When a recumbent person stands up, striking alterations in vascular physiology occur to accommodate for the alterations related to gravity and change of position. Is this injury? Somebody bumps you slightly so that you lose your balance. If you happen to have your feet firmly planted, you can quickly recover your balance without falling. If not, you may fall, and this may lead to a bruise or a broken bone, depending on where you are standing. The primary force is the same; the result may be anything from a reflexive rebalancing of muscular tension to severe damage or death.

2. There are a very few exceptions. For instance, in cellular infection by some RNA viruses, the RNA acts as a repository of genetic information, and a template for the synthesis of messenger or DNA. These have not yet been identified as functions of RNA in normal animal cells.

Can one say, then, that injury occurs whenever the "steady state" is forcibly unbalanced? The agents of injury include anything that is capable of causing unbalance, whether the degree of unbalance is minute or severe, and whether it is correctable or not. Injuries may originate inside or outside the cell. Any minor variation in the external environment requires an adjustment by the cell, and major variations, of course, require major adjustments. Injuries originating within the cell are mainly "genetic" mistakes, including those in transcription or translation. In general, external agents of injury fall into the following categories: drugs, parasites (e.g., viruses, bacteria, fungi, protozoa, metazoa), radiation, trauma, temperature, pH, nutrition, and immunologic phenomena.

The pattern formed by combinations of ultrastructural alterations in reaction to injury may occasionally be so characteristic that one can recognize the injury from the changes observed. The repertory of alterations is sharply limited, however, and usually a great many agents act through a common morphologic pathway. Specific diagnosis can rarely be made with the electron microscope.

At the light microscope level, tissues undergo a broader range of morphological alteration, and the permutations and combinations of these alterations are much more likely to give a characteristic diagnostic pattern. These alterations involve the relations between cells, the cell types, the direction of differentiation of cells, and various degenerative alterations in cells and extracellular materials. Recognition of the patterns formed by these microscopic alterations is the essence of diagnostic pathology, which enables the pathologist to differentiate on morphologic grounds between pneumonia due to pneumococcus and pneumonia due to staphylococcus, between arthritis due to infection and degenerative arthritis, and to detect the precise kind of liver disease which is causing the patient to become jaundiced.

Inflammatory and immunological reactions, both accorded considerable attention in this book, are natural properties of vertebrates. Both are complex combinations of interacting humoral and cellular forces, which contribute considerably to survival in the evolutionary struggle and help in coping with a variety of foreign agents, both living and inanimate. Both are subject also to occasional errors which pervert the reactions, so that considerable damage to host tissue ensues.

Only rarely does an injury lead to disability. It is what happens after the injury that usually causes disease. Certainly the severing of the head with an ax is an injury that in itself causes observable damage and disability. The injection of several million *Staphylococcus aureus* under the skin, however, is quite harmless in itself; it is the reaction of the body to the *Staph. aureus* that causes the development of inflammation, abscesses, and pus. In many diseases we do not even know what the injurious agent is. The vast group of diseases collectively called cancer, for instance, has been classified and subclassified and reclassified, but in only a very few cases do we have any clear understanding of the injurious agent. It is the hyperplastic-neoplastic responses to the injury that we see and that cause damage.

Most commonly, injuries are followed by homeostatic responses that restore normalcy. Sometimes a new steady state, differing from the normal but compatible with continued existence, is achieved. Sometimes the compensatory mechanisms used constantly by the cell or the body to maintain the status quo are insufficient, and balance is not restored. The cell, organ, or body can utilize a great variety of compensatory mechanisms, but in the face of overwhelming or continued injury, these may not be enough. Failure may occur (1) because of a greatly increased load on the cell's adaptive mechanisms or (2) because of damage to the adaptive mechanisms. In the case of energy metabolism, for instance, a cell may under certain circumstances be required to produce an extraordinary amount of ATP. The adaptive mechanisms will allow a mild increase in ATP production from existing structures and pathways, but substantially to alter energy production requires new mitochondria. To make mitochondria, however, takes time and ATP. The cell then can be said to be failing prior to the time when new mitochondria are available. The demands for energy may be so great in fact, that the cell is unable to make enough mitochondria to provide this energy. On the other hand, even normal energy requirements cannot be met by the cell exposed to cyanide, which by poisoning cytochrome oxidase prevents normal energy metabolism.

The broad areas of biological injury dealt with in this book have been traditionally known as general pathology. We have attempted to relate them more closely to the science of general biology in order to provide an anchor in modern biology for the student of pathology and an anchor in pathology for the student of biology.

References

Forbus, W. D. (1943), Reaction to Injury; Pathology for Students of Disease, Williams & Wilkins Co., Baltimore.

Weiss, Paul (1960), Deformities as cues to understanding development of form, *in* Disease and the Advancement of Science, H. K. Beecher, Ed., Harvard University Press, Cambridge, Mass.

2

CELLULAR REACTION TO INJURY

B. F. Trump, M.D., and Antti U. Arstila, M.D.

A. Introduction

The understanding of human disease and its treatment rests on an understanding of cellular reaction to injury, since the cellular and subcellular alterations that follow injury constitute the basis of all disease processes. All major manifestations of disease reflect altered cellular and subcellular physiology; indeed, it is at the organelle and macromolecular level that the most detailed correlation between structure and biochemistry is possible in disease states (see reviews by deReuck and Knight, 1965; Farber and Magee, 1965; Trump and Ericsson, 1965; Scarpelli and Trump, 1971; Trump *et al.,* 1971). From intensive investigations into both normal (Fig. 2-1) and abnormal cell biology in recent years, new concepts of disease are emerging. Thus it is possible to begin to speak of diseases as primarily affecting mitochondria, lysosomes, or cell membranes. It is the purpose of this chapter to review the basic concepts of cellular pathophysiology and, in specific instances, to relate them to known human disease processes.

To begin the study of cellular changes in disease, we need an over-all conception of cell injury and to define some terms used in its analysis. An injury is defined as any perturbation that upsets, even transiently, the normal homeostasis of the cell (Fig. 2-2). Injuries or injurious stimuli may be endogenous, often arising from defects in the genome; or they may be exogenous, involving such factors as nutritional deficiency, chemical toxins, microbiologic agents, physical agents, immunologic events, or deprivation of vital components such as occurs in hypoxia, ischemia, or starvation. Cells of different types, in different phases of the mitotic cycle, and at different points in their over-all life span may be affected

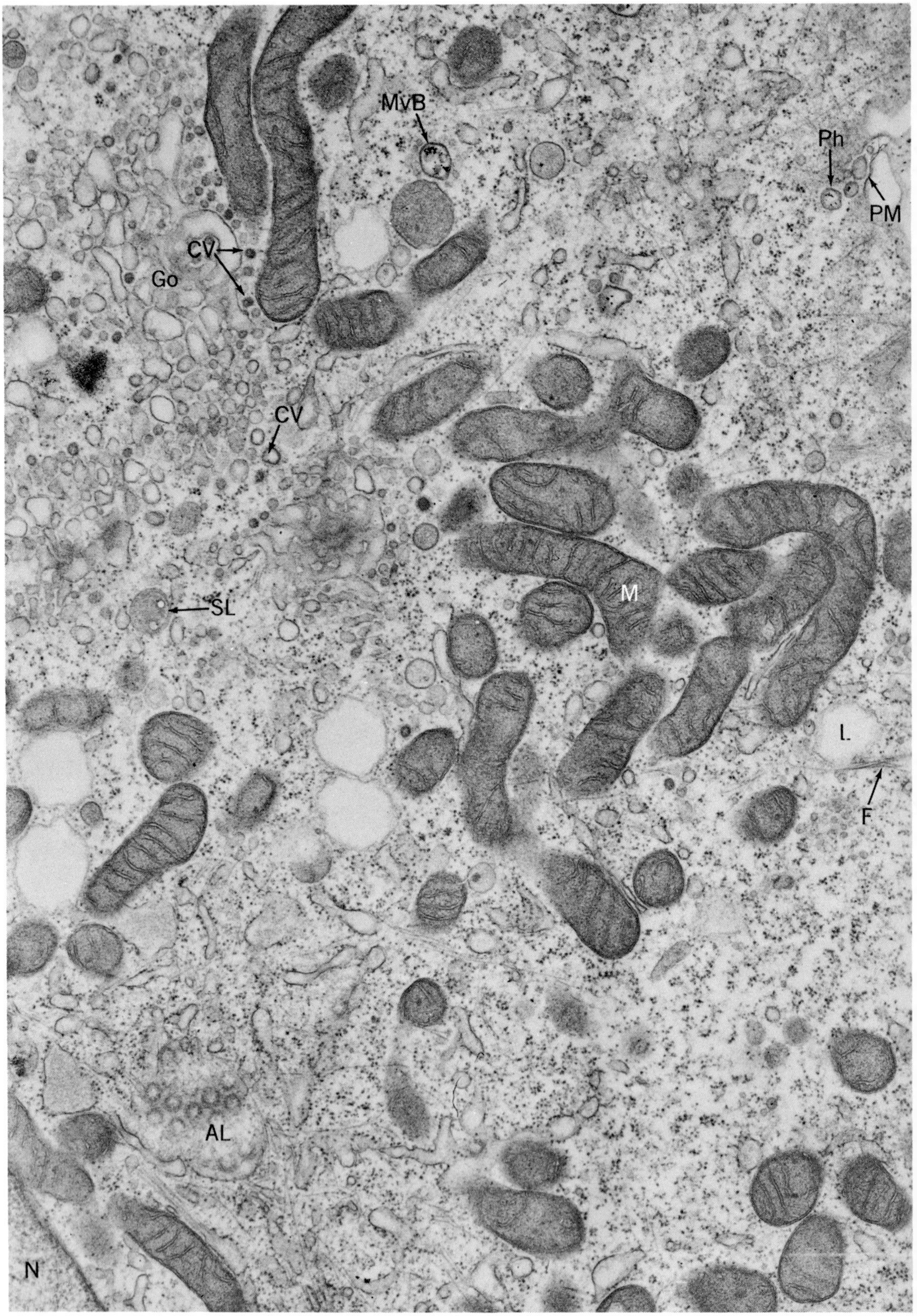
MvB
Ph
PM
CV
Go
CV
SL
M
L
F
AL
N

differently by the same injurious stimulus. A given injury may result in the instantaneous death of cells, or in prolonged survival ranging from minutes to years. Even when a cell survives the immediate effects of the injury, the life span of the cell may be reduced, although such reduction, if measured over months or years, may be difficult or impossible to assess. An example of virtually instantaneous lethal injury is that caused by sudden chemical treatment by fixatives such as formaldehyde or osmium tetroxide, which may kill the cell without substantially altering the morphology, even at the ultrastructural level. Few injuries occurring in human disease kill the cell, however; and when an injury is lethal, cell death is usually delayed.

1. Acute lethal injury

Complete ischemia is a rapidly lethal condition capable of producing irreversible damage in a neuron in 3 to 4 minutes, in a heart muscle cell in 15 to 20 minutes, or in a proximal convoluted tubule of the kidney in 1 to 2 hours at body temperature. If the injurious stimulus is removed by restoring the blood supply before the cell dies, however, it may recover and complete a normal life. If the ischemia persists, the cell becomes irreversibly injured and is said to die or to pass a "point of no return," then entering a phase called necrosis, in which its predominant reactions are denaturation and hydrolysis of cell components (see reviews by Majno *et al.,* 1960; Trump *et al.,* 1971). Death and necrosis are thus clearly distinguishable. Cell death means loss of reversibility; necrosis refers to the degradative reactions occurring after death. Direct chemical fixation, for example, would cause death without necrosis; ischemia would result in death followed by necrosis. Many of the degradative reactions of necrosis are the result of digestion by the cell's own enzymes, including the lysosomal hydrolases; hence, they are often collectively termed *autolysis.*

The term *autolysis* has been used to distinguish the degradative reactions occurring in cells after the somatic death of the entire body, from those occurring after the death of individual cells, groups of cells, or tissues in a live host. The

Figure 2-1. Electron micrograph of a portion of a HeLa cell, illustrating characteristic features of the cytoplasm of mammalian cells. This cell was grown in a medium containing colloidal thorium dioxide, which was phagocytosed by the cells and is now present within phagocytic vacuoles and lysosomes. Note the prominent Golgi apparatus (Go) and the appearance of the mitochondria (M), lipid droplets (L), annulate lamellae (AL), phagosomes (Ph), and a multivesicular body (MvB). Coated vesicles (CV) are present near the Golgi apparatus. Cytoplasmic filaments (F) course through the cytoplasm. A secondary lysosome (SL) can be seen. PM, plasma membrane; N, nucleus.

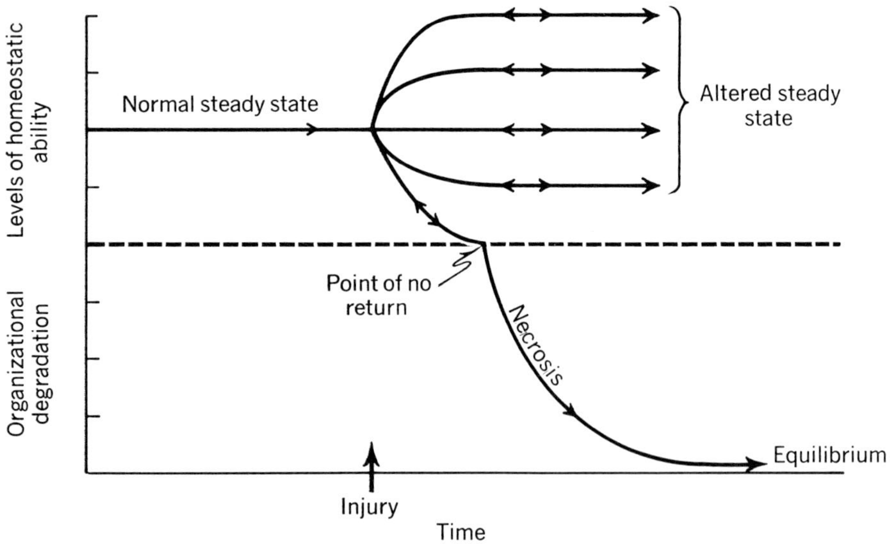

Figure 2-2. Conceptualization of cell injury. Following sub-lethal injury, a cell previously in a normal steady state can be considered to enter a phase in which the homeostatic mechanisms are altered, resulting in new steady states such as fatty metamorphosis, hypertrophy, or atrophy. The cell may remain in such new steady state for long periods while the injury is prolonged. In the case of lethal injuries, on the other hand, the cell can eventually be assumed to pass a point (shown as zero level of homeostatic ability) beyond which it is unable to restore equilibrium even if the injury is eliminated. The zero level of homeostatic ability may be referred to as the **point of no return** or the **point of cell death.** Beyond this, the cell undergoes a series of degradative reactions leading to the production of cell debris or a state of physicochemical equilibrium. (From Trump, B. F., and Ginn, F. L., **Methods and Achievements in Experimental Pathology,** vol. 4, E. Bajusz and G. Jasmin, Eds., Yearbook Medical Publishers, Chicago, 1969)

distinction is, however, artificial, since the same degradative reactions occur in both situations.

2. Somatic death versus cell death

Considerable confusion attends the term "death," mainly because it is currently impossible to define life. The phrase "somatic death" refers to the death of the entire body; it is largely a legal conception that has evolved over the years, defined by physical or electrical signs that correlate with loss of reversibility. Absence of heart beat, pulse, respiration, or brain waves have been used to define death. Somatic death is clearly different from cell death, since after cessation of heart beat and blood flow the cells become ischemic, and survive for various periods of time, depending on the cell type, the decreasing temperature of the body, and other factors. For this reason it is possible to remove organs for transplantation from individuals who have been pronounced dead; some cells, such as fibroblasts, may be successfully cultured many hours after somatic death.

3. Chronic (sub-lethal) injury

Some types of injury are not immediately lethal to the cell but result in changes of structure and function which, though rendering the cell different from its normal counterpart, are compatible with maintenance of cellular homeostasis over long periods of time, measured in months or years. These alterations include lipid accumulation in cells, formation of autophagic lysosomes and pigmented residual bodies within the cytoplasm, several kinds of watery vacuolation ("cloudy swelling") including dilatation of the endoplasmic reticulum (ER) or of the phago-lysosomal system, modifications in the microtubules with inhibition of mitotic division and cell migration, formation of cytoplasmic or nuclear inclusions, atrophy or reduction in size, and hypertrophy or increase in size. Special cases of adaptation of cells with alteration in the mitotic cycle, as well as striking cell surface changes, occur in the case of neoplastic transformation.

B. Light Microscopy of Injured Cells (Figures 2-3 and 2-4)

Ever since Virchow proposed the cell theory of disease–shortly after Schleiden and Schwann's introduction of the cell theory of life–light microscopy has been the principal technique used to study cell injury. At present the light microscope remains one of the most widely used instruments for studying cells and classifying disease. Many innovations have broadened its range of use, including phase, interference, fluorescence, and polarization microscopy, histo- and cytochemistry, time-lapse cinematography, autoradiography, and microspectrophotometry. What follows is an account of certain alterations in injured cells that can be seen with the light microscope.

1. Lethal reactions

Reactions that indicate that necrosis is occurring–i.e., that the cell has passed the "point of no return"–are the most dramatic. An early cytoplasmic change is increased eosinophilia. This reaction results partially from increased binding of eosin by cytoplasmic proteins. At the pH conventionally used in stain-

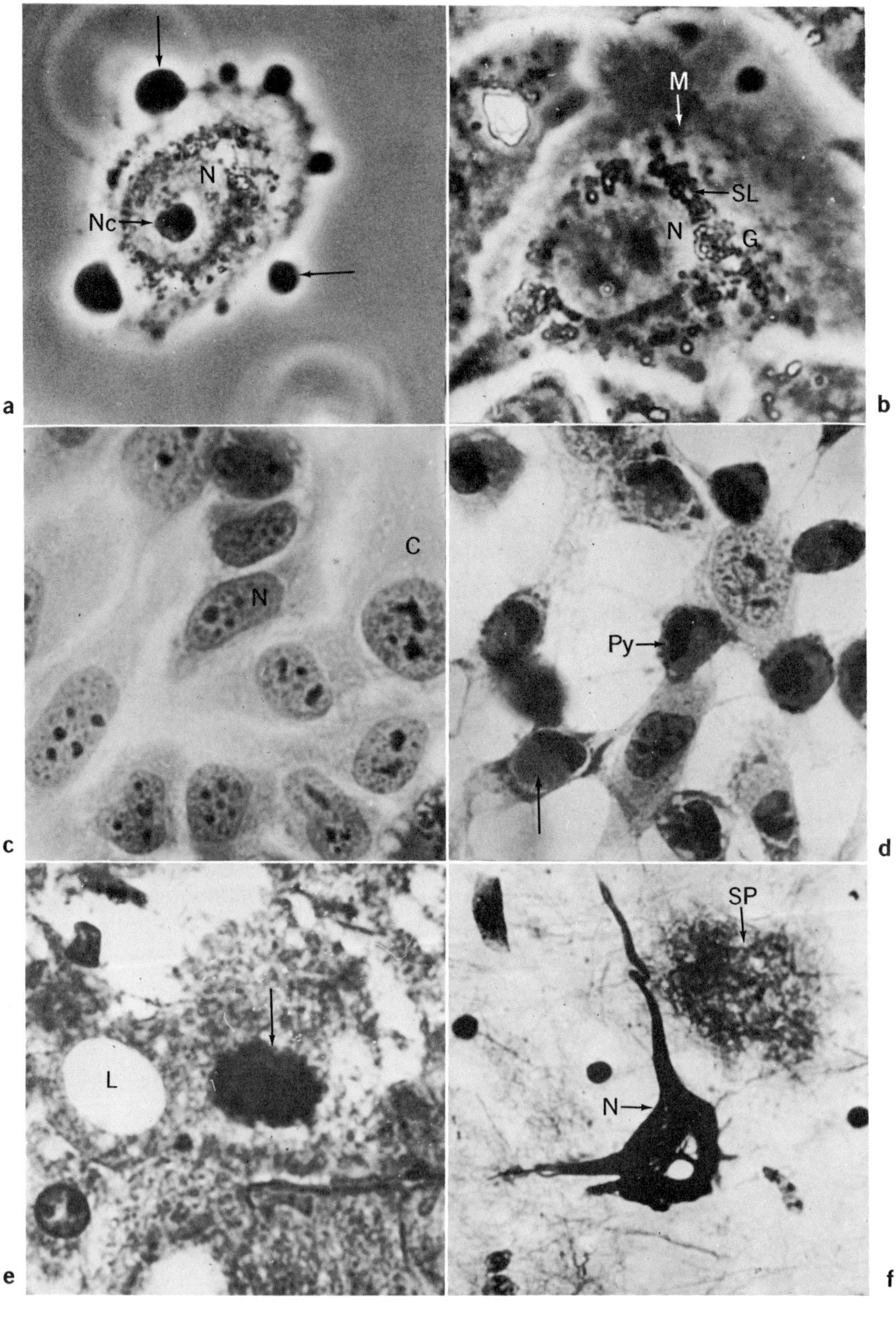
N
Nc
M
SL
N
G
C
N
Py
L
SP
N
a
b
c
d
e
f

ing, eosin is negatively charged; the increased binding has been interpreted as a result of greater exposure of positively charged reactive sites along polypeptide chains after their denaturation. Another cause of the increased eosinophilia is the loss of cytoplasmic basophilia (loss of binding of hematoxylin, a positively charged dye), which usually reflects detachment and scattering of polysomes from rough-surfaced endoplasmic cisternae. Another change that can be seen in the cytoplasm in good preparations is swelling of mitochondria, visible as eosinophilic globules because of their high content of basic proteins. The cell margins may show irregularities and protrusions related to the blebs of the membranes (Fig. 2-3a). Late in the course of necrosis, granulation and irregular spaces in the cytoplasm represent the effects of denaturation and digestion of cytoplasmic organelles. A common change in the necrotic phase is deposition of complex calcium phosphates within the cytoplasm, often related to mitochondrial damage.

In the nucleus the initial changes often include accentuation of the chromatin clumps. Because of the variations produced by fixation, which itself may induce chromatin clumping, this alteration is often difficult to assess. Later changes in the nucleus consist of coarsening, increased basophilia, and shrinking of the

Figure 2-3. a. HeLa cell 15 minutes after addition of potassium cyanide (10^{-3}M) and iodoacetic acid (10^{-4}M) to the medium. When given together, these compounds inhibit both glycolysis and respiration. Blebs (arrows) have appeared at the cell surface. The nucleus (N), the nucleolus (Nc), and the cytoplasmic organelles, visualized as granules in the perinuclear area, have a normal appearance. Phase contrast.

b. Untreated living HeLa cell photographed under phase contrast. Note the thin cytoplasm and cytoplasmic processes. N, nucleus; G, Golgi; SL, secondary lysosomes; M, mitochondrion.

c. Untreated HeLa cells photographed after fixation, sectioning, and staining. The nucleus (N), nucleoli, and cytoplasm (C) appear quite different from those of the unfixed cell in Figure 3b. H & E stain. (Courtesy of Dr. C. A. Daniels)

d. HeLa cells 12 hours after infection with polio virus. Note the necrotic cell with shrunken pyknotic nucleus (Py) and eosinophilic cytoplasmic inclusion (arrow). Long cytoplasmic strands emerge from the cell surface. An adjacent nucleus is less altered. These are fixed cells viewed with conventional light microscopy. H & E stain. (Courtesy of Dr. C. A. Daniels)

e. Liver cell from a patient with alcoholic cirrhosis. The arrow indicates a mass of alcoholic hyalin in the cytoplasm of a hepatic parenchymal cell. A lipid droplet (L) is present also. Trichrome stain.

f. Neuron (N) from brain of elderly person, showing cytoplasmic staining characteristic of neurofibrillary tangles. A senile plaque (SP) is seen in the upper right. Trichrome stain.

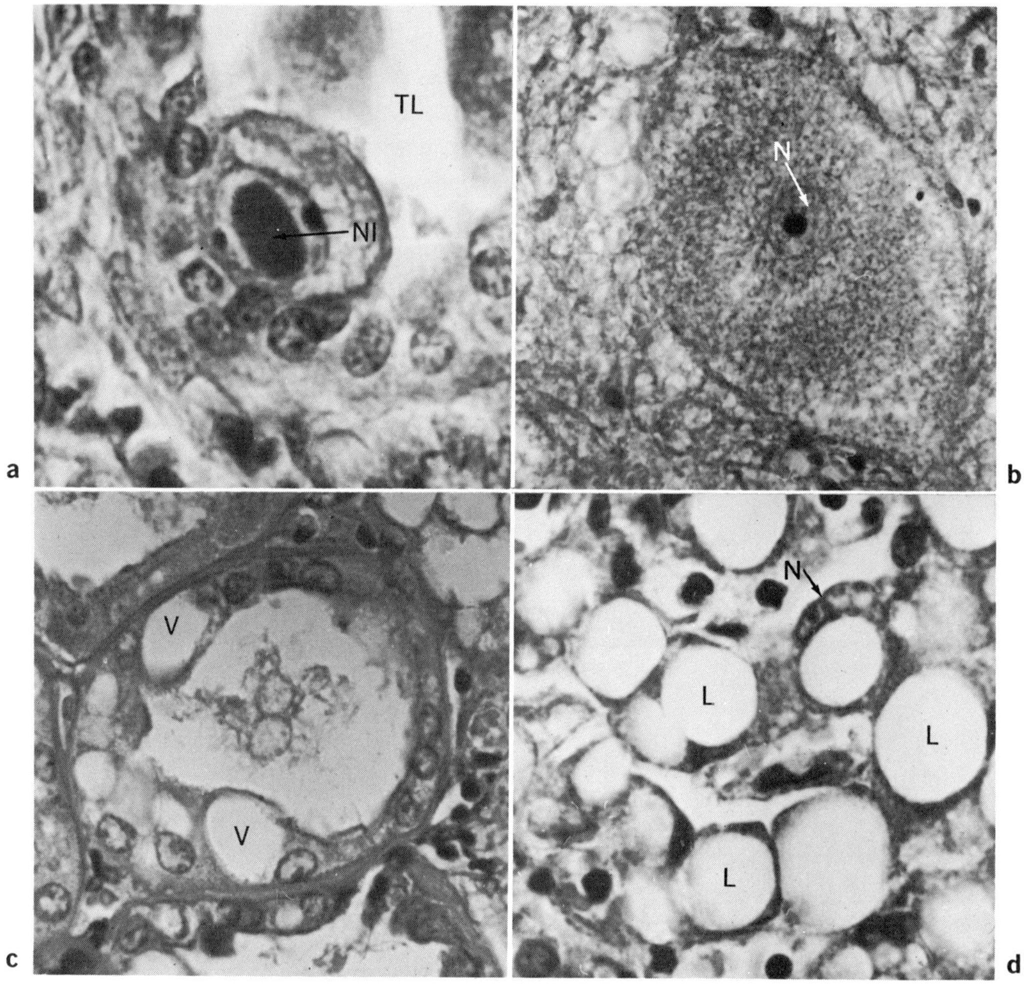

Figure 2-4. **a.** Kidney tubule cell from a patient with cytomegalic inclusion disease. The large nucleus contains an inclusion body (NI), which consists of virus particles. TL, tubular lumen. H & E stain.

b. Spinal neuron from a patient with Tay Sachs disease. The fine, scattered lipid inclusions are basophilic and consist principally of gangliosides. N, nucleus. H & E stain.

c. Kidney tubules from a patient with hypokalemic nephrosis. Scattered large vacuoles (V) appear in the proximal tubular epithelium in such patients. H & E stain.

d. Liver cells from a patient with alcoholic cirrhosis. The hepatic parenchymal cells contain large triglyceride droplets (L). Nuclei (N) are indented by the lipid. H & E stain.

chromatin clumps (pyknosis) (Fig. 2-3d), fragmentation of chromatin clumps or nuclei (karyorrhexis), or disappearance of stainable chromatin material (karyolysis). The nuclear changes observed depend in part on the cell type and phase of the cell cycle.

2. Pre-lethal or sub-lethal reactions

VACUOLES. Clear "vacuoles," frequently seen in conventionally stained preparations of injured cells, are diverse in origin, and the cause is often difficult or impossible to identify with conventional stains. Accumulations of triglyceride within the cell commonly appear as vacuoles (fatty metamorphosis) (Figs. 2-3e and 2-4d) because of their solubility in the materials used for preparing the sections. In tissues prepared without lipid solvents–e.g., frozen sections–the lipid may be stained by fat-soluble dyes such as Sudan IV or oil red O. Removal of acid mucopolysaccharides accumulating in storage diseases such as Hurler's disease may also give rise to vacuoles. Other types of irregular clear areas in cells stained with hematoxylin and eosin may be due to accumulations of material such as glycogen, which is not stained with this technique. In these cases other staining methods may be used. Glycogen, for example, can be readily identified with the periodic acid-Schiff (PAS) technique, without prior amylase digestion. Glycogen depletion, an early manifestation of ischemia, is followed by the disappearance of these unstained areas, and PAS staining will confirm the absence of glycogen.

Many vacuoles, however, represent accumulations of watery fluid (usually isosmotic with plasma) in such intracellular compartments as the endoplasmic cisternae, the mitochondria, the digestive vacuoles (lysosomes), the cell sap, or the nucleus. This cell swelling has been known as *hydropic degeneration.* The nature of the vacuoles cannot be established unless specific histochemical or electron microscopic methods are used. Such vacuoles occur in renal proximal tubular cells in patients with low serum potassium (Fig. 2-4c), in foamy liver cells as a result of the massive enlargement of endoplasmic cisternae caused by chemical or viral injury, and in the nucleus after clumping of the nuclear chromatin.

INCLUSIONS. The term *inclusion* is commonly used to refer to stainable accumulations of material within the nucleus (Fig. 2-4a) or cytoplasm (Fig. 2-4b). Inclusions may be spherical or irregular, homogeneous or granulofibrillar. Precise identification depends, again, on detailed analysis by histochemistry and electron microscopy and may require isolation of the inclusions by differential or density-gradient centrifugation. Many inclusions represent accumulations of ma-

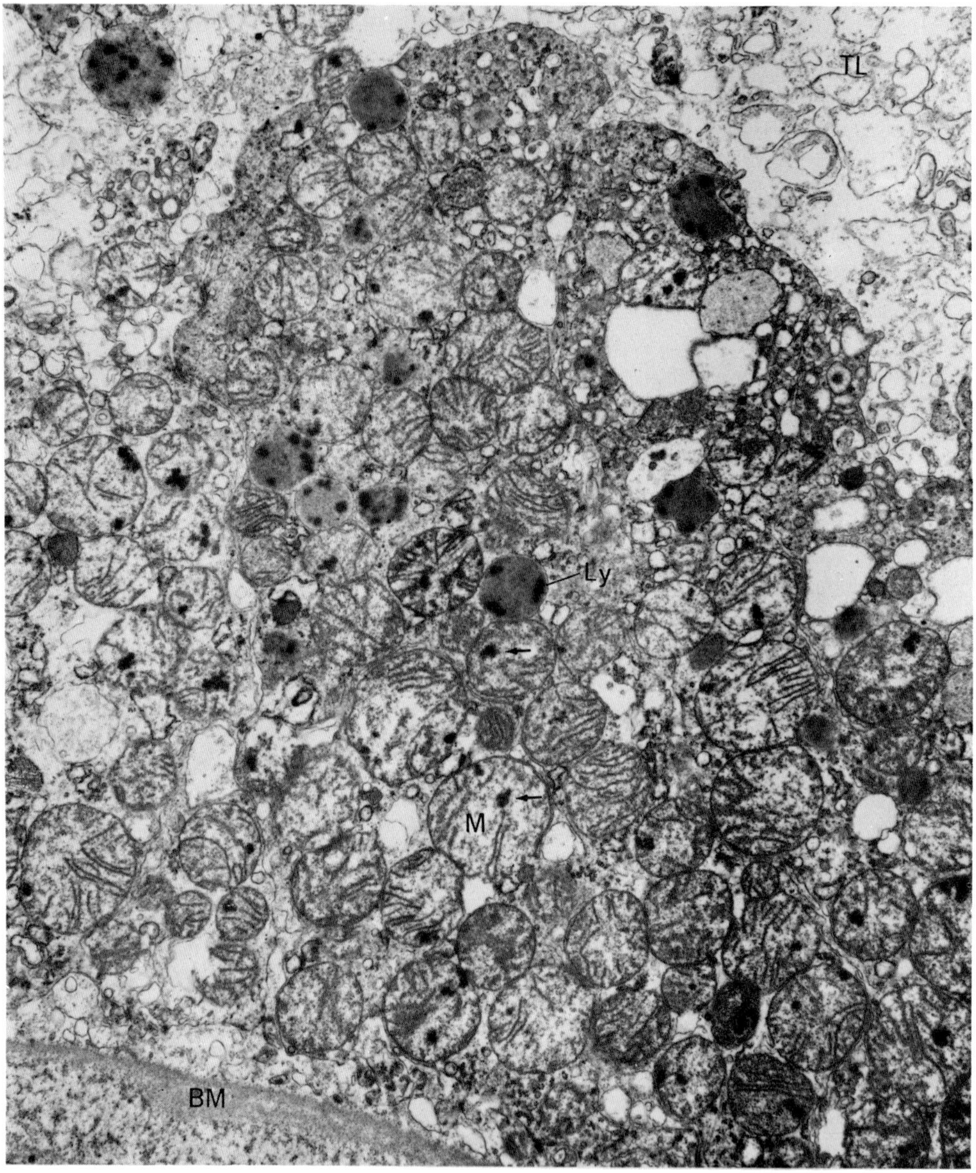

Figure 2-5. Electron micrograph showing a proximal kidney tubule in stage 5 from a patient in acute shock. The changes include high-amplitude swelling of mitochondria (M) with flocculent densities (arrows), dilatation and fragmentation of endoplasmic reticulum, distortion of cell membrane contour, fragmentation of other cells as indicated by cell debris in the tubular lumen (TL) at the top, and intact lysosomes (Ly). The basement membrane (BM) is at the lower left.

terial within heterophagic or autophagic digestive vacuoles. This, for example, is the nature of the hyaline droplets of the renal proximal tubules associated with proteinuria. Masses of virus particles may also be visible as inclusions within the nucleus or cytoplasm (Fig. 2-4a). Inclusions may result from specific synthesis, as in the case of the neurofibrillary filaments seen in neurons of the elderly or in Alzheimer's disease (Fig. 2-3f), or from obscure degenerations, as in the case of Mallory's alcoholic hyalin (Fig. 2-3c) in the liver cells of alcoholics.

PIGMENT. Many types of pigment may accumulate in cells. These may be endogenous, such as lipofuscin ("aging" pigment) and ferritin, or exogenous, such as tattoo pigments, phagocytosed carbon, or other colored indigestible particles. In most cases pigment accumulations are found in digestive vacuoles. Accumulation of lipofuscin pigment commonly occurs in cells as a general manifestation of sub-lethal injury, and often represents a residuum of autophagocytosis.

INORGANIC DEPOSITS. Abnormal depositions of inorganic material such as calcium phosphate may occur in pathologically altered cells. In Wilson's disease, copper-containing deposits are often seen in digestive vacuoles of the liver and other organs. Crystalline masses are sometimes found in or about the injured cells. These may be exogenous, as in the case of foreign bodies, but they may also originate in the accumulation of abnormal amounts of metabolites such as oxalate or cystine.

C. Acute Lethal Injury

In this and the following sections the effects of injury on cells will be discussed in the context of patients' case histories. Cellular derangements, of course, have effects on function in the body as a whole. The resulting changes in body function are expressed in the history, the physical findings, and the results of laboratory examinations of body fluids such as the blood or urine.

1. Ischemic and hypoxic injury

Acute injury of cells by ischemia is very common in human disease. It plays an important role in three of the four major causes of death in the United States—namely, heart disease, stroke, and trauma. *Ischemia* is defined as reduction of blood supply, either partial or complete, to cells or tissues. *Hypoxia* is defined as partial reduction in the oxygen concentration supplied to cells or tissues, and a complete reduction is referred to as *anoxia*. Ischemia differs from hypoxia in that not only is the supply of oxygen reduced in ischemia, but also the supply of substrates and the processes of perfusion, permitting accumulation of products of cell metabolism.

CASE 1 A 16-year-old girl was thrown from a car and pinned beneath the overturned vehicle in brackish water, her head immersed, for about 10 minutes. When rescued, she was not breathing, had no palpable pulse, and did not respond to any stimuli. Resuscitation was begun immediately, and she was admitted to the hospital within 20 minutes after the accident. En route to the hospital she received three epinephrine injections and was given external cardiac massage. At the hospital, electrical cardiac stimulation was performed with return of a spontaneous heart beat and rise of the systolic blood pressure to 170 mm Hg. The patient did not respond to any stimuli, however, and there were no spontaneous respirations. With the passage of a nasogastric tube, large amounts of fluid and gas were removed from the stomach. Arterial blood gas analysis revealed a PaO_2 of 47 mm Hg, pH 6.86, a $PaCO_2$ greater than 100 mm Hg, and a base excess of 22 mEq per liter. The serum osmolality was 332 mOsmoles per kg, and the serum water concentration was 95.3 per cent.* The patient failed to respond to therapy, and her condition degenerated rapidly. She never produced any urine, became hypotensive, and died five and one-half hours after admission.

This case illustrates the effects of sudden severe hypoxia on cells, chiefly those of the liver and kidney. When examined immediately after the patient's death, the hepatic parenchymal cells and the renal tubular and glomerular cells showed massive changes (Fig. 2-5). The cells themselves were markedly swollen, the mitochondria exhibited high-amplitude swelling with flocculent matrix densities, the endoplasmic reticulum was dilated with dispersal of polysomes, the cell membrane contours were distorted and fragmented, there was marked clumping of nuclear chromatin, and the lysosomes, though apparently intact, were dilated and lucent. Cells altered to this degree clearly are irreversibly damaged and in the phase of necrosis. Mitochondria isolated from the liver or kidney were shown to have retained respiratory activity but were unable to phosphorylate, so that they could not have supported ATP formation. These cells are nonfunctional as units.

These findings serve to illustrate three important features of irreversibly injured cells which need further elaboration: (a) altered cell volume regulation; (b) altered energy metabolism; and (c) the suicide bag concept of lysosomes.

a. Altered cell volume regulation

In mammalian cells the intracellular ionic composition differs markedly from that of extracellular fluid and includes a high concentration of negatively charged protein. Since the plasma membrane can be shown to be permeable to cellular and extracellular ions but not to protein, the maintenance of these

* Normal values: PaO_2: 100 mm Hg; $PaCO_2$: 40 mm Hg; pH 7.35–7.45; serum osmolality 285–93 mOsmoles per kg; serum water 93.5–94.5 per cent.

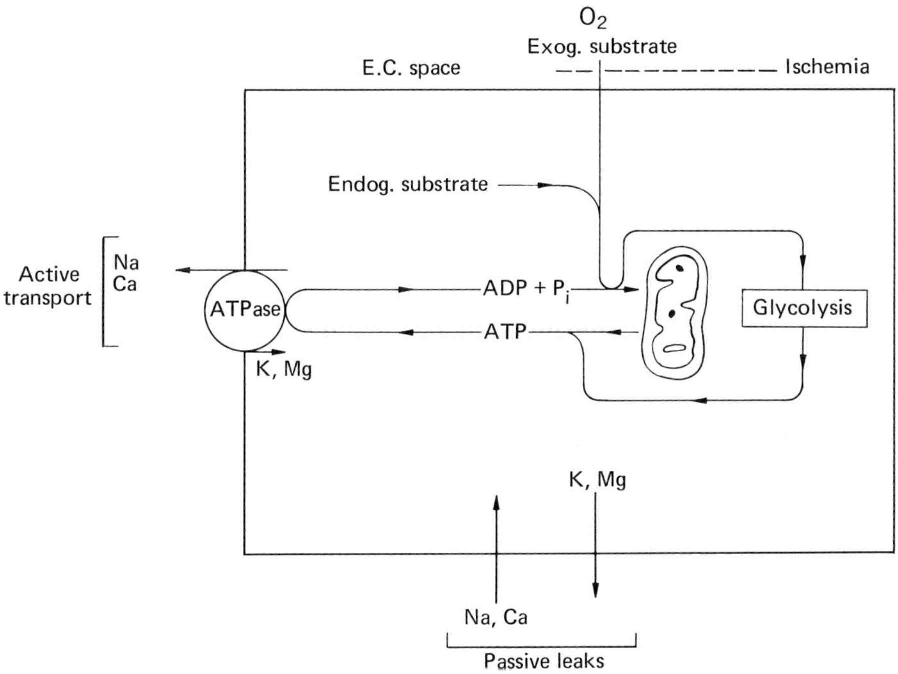

Figure 2-6. Diagram showing some important factors in cell volume and ion regulation in mammalian cells. For explanation see text.

differences in composition represents a delicate balance between diffusion and active transport of ions. Active transport of ions is energy-dependent and is associated with membrane-bound enzyme systems or carriers such as the sodium-potassium dependent, ouabain-sensitive ATPase, which is responsible for at least some of the sodium and potassium movements at the cell membrane (Fig. 2-6).

Clearly, the sensitive balance between the intracellular and the extracellular milieu depends on the integrity of plasma membrane structure, membrane-associated enzyme or carrier systems, the electrochemical gradient, and the energy supply. Changes in each of these factors have been demonstrated to occur in various cell injuries and to account for a wide variety of structural and functional alterations of cells in disease states.

The control of cell volume, depending largely on the control of water content, is a fundamental characteristic of mammalian cells (see review by Tosteson, 1964). Water movements, however, are not under direct control but are passively determined by such factors as differences in hydrostatic pressure, chemical activity of water, electrical potential, temperature, and chemical potential. Since the activity of water and the hydrostatic pressure are essentially equal in the cell and the extracellular fluid, water at the normal steady state of the cell is at equilibrium. Cells are not at Gibbs-Donnan equilibrium, in which the osmolality inside the cell and the intracellular pressure would significantly exceed those in the extracellular fluid. Sodium and potassium transport mechanisms are the key to regulation of intracellular volume; small *anions* such as chloride and bicarbonate exist at equilibrium.

If the operation of these transport mechanisms is interfered with by any means, the cells tend to approach Gibbs-Donnan equilibrium by taking on fluid with dissolved solute at a concentration equal to that in the extracellular phase, leading to an increase in intracellular volume and hydrostatic pressure. If this is permitted to continue, cell volume will increase until either the membrane bursts or its volume is constrained by some external force that equals the internal hydrostatic pressure. This increase in cell volume, known as *isosmotic swelling* or colloid osmotic lysis, is the most common type of volume change observed in injured cells *in vivo* (see review by Trump *et al.,* 1971). It has been especially well studied in the red cell, where swelling and rupture (hemolysis) occur frequently as a result of injury to the plasma membrane and/or its associated transport functions. Such injury may involve direct modification of membrane permeability, damage to transport systems within the membrane, or interference with the supply of energy (possibly ATP) for the membrane transport systems.

It is possible also to observe osmotic types of volume changes if the osmolality of the extracellular fluid is increased or decreased. This occasionally occurs in clinical conditions such as diabetes or severe dehydration, on the one hand, or in patients infused with dilute solutions or distilled water, on the other. Isosmotic swelling may occur also when extracellular sodium is replaced with a penetrating cation such as potassium.

b. Altered energy metabolism

The principal function of mitochondria is the supply and storage of energy in the form of high-energy compounds, resulting from the production of an energized state in the presence of substrate and oxygen. The electron transport system and associated coupling factors responsible for these reactions reside in intimate association with the cristae and other subunits of the inner membrane.

Mitochondrial structure is closely linked with mitochondrial function (see review by Parsons, 1965). Differences in rate of respiration, phosphorylation, ion uptake, and water uptake are reflected by changes in ultrastructure.

MITOCHONDRIAL VOLUME CHANGES. Mitrochondria, like other organelles, move, swell, and contract continually in the living cell. We may speculate that

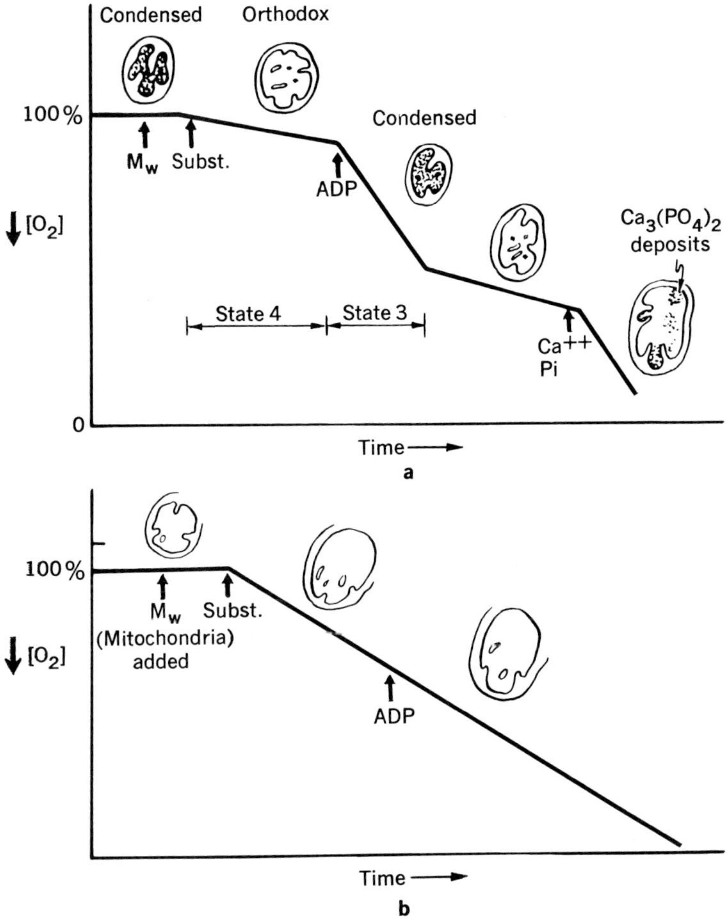

Figure 2-7. a. Metabolic transformations in normal mitochondria. When mitochondria are isolated in 0.25 M sucrose, the inner compartment appears condensed. After addition of substrate in the presence of oxygen, they transform to the "orthodox" conformation, State 4. When a phosphate acceptor, ADP, is added, mitochondria enter a phase of rapid respiration (State 3) and change to the condensed conformation. The cycle can be repeated if substrate and oxygen are present; the condensed-to-orthodox transformation, however, is prevented by addition of electron transport inhibitors such as cyanide. If calcium and phosphate are added, mitochondria undergo marked swelling, and calcium phosphate accumulates along the inner membrane. Oxygen concentration in the medium is shown along the ordinate.

b. Similar tracing of the behavior of mitochondria from ischemic cells. Swelling of the inner compartment is present at zero time. When substrate is added, further swelling occurs; whereas, contraction does not occur following addition of ADP. Mitochondria are said to be "uncoupled" and to have lost respiratory control.

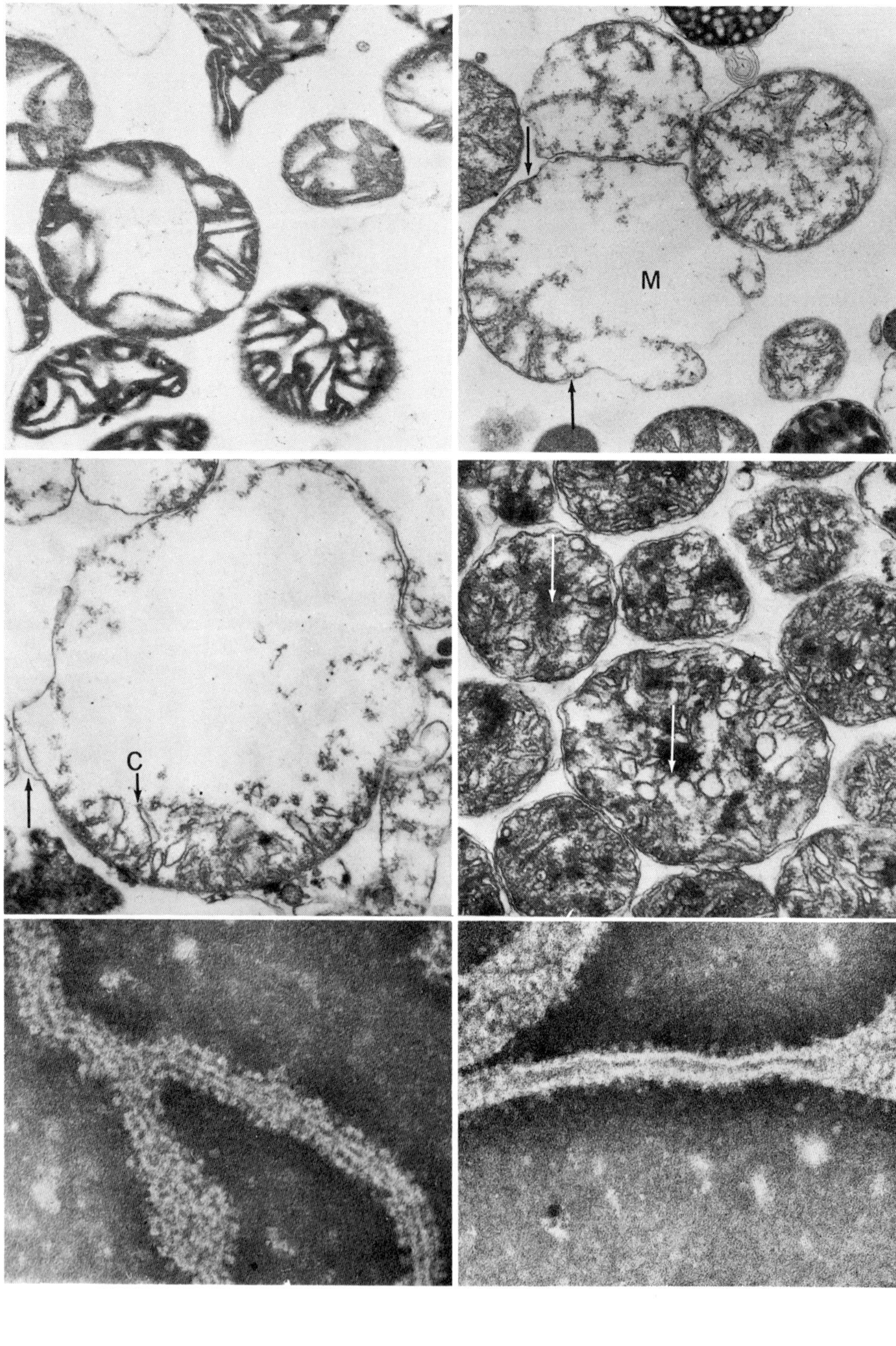

a b c d e f

these movements can exert control over local aspects of the intracellular microenvironment and that accumulation of water and/or ions by mitochondria could provide sensitive local control and even functional compartmentation within the protoplasm. A mitochondrial role in the compartmentation of ATP, for example, has been suggested.

Mitochondrial swelling is defined as an increase in mitochondrial size due to uptake of water, and thus is to be distinguished from true mitochondrial enlargement due to increase in membranes and cristae. It has often been studied in isolated mitochondria by morphologic examination, measurement of packed mitochondrial volume (mitocrit), or measurements of light scattering. Light scattering is inversely proportional to the degree of swelling, since a suspension of swollen mitochondria is relatively transparent. Mitochondrial swelling can be seen within cells by electron microscopy or by utilizing phase contrast microscopy in conjunction with time-lapse cinematography.

Swelling of mitochondria is a phenomenon that has for many years been known to occur in injured cells. This increase in mitochondrial volume imparts a granular appearance to the cytoplasm in light microscopic preparations and is one basis of "cloudy swelling" or *hydropic degeneration.* Mitochondrial swelling and contraction have also been observed in normal, uninjured cells by time-lapse photography. Two patterns of mitochondrial swelling, known as *low-amplitude* and *high-amplitude* swelling, are recognized.

MITOCHONDRIAL SWELLING IN VITRO. Low-amplitude volume changes (less

Figure 2-8. Alterations in isolated mitochondria.

a. Mitochondria from control kidney incubated in isosmotic potassium chloride. The condensed conformation is maintained.

b. Mitochondria (M) isolated in the same medium but from a kidney that had been ischemic for two hours. High-amplitude swelling occurs, with interruption of outer membrane (arrows).

c. Hypotonic swelling of mitochondria in distilled water. Note the massive expansion of inner compartment. Cristal residues (C) appear attached along one pole, as does a remnant of the outer membrane (arrow).

d. Mitochondria aged in sucrose for 24 hours, showing fragmentation of cristae and appearance of fluffy intramatrical deposits (arrows).

e. Micrograph showing inner membrane fragments of normal rat kidney mitochondria visualized by negative staining. Note the appearance of the membrane or inner membrane spheres (ATPase or F_1 particles) along the membrane fragment.

f. Same as Figure 8e, but after 4 hours of ischemia. Note the absence of the ATPase particles; this correlates with a decreased chemical activity of the enzyme. (Courtesy of Dr. Wolfgang J. Mergner) than 20 per cent) in isolated mitochondria accompany transitions between different respiratory steady states (Fig. 2-7a), and seem to reflect movement of water between the inner and the outer compartment. When mitochondria pass from the energized to the de-energized condition—as for instance when ATP and magnesium are added—there is a rapid contraction as measured with optical density techniques, reflecting the movement of water from inner to outer compartment. This contraction is thought to result from changes in protein conformation, similar to changes in the actomyosin filaments during muscle contraction. In this de-energized, contracted state (Fig. 2-8a), mitochondria appear condensed with a dense matrix and an expanded outer compartment, including the envelope and the intracristal spaces. In the energized state, mitochondria undergo low-amplitude swelling, with water moving from the outer to the inner compartment.

By contrast, in high-amplitude swelling, the inner compartment appears to expand by unfolding of the cristae (Fig. 2-8c); later, the outer compartment expands after rupture of the outer membrane (Fig. 2-8b). High-amplitude swelling implies an increase in the permeability of the inner membrane to the solute in the medium in which the mitochondria are suspended, and is accompanied by a large change (up to 10-fold) in optical density. In the early stages, high-amplitude swelling is reversed by addition of ATP and magnesium (Fig. 2-9).

There are many categories of agents that cause swelling *in vitro*. These include ions such as calcium, natural products such as fatty acids, hormones such as thyroxine, and membrane-damaging events or agents such as phospholipases. Prolonged reduction of ATP levels within mitochondria appears to promote breakdown or deterioration of inner membranes with high-amplitude swelling (Fig. 2-8d); certain ionophorous antibiotics such as valinomycin also promote it. High-amplitude swelling is associated with loose coupling of oxidative phosphorylation during the early stages and, if prolonged, with complete loss of phosphorylating ability. This may reflect the need of an intact membrane for ion-gradient conditions required for ATP synthesis.

MITOCHONDRIAL SWELLING AND CONTRACTION IN CELLS. Low-amplitude changes resembling those seen *in vitro* occur also in intact cells under conditions that change the respiratory steady states. Especially important in this regard are changes in the ADP/ATP ratio associated with increased ATP utilization. Conditions associated with increased ATP utilization include increased transport of sodium and increased uptake of amino acids, all of which use ATP and thus increase the ADP/ATP ratio. Mitochondria then appear condensed, with expansion of the outer compartment. Other conditions associated with low-amplitude changes and condensation, indicative of the de-energized state, are those asso-

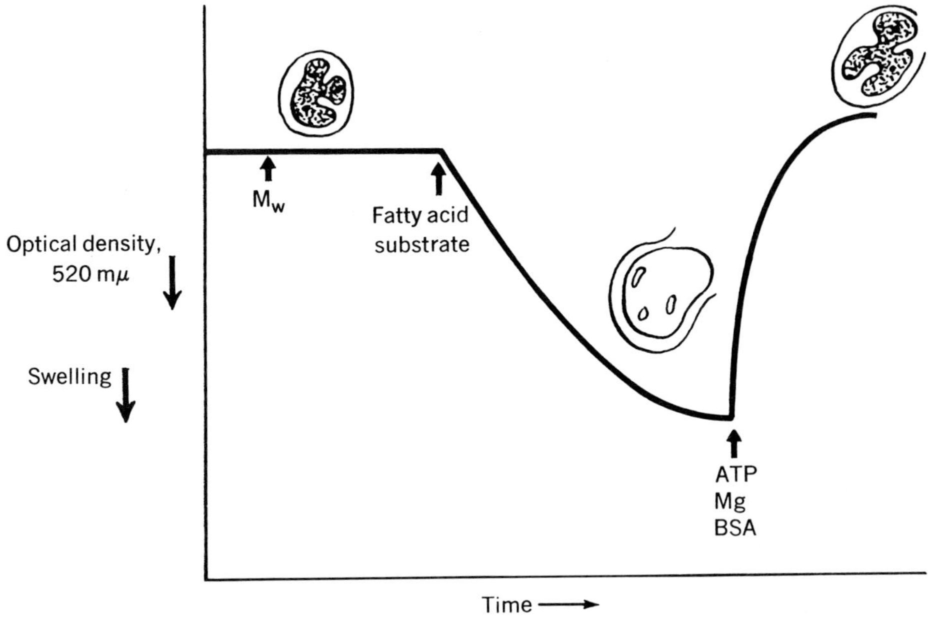

Figure 2-9. Optical density or light-scattering trace of a swelling and contraction cycle. This represents "energized" swelling. When isolated, mitochondria have the condensed configuration; however, following addition of a swelling agent such as phosphate in the presence of substrate, high-amplitude swelling of the inner compartment occurs with rupture of the outer membrane. The swelling is readily reversed by addition of ATP, magnesium, and albumin; the mitochondria again become condensed, and the optical density increases. Mitochondria are added at Mw.

ciated with inhibition of the energizing process, such as anoxia or treatment with electron transport inhibitors. A delicate balance seems to exist between the low-amplitude swelling of the de-energized state and high-amplitude swelling, since the integrity of the inner membrane is apparently dependent on ATP. With prolonged anoxia or prolonged treatment with respiratory inhibitors, the inner membrane deteriorates, and soon mitochondria pass from a condensed phase to a phase of high-amplitude swelling.

High-amplitude swelling identical with that observed in mitochondria *in vitro* occurs also *in vivo,* especially after lethal injuries. Initially, high-amplitude swelling occurs during the phase of altered homeostasis, and the changes, which include permeability to normally impermeant salts, are reversible. Later, however, the mitochondria lose the ability to contract, even if ATP and magnesium are added. In electron micrographs, high-amplitude swelling in intact cells begins

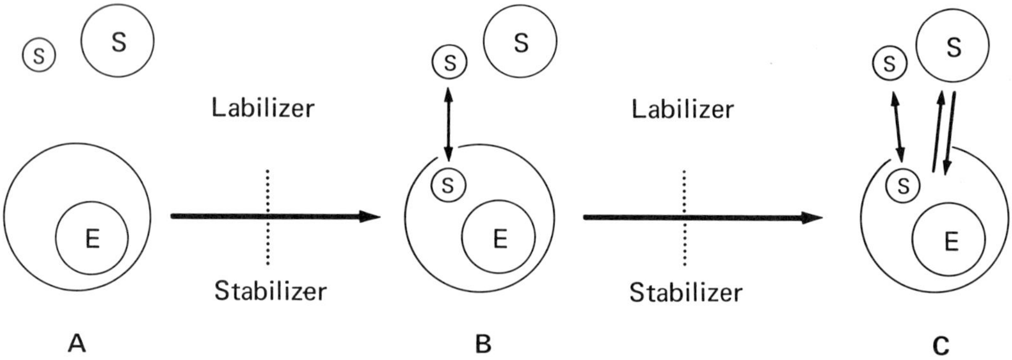

Figure 2-10. Diagram illustrating concepts of lysosome integrity in relation to enzyme activity and release.

In "A" lysosomal hydrolases (E) reside within the particles protected by the membrane from the surrounding medium containing substrate (S). Under these conditions the enzyme activity measured in the total system will be nil or very low, since substrate access to the enzyme is prevented by the limiting membrane. In the presence of agents resulting in mild damage to the lysosomal membrane known as lysosomal labilizers, membrane permeability may be increased, thus permitting access of substrate to enzyme. At this stage enzyme is still retained within the particles, as leaks are too small to permit enzyme release. Agents known as lysosomal stabilizers can counteract the effects of labilizers. In "C" more severe damage has occurred, with result in defects permitting both substrate entry and enzyme release. In "B" the increase is known as free activity, as the enzyme activity remains with the particles and can be sedimented with them; in "C" release of enzyme results in soluble enzyme, so-called unsedimentable activity.

with loss of matrical granules, pallor of the matrix, and appearance of a dense flocculent material within the inner compartment. Later, fluffy densities appear with the matrix. The outer membrane is interrupted, and this permits further expansion. Ultimately the inner membrane deteriorates also (Fig. 2-8e, f), and the process terminates with the development of non-functional tubular structures derived from the inner membrane.

c. Suicide-bag hypothesis

It has been proposed that the event that sends the cell beyond the "point of no return" is the bursting of hydrolase-laden vacuoles or granules, the lysosomes, and the consequent destructive release of enzymes (Fig. 2-10). This was an attractive hypothesis, and there is little doubt that digestive vacuoles do in fact break during the necrotic phase and release hydrolases into the cell sap; but this appears to be the result, not the cause, of cell death. Changes characteristic of lethally altered cells do not usually appear first in that region of the cell which is rich in acid-hydrolase-containing structures. In fact, the presence of intact di-

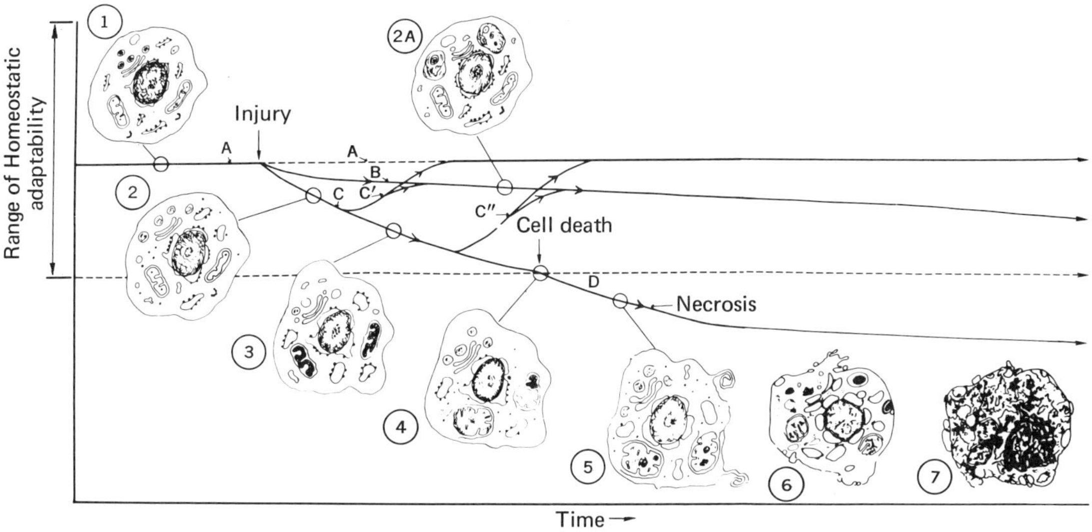

Figure 2-11. Stages of cell injury. Plotted along the abscissa is time, and along the ordinate is range of homeostatic ability.

Stage 1 shows a cell in a normal steady state (curve A). At the arrow an injury is applied and it may be acutely lethal or sub-lethal. In the case of the lethal injury, the cell loses homeostatic ability along curve C. Prior to the point of cell death, however, recovery can occur if the injurious stimulus is removed. Such recovery might proceed along curve C′ or curve C″. In stage 2 the principal change consists of dilatation of the ER and slight clumping of the nuclear chromatin, though some ribosomes may be detached from the endoplasmic reticulum, and the entire cell may be slightly swollen. In stage 3 the mitochondria are condensed, the cell is more swollen, and blebs begin to appear along the cell membrane. After the point of cell death, recovery cannot occur, even if the injurious stimulus is removed; the cell is said to enter the phase of necrosis. During this transitional period, stage 4 is seen, and in it changes similar to those in stage 3 occur, except that some mitochondria are markedly swollen, while in others portions of their inner compartments are condensed and other portions are swollen. The lysosomes remain intact; there is increased ribosomal scattering and increased cell swelling. During the phase of necrosis the cell undergoes degradation by autolysis and denaturation, and a typical morphologic picture occurs as in stage 5. In stage 6 the secondary and primary lysosomes in the cell begin to disappear, and large gaps and irregularities in the cell surface membrane can be seen.

In stage 7 the membrane debris resulting from fragmentation and distortion of organelles begins to be converted to large myelin figures that occupy large areas of the cytoplasm and represent formation of bi-layer configurations from the altered and hydrated lipid derivatives.

Stage 2A represents a common sub-lethal adaptation, one in which numerous secondary lysosomes filled with digestive debris can be seen. Note that the other organelles appear well preserved. Note also that incomplete recovery during the reversible phases after a lethal injury might result also in a new steady state depicted by the right hand limb of curves C′ and C″. (Modified from Trump **et al.**, Hum. Pathol., **4**:89, 1973).

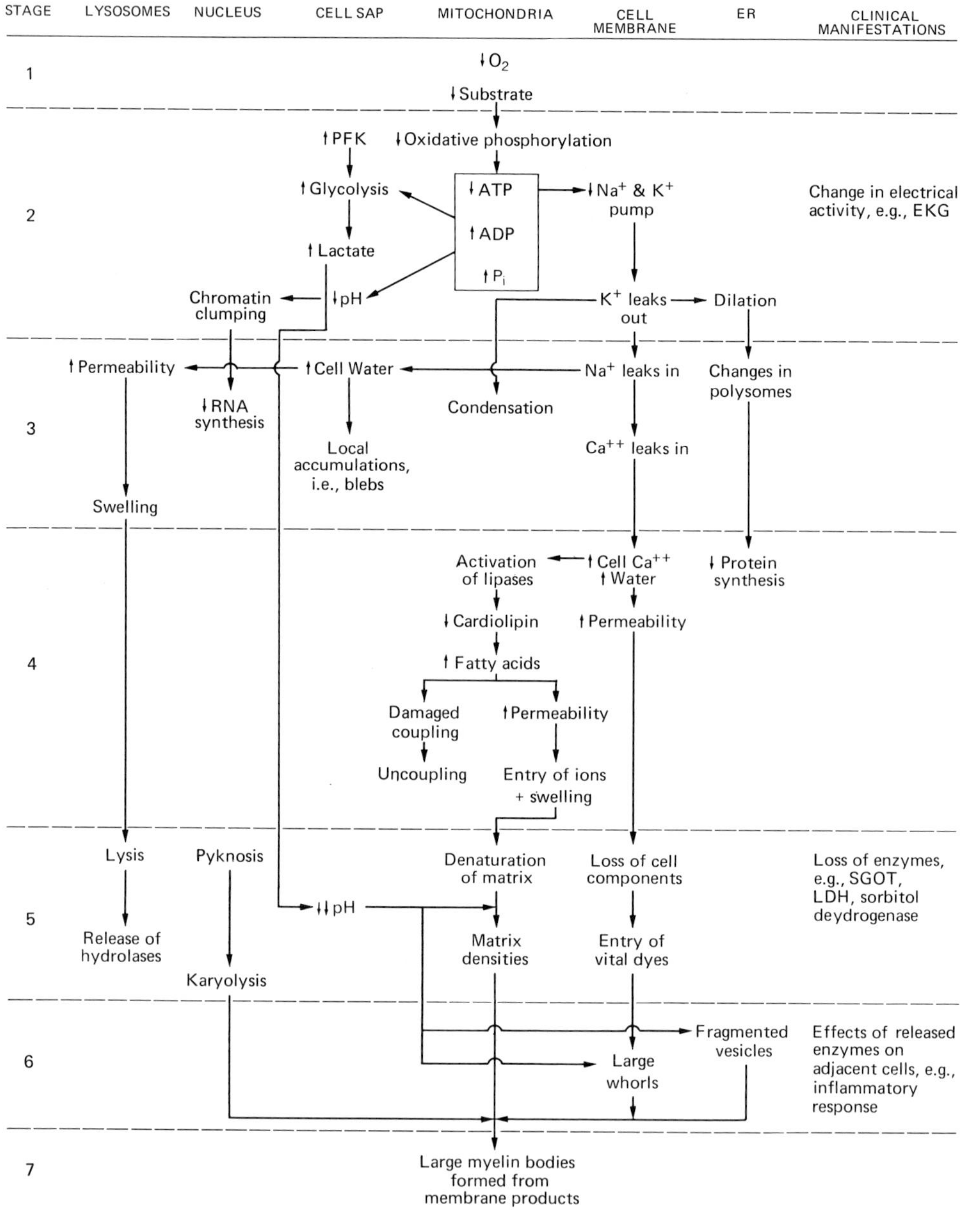

Figure 2-12. Hypothetical sequence of events leading from a normal to a necrotic cell following ischemic cell injury. The stages referred to in the text and diagrammed in Figure 11 are indicated along the left in relation to the progression of cellular change. At the right are shown clinical manifestations correlating with stages of subcellular alteration.

gestive and endosecretory vesicles can be demonstrated well into the necrotic phase (see reviews by Trump *et al.,* 1971; Scarpelli and Trump, 1971).

d. Pathogenesis of acute ischemic injury

A sequence of changes following acute ischemic injury can be postulated as a working hypothesis on the basis of observations in both humans and experimental animals (Figs. 2-11, 12) (Trump *et al.,* 1971). This sequence can be divided into several characteristic stages.

In the first stage, complete ischemia results in a sudden decrease in the oxygen tension within the cell and extracellular fluid. As the oxygen concentration falls, mitochondrial phosphorylation decreases rapidly, and contraction of the inner compartment starts. The drop in cellular ATP stimulates the activity of phosphofructokinase in many cells, and this results in an increased rate of anaerobic glycolysis. Accelerated glycolysis leads to the accumulation of lactate, which, together with the increased inorganic phosphate, soon reduces the intracellular pH. Since the circulation has ceased, metabolites such as lactate and hydrogen ions also tend to accumulate in the extracellular microenvironment, depressing the extracellular pH. The decreased pH may also be protective in that it seems to have a "stabilizing" effect on the cell membrane. The change in intracellular pH is probably reflected by the clumping of nuclear chromatin - which occurs very rapidly but is clearly reversible. Clumping of nuclear chromatin is known to be associated with decreased nuclear RNA synthesis; this, however, is of no immediate consequence to the cell, since, if the circulation is not restored, the cell will die and undergo necrosis long before the decreased RNA synthesis has any effect.

This chromatin clumping can easily be observed in living cells by phase contrast microscopy, and in cultured cells it can be induced and reversed by alternately lowering and restoring the pH of the medium. This can be done several times without interfering with the subsequent mitotic activity of the cells. Clumping of chromatin in nuclei that have shrunk because of injury may give the entire nucleus a uniform densely basophilic appearance known as *pyknosis* (Fig. 2-3d).

Meanwhile, the cell also begins to show the effects of reduced ATP concentration. As a result of interference with the sodium-potassium pump at the cell membrane, ion shifts begin to occur, sodium leaking into the cell, potassium leaking out.

An early expression of the ion shifts is dilatation of the endoplasmic reticulum, reflecting a loss of volume regulation, a sign of stage 2 injury (Fig. 2-10a). The mechanism of the dilatation is not known, and the ion moving into the reticulum has not been identified. At this stage the mitochondria, Golgi apparatus, lysosomes, and other organelles show few alterations. The cell sap may be slightly diluted. The polysomes remain attached to the rough endoplasmic reticulum, though dissociation into ribosome monomers is beginning to occur.

The twin phenomena of detachment of polysomes from the membranes of the endoplasmic reticulum and scattering or disaggregation of both free and bound polysomes into monomeric ribosomes occur soon thereafter (Fig. 2-10b), presumably reflecting modifications of the energy-dependent maintenance of interactions between membranes and ribosomes, and between messenger RNA and ribosomes. This fragmentation of polysomes is accompanied by defective protein synthesis. Both the structure and function of the protein-synthetic apparatus revert to normal with restoration of oxygenation and synthesis of ATP.

In stage 2, blebs may form at the cell surface (Fig. 2-3a). Typically, the cytoplasm in these blebs is of low viscosity, and in time-lapse movies the blebs can be observed to appear and disappear. As the cell approaches the "point of no return," the rate of appearance and disappearance of the blebs increases markedly. Also seen at this stage are bizarre alterations of other cell surface structures such as microvilli.

In stage 3, the mitochondria are further condensed, and the endoplasmic reticulum remains dilated; at this stage the entire cell is often swollen with increased sodium, chloride, and water content and decreased potassium. Mitochondrial function is of course inhibited because of the continued lack of oxygen, and as a consequence ATP levels are low. Because of the decreased ATP values the ADP, AMP, and inorganic phosphate levels are high. If cells in this state are restored to normal conditions, the mitochondrial inner compartments re-expand, the endoplasmic reticulum contracts, and the cells extrude sodium along with water and later chloride. Thus, we can conclude that although the mitochondria are dramatically changed in form, they retain the ability to respire and phosphorylate as well as to regain their normal internal compartment volume following restitution of a normal microenvironment.

At this stage, protein synthesis is severely inhibited, and both free and bound polysomes are present as monosomes, some of which may still maintain their membrane attachments. The cell sap is swollen because of the increased water content, and the lysosomes are clear and often swollen, although leaks in the lysosomal membranes apparently do not occur.

Stage 4 begins the transition across the "point of no return." In this stage the mitochondria begin to show high-amplitude swelling, which seems to indicate an irreversible loss of the inner membrane function. In consequence, some mitochondrial profiles show high-amplitude inner-compartment swelling while others remain condensed; in some cells such as renal tubular epithelium, where two or more inner compartments are present in a given mitochondrion, one compartment may be condensed and the others swollen. Otherwise, the organelles resemble those seen in stage 3. The lysosomes are swollen, though again no evidence of acid hydrolase leakage can be observed.

In stage 4a, in addition to the above, all mitochondria are swollen, and the inner compartments are expanded, often with interruption of the outer membrane. Stages 1 through 4a appear to be reversible; stages 5, 6, and 7 appear to be irreversible.

In stage 5, all the mitochondria exhibit high amplitude swelling with flocculent matrical densities, the cell is swollen, and the membranes in the cytocavitary network are fragmented. Though the lysosomes are swollen they retain macromolecular particles. In this stage the chromatin begins to undergo enzymatic attack, and in later stages chromatin is dissolved completely (karyolysis). The denaturation of protein that becomes prominent at this stage changes the light-scattering properties of the cell. Such changes are probably related to what Virchow described as "cloudy swelling." Because of the confusion that attended the use of that term, it has essentially been discarded.

In stage 6, digestion of cell components is most striking, and equilibration of cell components with the extracellular space occurs. Thus, particles such as vital dyes, when added to the extracellular fluid, readily leak into the cell, and both organelle and cell sap enzymes begin to leak into the cytoplasm while substrates enter the lysosomes.

In stage 7, the cell is virtually completely degraded; yet large new structures, often striking in appearance, begin to form. Large laminated masses, often greater in diameter than the nucleus, appear. Such multilaminated configurations apparently represent phospholipid myelin figures forming from complex parallel membrane infoldings. Simultaneously, vermicular tubes protrude from the membrane, visible in unfixed cells as long, undulating, thread-like extensions of the membrane into the extracellular medium. Finally, increased calcium binding to various cell fragments also begins to appear. This is a non-energy-dependent process in which calcium binds to phospholipids and to fatty acids released from phospholipids forming calcium soaps. In lethal injury of adipose tissue cells this calcium soap formation, known as fat necrosis, can be very striking.

At this point we may return to Case 1. Hepatic and renal cells were found to exhibit stage 5, irreversible changes indicative of non-function, and the lack of urinary output reflected the kidney damage. Moreover, the patient's deep coma indicates that central nervous system function was severely damaged. Yet her heart was able to beat effectively, an activity requiring large quantities of ATP;

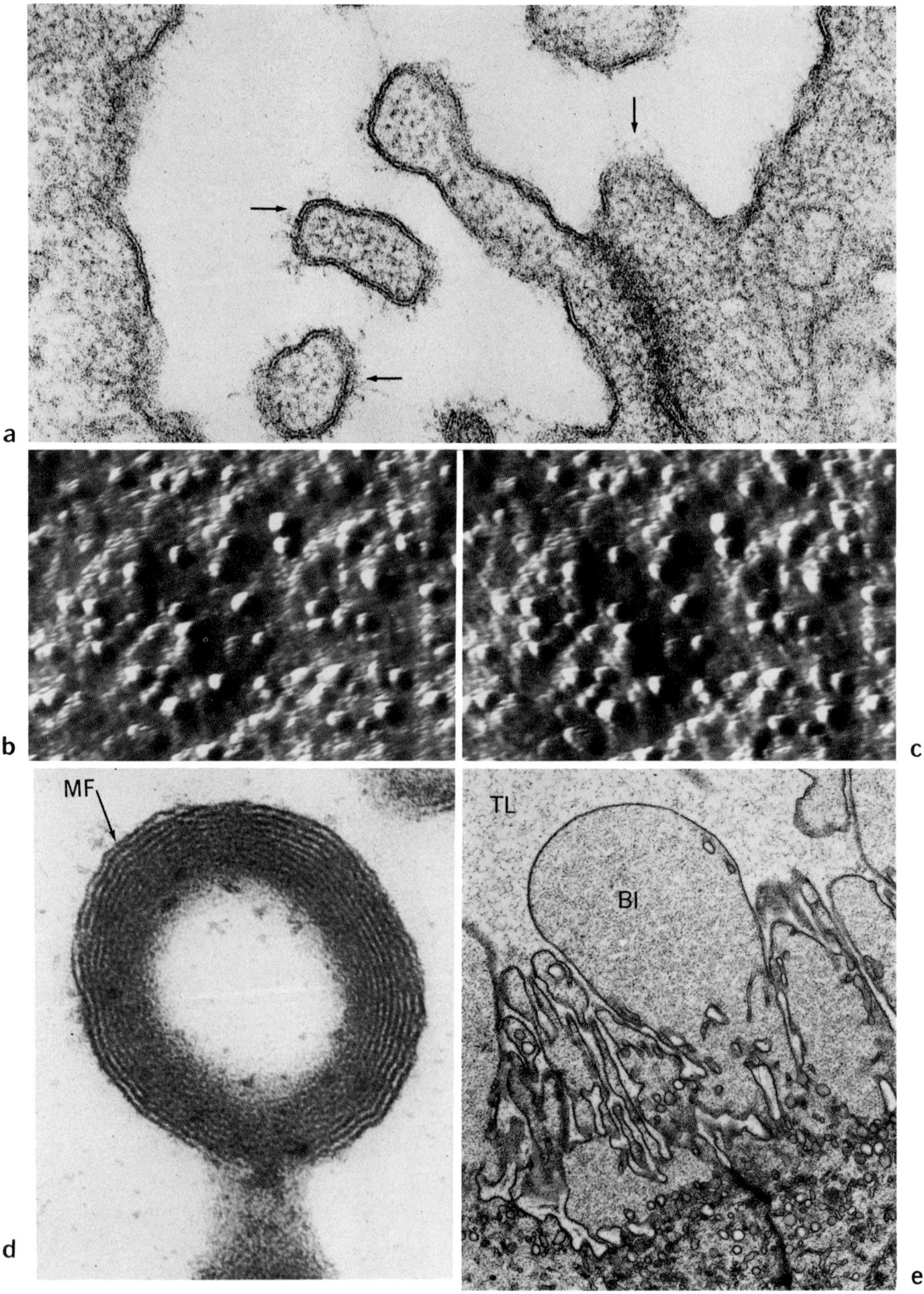

a
b
c
MF
d
TL
Bl
e

and therefore we can safely assume that the myocardial cells were not irreversibly damaged by the initial event. This example dramatically illustrates the variability among different cell types in their susceptibility to anoxic damage, and points clearly to those tissues that must have priority in the treatment of patients with anoxic injury.

2. Direct damage to cell membrane

After ischemia the most common type of acute lethal injury results from events at the cell membrane (Fig. 2-13) that either increase its permeability or block membrane transport sites. In many instances both changes occur simultaneously.

CASE 2 A 67-year-old woman was admitted to the hospital for resection of an adenocarcinoma of the rectosigmoid colon. The operative procedure for removal of the tumor was uneventful; on the first post-operative day, however, she developed a temperature of 105° F, and the urinary output dropped dramatically. On the second post-operative day, jaundice, stupor, and severe metabolic acidosis were observed. By the third post-operative day she was in coma, bowel sounds were absent, crepitance was evident in the lower left quadrant of the abdomen, and the entire abdominal skin had a purple-brown discoloration. Her systolic blood pressure had dropped to 40 mm Hg. Laboratory examination of the blood revealed a pH of 7.3 and a base excess of −12.8 mEq/liter. The hemo-

Figure 2-13. **a.** Normal distal tubule from rat kidney, showing apical region of cell and illustrating the structure of plasma membrane. Note the bilaminar appearance and the attached filaments to the outside surface forming the so-called glycocalyx (arrow). Note also the area of the junctional complex, which is cut tangentially in this picture.

b and **c** are stereo views of a freeze-etched preparation of human erythrocyte plasma membrane. These micrographs show the outside of the inner membrane surface. The membrane particles are thought to be related to the trans-membrane protein glycophorin. These particles are more numerous on the inner aspect. A cleavage plane in this membrane passes between the inner and outer leaflets of the cell membrane, permitting visualization of the outer aspect of the inner leaflet. This is a stereo pair and for three-dimensional effects view **b** and **c** with a stereoscopic viewer. (Courtesy of Mr. Gary Cohen)

d. Complex myelin figure at the surface of microvilli in a toad bladder treated with the detergent, cetyl pyridinium chloride. (Courtesy of Dr. Hal K. Hawkins)

e. Apical blebs of plasma membrane in fish (flounder) kidney tubule exposed for 5 minutes to 3×10^{-3}M potassium cyanide. The blebs (Bl) protrude into the tubular lumen (TL). The low density of the cell sap within the blebs correlates with low viscosity in this region.

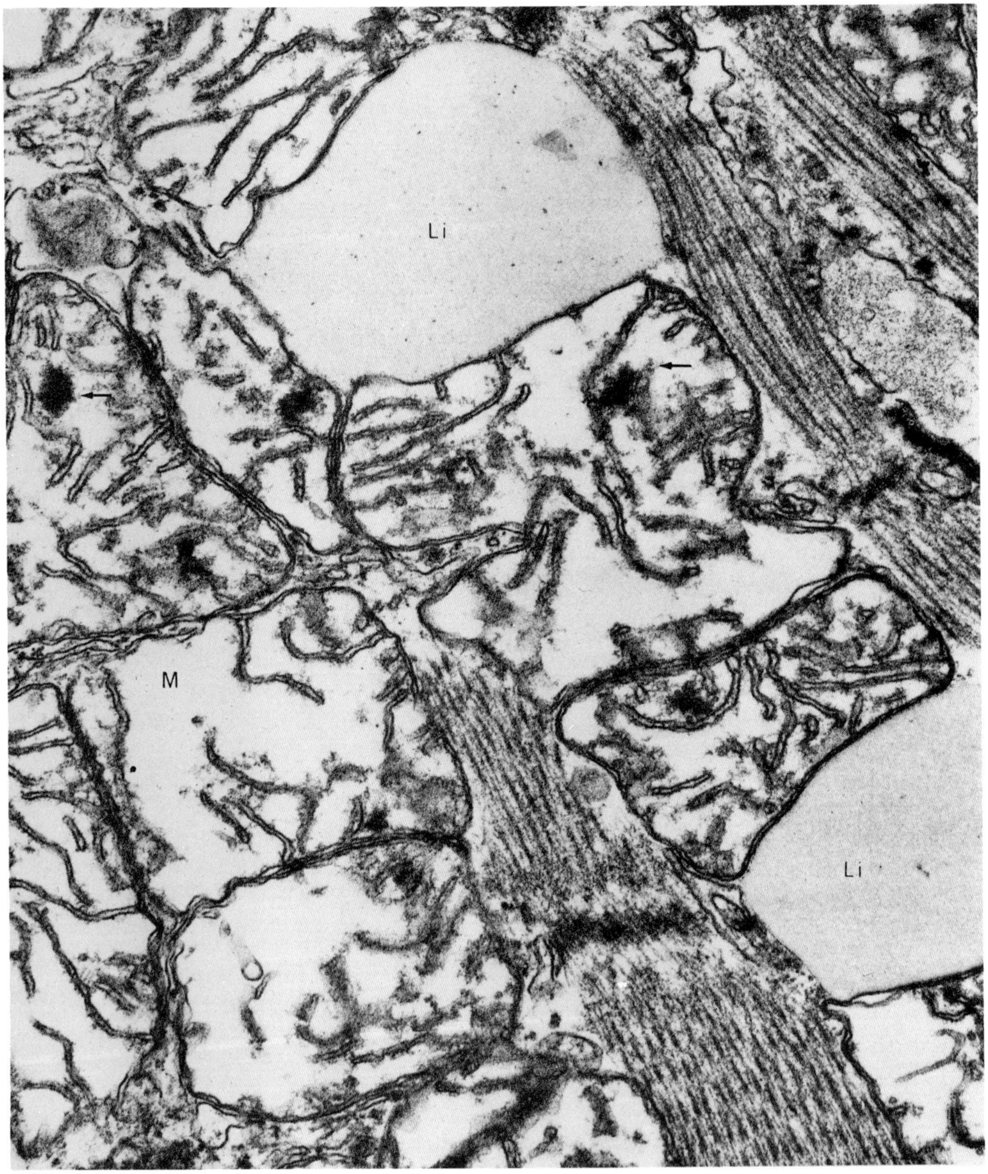

Figure 2-14. Myocardium from patient dying of gas gangrene showing stage 5 changes of cell injury. The mitochondria (M) are markedly swollen, and contain flocculent densities (arrows). Note also lipid droplets (Li), Z-band, and myofibers.

globin was 7.7 gm per dl, platelets 44,000 per cu mm, fibrinogen 156 mg per dl* but the prothrombin time was normal. Despite rigorous therapy with ventilatory assistance and the administration of antibiotics, steroids, and whole blood, neither the metabolic acidosis nor the shock could be reversed. The patient was placed in a hyperbaric chamber to treat a clostridial infection, but she died twelve hours later of profound shock and acidosis. Autopsy revealed massive, generalized peritonitis and gangrenous necrosis. Organisms recovered from the affected tissues included *Clostridium perfringens* and anaerobic streptococci.

Electron microscopic examination of tissues removed within twenty minutes of death revealed stage 5 and 6 changes in myocardial (Fig. 2-14), renal, hepatic, and pancreatic tissues. In addition, the kidney showed large foci of calcification in the necrotic tubules.

This case illustrates the massive cell damage that can occur with clostridial infections. A common causative organism of gas gangrene is *Clostridium perfringens,* a bacterium that produces a number of toxins, including phospholipase C, which interacts with phospholipids to release diglycerides. When applied to cells or subcellular organelles, this toxin directly attacks membranes, causing rapid permeability changes, liberation of diglycerides accumulating within the membrane, modification of membrane-bound proteins, and changes in both membrane structure and function (Fig. 2-15a, b) (Trump *et al.,* 1970). In gas gangrene patients, there occur rapid changes due to rapid ionic leaks, with influx of water, massive swelling, release of cellular enzymes, and interference with organelle functions, especially the mitochondrial synthesis of ATP. Necrosis occurs very rapidly. In many respects the cell stages en route to irreversible damage resemble those described for ischemia, but model experiments with cells cultured *in vitro* indicate that the rate of progression through the stages in cell membrane damage is much more rapid.

Injury involving primary attack on the cell membrane commonly causes mitochondrial calcification. Presumably the influx of calcium and phosphate results in their active accumulation by the mitochondrion, a process inhibited by total ischemia (Fig. 2-15c–e). This is referred to as stage 5A. Cell calcification is well illustrated by the following case.

CASE 3 A 42-year-old laboratory worker drank an unspecified amount of mercuric chloride solution. Nausea and severe vomiting occurred. Upon admission to the hospital she was given dimercaprol intramuscularly to bind the heavy metal. She had severe watery and bloody diarrhea, for which she was given

* Normal values: Hemoglobin 12–16 gm per dl; platelets 150,000–400,000 per cu mm; fibrinogen 200–400 mg per dl.

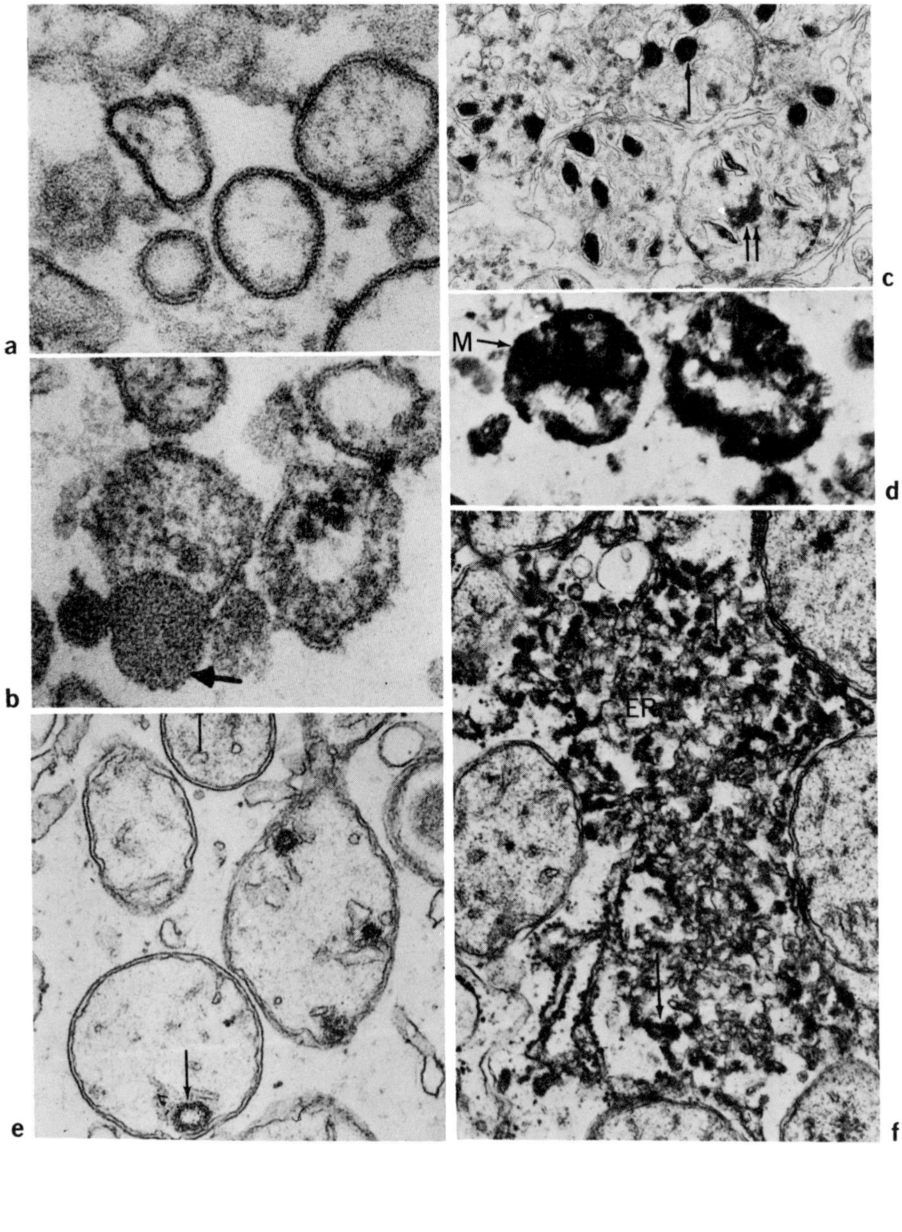
a
b
e
c
M
d
ER
f

fluid and serum replacement. On the second day, serum levels of urea and potassium were elevated. The urine contained 8 gm of protein per 24 hours,* casts, desquamated tubular epithelial cells, and blood. Urinary output ceased, and the patient died in shock on the fifth hospital day.

Examination of the kidneys at autopsy revealed widespread necrosis of proximal tubular epithelial cells and detached, necrotic tubular epithelium was present within tubular lumens. In many areas, calcification of the necrotic cells was observed. Electron microscopic study of these cells revealed typical stage 5A and stage 6 changes, with widespread mitochondrial calcification. Between the necrotic cells, regeneration of spared epithelium was noted.

The necrosis with calcification and regeneration observed in this case is typical of the nephrotoxic action of mercury in both humans and experimental animals. When mercury is administered as an inorganic salt–usually mercuric chloride–the principal toxic effects involve the kidney. Organic mercurials such as methyl mercury, on the other hand, involve the central nervous system. In both cases the effect is cellular necrosis. Methyl mercury is probably more important in terms of our environment, since industrial effluents of inorganic or metallic mercury are methylated by aquatic organisms.

The pathogenesis of the cell necrosis is apparently similar to that of necrosis resulting from the gas gangrene toxin, except that mercury binds to cell mem-

* Normal value: 10–150 mg per 24 hr.

Figure 2-15. a. Normal rat liver microsomes representing fragments of ER. The vesicles are enclosed by a trilaminar membrane.

b. Microsomes treated with phospholipase C. Note eccentric density, probably representing diglyceride accumulations in the hydrophobic interior of the membrane. The trilaminar membrane is about 50 per cent increased in thickness, and glucose-6-phosphatase is inactive.

c. Kidney tubule mitochondria 24 hours after administration of mercuric chloride. There are two types of deposits: (1) flocculent intramatrical densities (double arrow), and (2) microcrystalline deposits in apposition to the inner membrane (arrow).

d. Mitochondria in kidney tubule 48 hours after mercuric chloride administration. Complete calcification of mitochondrial profiles is seen.

e. Mitochondria in a kidney tubule cell irradiated with ultraviolet light for 4 hours. The cell sap is pale, and calcification is seen along the inner membrane in the form of microcrystalline material. The calcium has entered the cell through the damaged plasma membrane. (Courtesy of Dr. Fred L. Ginn)

f. Cytoplasm of a hepatic parenchymal cell after administration of carbon tetrachloride. Clusters of collapsed endoplasmic reticulum appear (ER). The densities (arrows) are characteristic of peroxidation lesions.

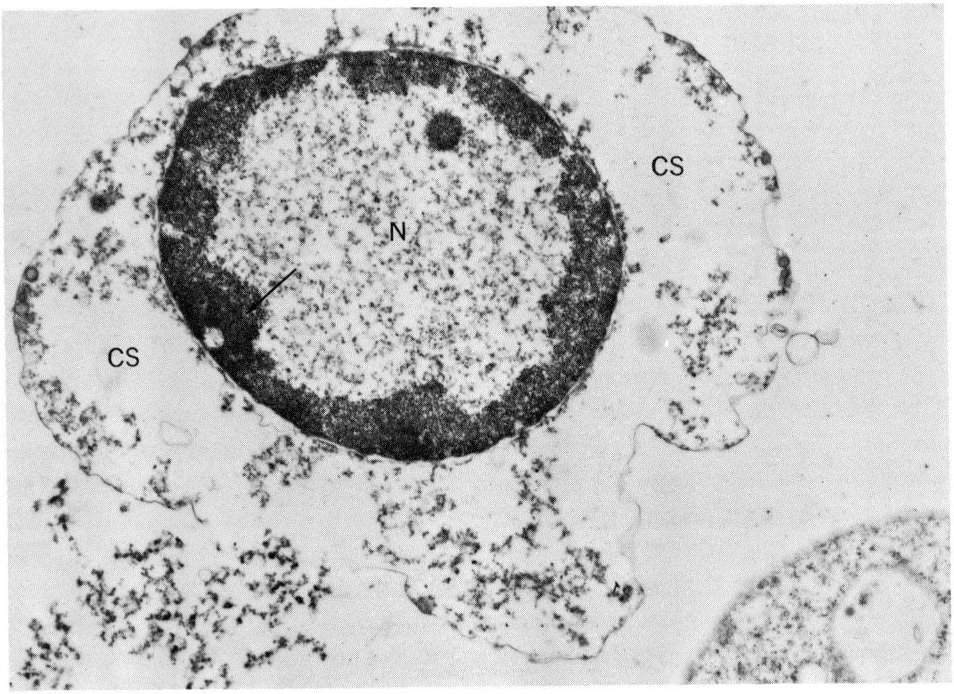

Figure 2-16. Necrotic Ehrlich ascites tumor cell after treatment with sulfhydryl reagent, **p**-chloromercuribenzoate. The chromatin of the nucleus (N) is severely clumped (pyknosis), and organelles have completely dissolved. The cell sap (CS) is expanded and pale.

brane protein sulfhydryl groups, causing rapid increase in permeability with subsequent ion shifts and inactivation of membrane transport systems (Fig. 2-16). Once again, since the mitochondria are not primarily affected, they proceed to accumulate the entering calcium; the electron microscope is not needed to see the massive mitochondrial calcification that results.

Evidence of tubular regeneration was also seen in the third case. As the tubule cells die, they detach from each other and from the basement membrane and slough into the urine. Other cells, which have successfully resisted the injury, are stimulated to re-enter the mitotic cycle and thus cover the defects left by the dead cells. The new cells then proceed with differentiation, and over a 2–4 week period normal epithelium again covers the tubule.

Other common agents or processes associated with membrane damage—such as amphotericin, complement lysis, and direct mechanical trauma—presumably act in a similar fashion. Particularly striking is the lytic action on the structure

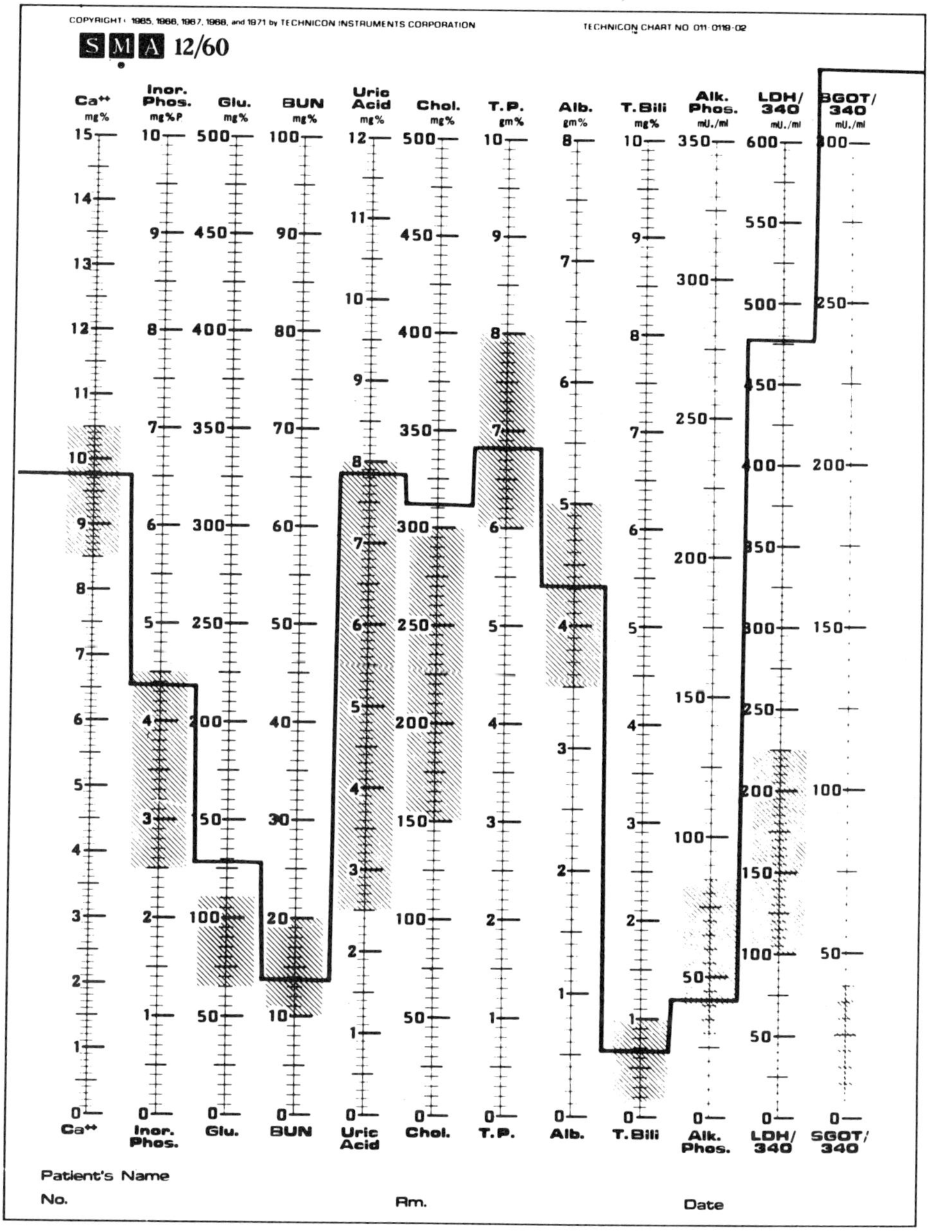

Figure 2-17. Biochemical profile of serum findings in acute myocardial infarction. These results are the recorder tracing from an SMA-12 autoanalyzer. Solid line indicates the findings in the patient; hatched areas indicate the range of normal. (Reproduced from J. A. Preston and D. B. Troxel (1971), **Biochemical Profiling in Diagnostic Medicine,** New York, Technicon Instruments Corp.)

of the membrane, an action produced by complement-mediated hemolysis in human red blood cells.

3. Clinical pathological correlation of acute injury

When there is injury to a group of cells in the human body—myocardial, skeletal muscle, liver or kidney cells, for instance—materials are released from these cells which produce characteristic clinical manifestations. These manifestations represent both the direct effects of the released materials and the response of the body, e.g., the inflammatory process and fever. In addition, many released substances such as potassium, magnesium, and adenine nucleotides are usually harmless; these are rapidly diluted, or go into large body pools, or are excreted.

On the other hand, some substances released from damaged cells are useful in the diagnosis of cell damage. Among these are enzymes, which can be detected in very low concentrations (Fig. 2-17). After reaching a peak level in the plasma, the activity of enzymes released from damaged cells declines gradually. In general, enzymes located within the cell sap, such as lactate dehydrogenase, tend to be released before organelle enzymes such as lysosomal acid phosphatase or mitochondrial glutamic dehydrogenase; and membrane-bound enzymes seem to be

Figure 2-18. **a.** Hepatic parenchymal cell 4 hours after administration of carbon tetrachloride. Marked dilatation of the endoplasmic reticulum (ER) is seen. Polysomes appear intact, and mitochondria (M) show no change.

b. HeLa cell 6 hours after infection with Herpes simplex virus, showing dissociation of polysomes into ribosome monomers (R). M, mitochondrion; N, nucleus.

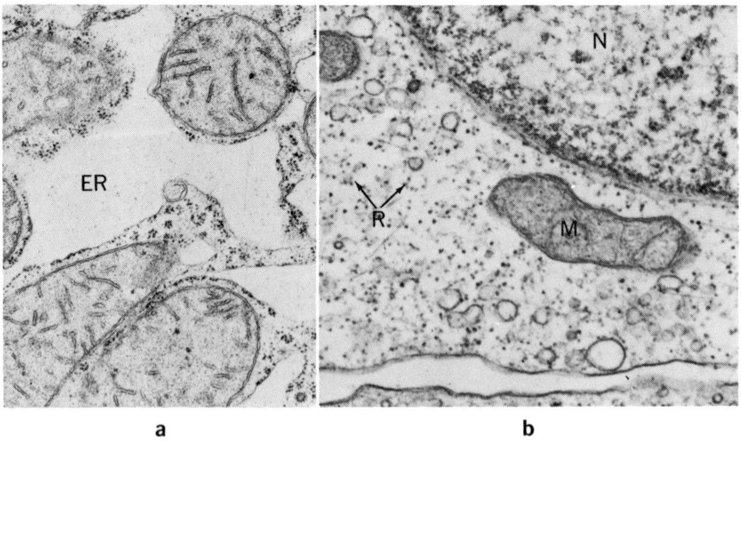

a b

less easily released than those not tightly associated with membranes. Although all cells have similar intracellular enzymes with similar organelle localizations, there are some variations that allow prediction of organ involvement; and because of its diagnostic power in puzzling cases, this technique has been pursued with vigor. The recent discovery of organ-specific isoenzymes has greatly increased specificity in locating organ involvement. Another diagnostic indicator of necrosis is altered cellular electrical activity, as revealed by the electroencephalogram and the electrocardiogram. Electrical abnormalities are related to the ion shifts and membrane alterations mentioned above.

Decreased protein synthesis in damaged cells may produce clinical manifestations useful in diagnosis and prognosis. This is especially true in the case of liver cell injury, since the liver normally synthesizes large amounts of protein, notably albumin and fibrinogen. In the presence of liver damage the serum concentration of these proteins decreases as turnover proceeds in the absence of synthesis. This may be associated with scattering of polysomes and dilatation of endoplasmic reticulum and Golgi apparatus (Fig. 2-18).

D. Chronic Cell Injury

1. Alterations of intracellular digestion

a. The cytocavitary network

The application of the electron microscope to the study of cells has revealed that the various membrane systems that permeate virtually the entire cytoplasm are anatomically and physiologically related (Fig. 2-19). These cytoplasmic structures are referred to as endoplasmic reticulum (ER), Golgi apparatus, lysosomes, microbodies, and nuclear envelope. It is evident that all of these components form a functionally interconnected system of cavities that is separated from the cell sap by membranes. This system is called the *cytocavitary network.*

It has become conventional to divide the cytocavitary network into two parts, exoplasmic and endoplasmic. The exoplasmic portion includes phagosomes, lysosomes, multivesicular bodies, secretory granules, and the maturing face of the Golgi apparatus; the endoplasmic portion includes the forming face of the Golgi apparatus, endoplasmic reticulum, microbodies or peroxisomes, and nuclear envelope. The membranes of the exoplasmic side are thicker, measuring about 100 Å; endoplasmic membranes are about 60 Å. In addition, exoplasmic membranes have high lipid/protein ratios and larger amounts of cholesterol.

The Golgi apparatus appears to contain the transition between the two portions. Movement of particles occurs from the outside of the cell into the exoplas-

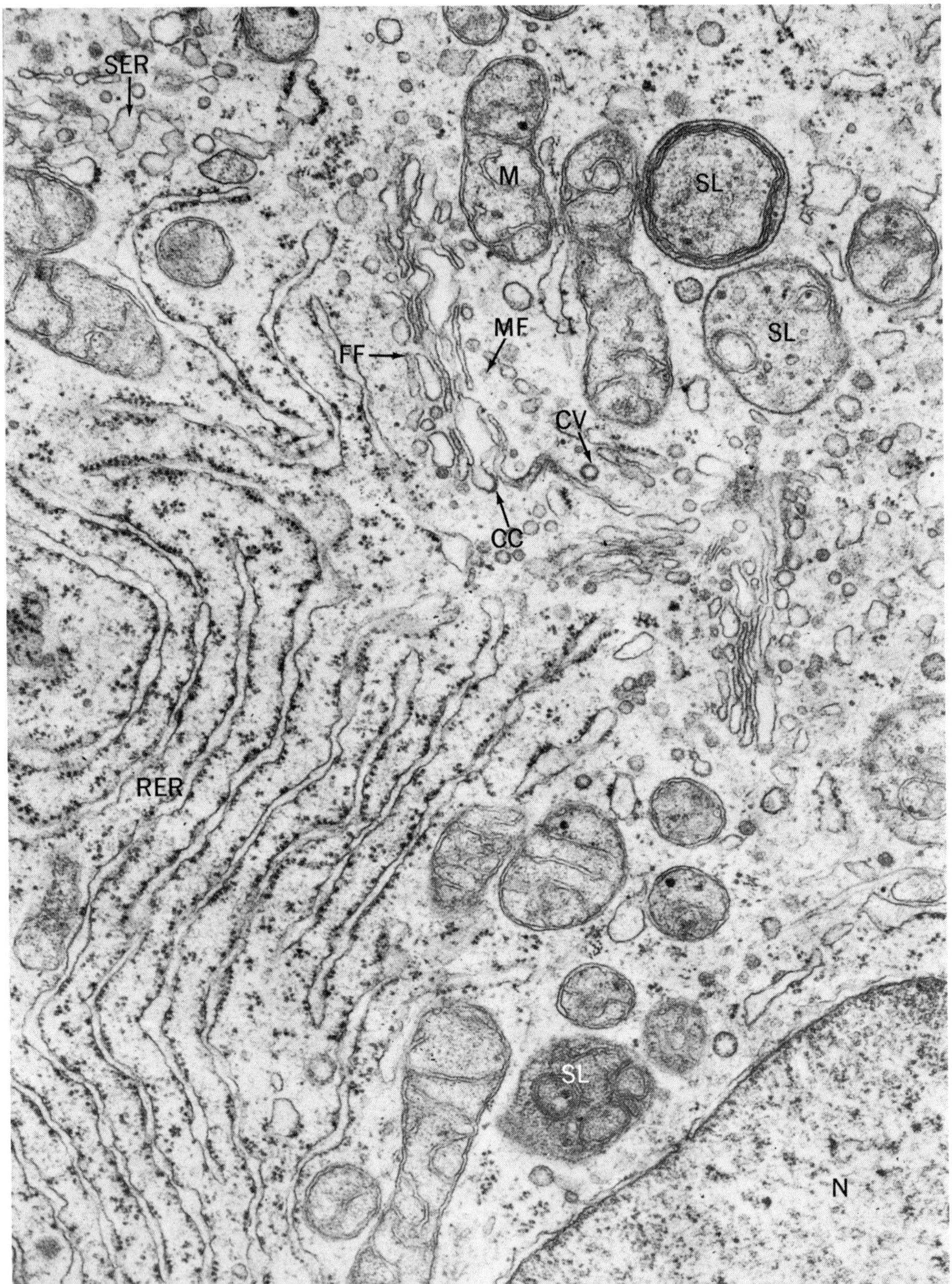
SER
M
SL
SL
MF
FF
CV
CC
RER
SL
N

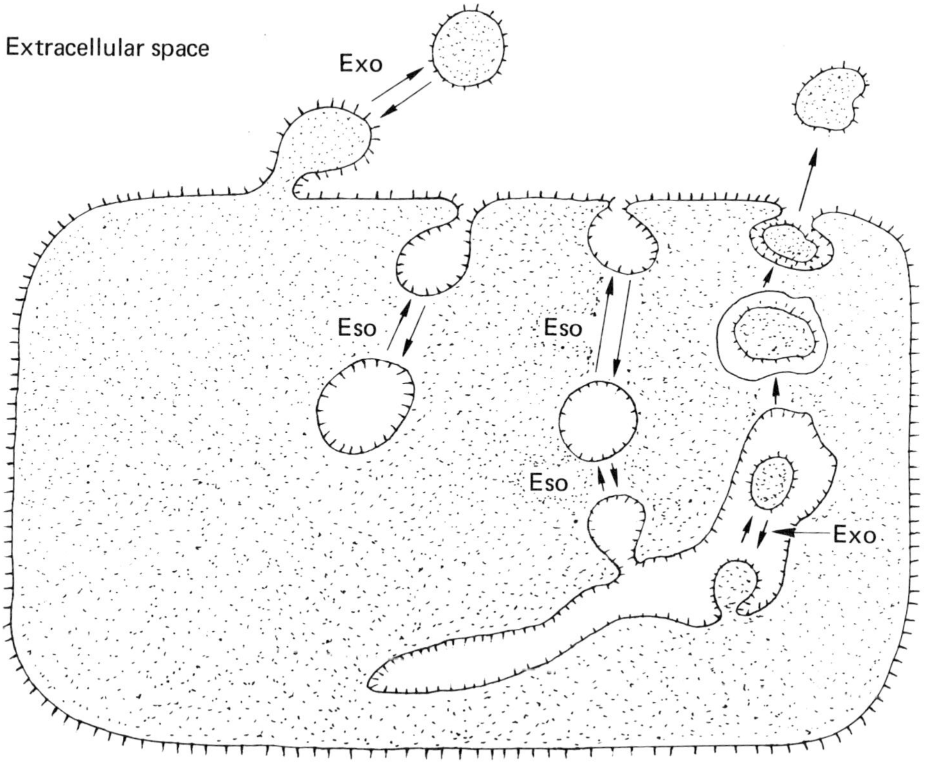

Figure 2-20. Diagram illustrating the principles of exotropy and esotropy. For more information see text.

mic side and again out of the cell, but particles entering the exoplasmic side from the cell exterior do not enter the endoplasmic portion. On the other hand, proteins that are synthesized for secretion enter the endoplasmic side, pass through the Golgi apparatus region into exoplasmic membrane-bound vacuoles, and are secreted to the cell surface or into secondary lysosomes. The Golgi apparatus may also have a key role in modifying the membrane through changes in lipid composition and addition of the glycocalyx. This could be of great importance

Figure 2-19. Region of Golgi apparatus in normal human kidney tubule cell. The cisternae of rough-surfaced endoplasmic reticulum (RER) are in transition to Golgi apparatus at the forming face (FF). Some coated vesicles (CV) and coated caveoli (CC) are present in the Golgi region. Note the vesicles along the maturing face (MF) of the Golgi apparatus and the adjacent digestive vacuoles (SL) containing debris. Mitochondria (M) and cytoplasmic filaments can be seen. SER, smooth-surfaced endoplasmic reticulum; N, nucleus.

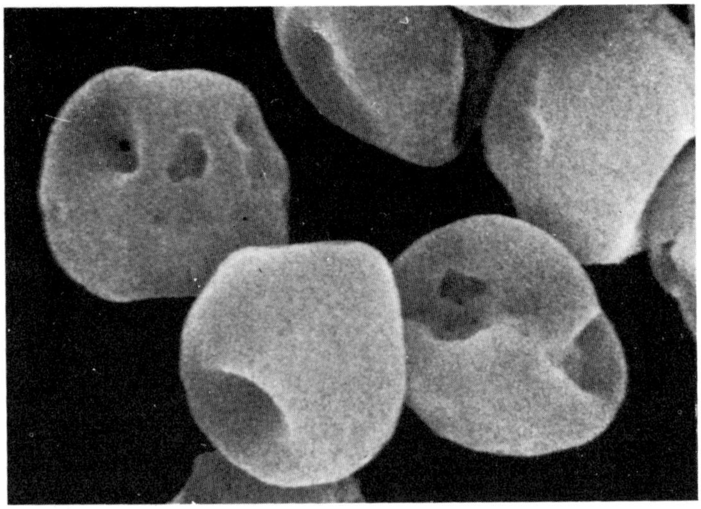

Figure 2-21. Human red blood cells treated with 1×10^{-3}M primaquine in the presence of glucose, which induces estropy of the plasma membrane. Note that the cells have rounded up; note also the numerous single and compound esotropic invaginations.

in specifying the identity of the cell surface, and might exert critical control over differentiation and malignant transformation.

The space within these cavities is topologically equivalent to the extracellular space, and the membranes are topologically equivalent to the plasma membrane. Transport between various portions of the cytocavitary system, as well as to and from the cell sap and the extracellular space, often occurs by means of vesicle formations and fusions. Although these may initially seem complicated, they can be reduced to two geometrically simple processes termed *esotropy* and *exotropy* (Fig. 2-20).

Esotropy (Figs. 2-20, 21) (*Greek:* "a turning in") refers to a membrane movement wherein the membrane turns in, so that the original outer (exoplasmic) surface becomes the inner surface of a new membrane-bound vesicle. If one remembers that the space within the cytocavitary network is topologically equivalent to the extracellular space, it is apparent that esotropy may occur by budding from either the cell membrane or the cytocavitary membrane *into* the cyto-

Figure 2-22. Micrograph of HeLa cell after infection with Herpes simplex virus. Several virions in the cytoplasm are undergoing exotropic budding into membrane-limited cisternae. **1.** indicates a virion in the cell sap approaching a cisterna. **2.** indicates a bud with a slender stalk into a membrane-bound cisterna. **3.** indicates two virions in a fairly completely formed bud. **(courtesy of Dr. Bernard B. Poeschel)**

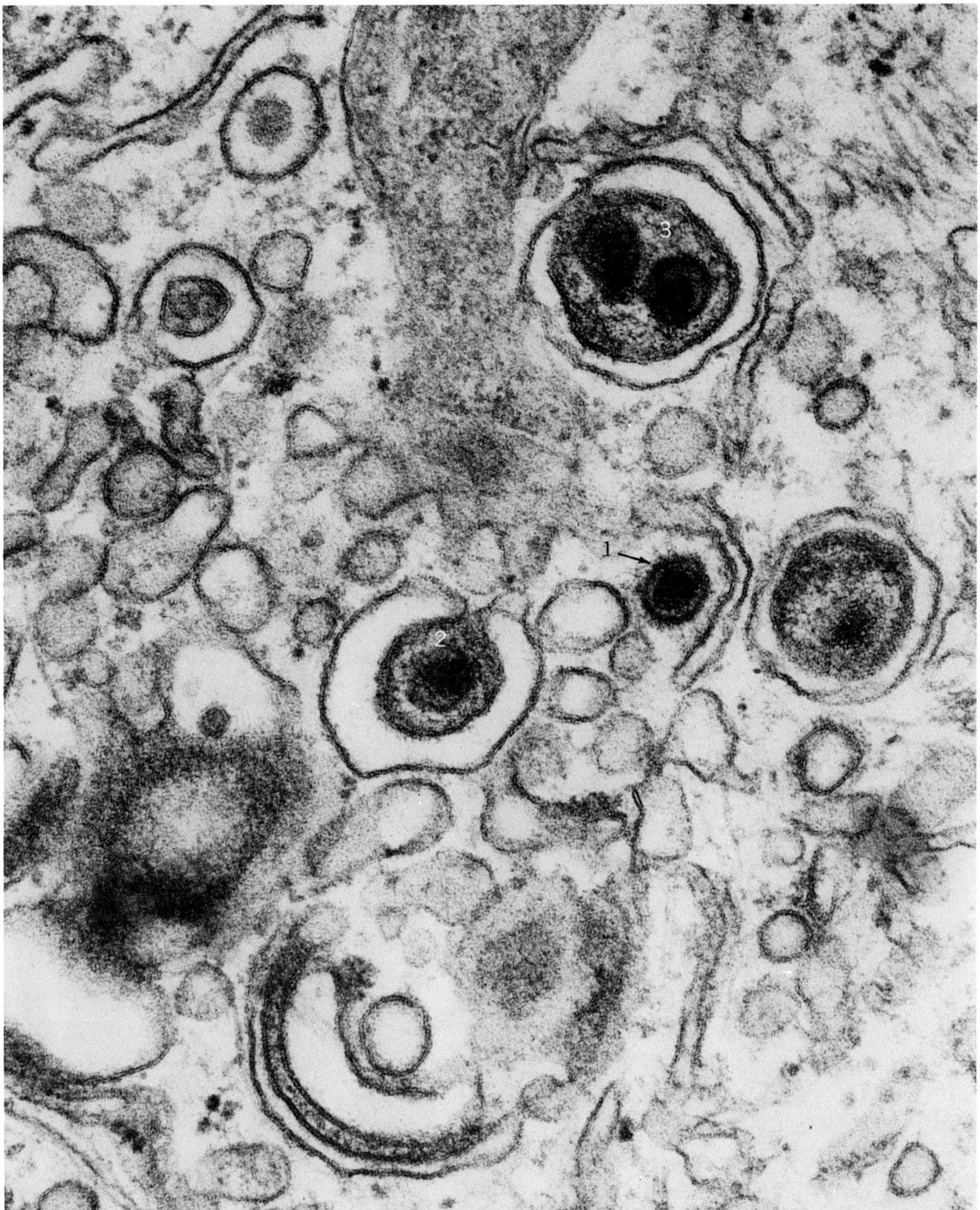
1
2
3

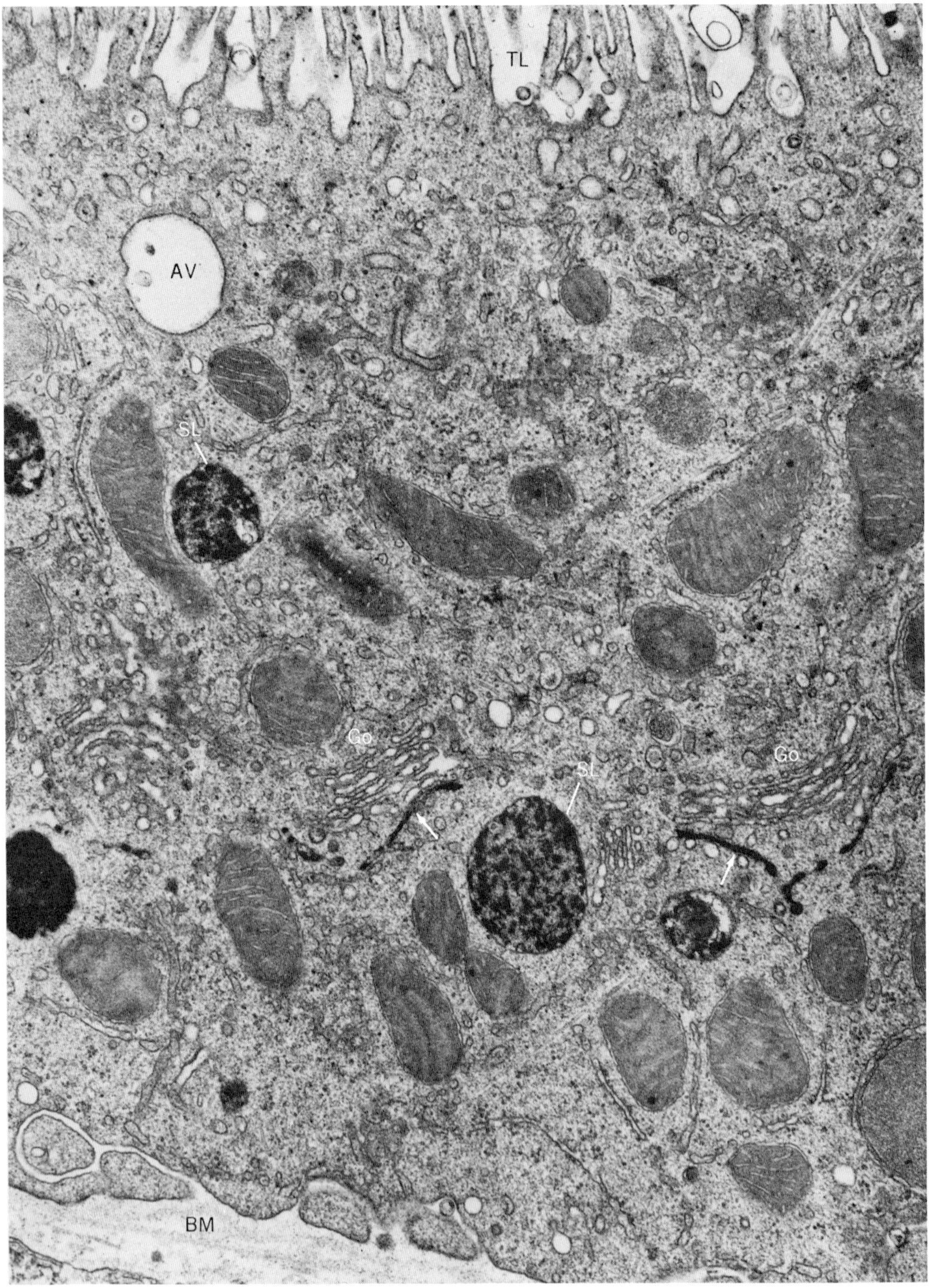
TL
AV
SL
Go
SL
Go
BM

plasm. Topologically, an esotropic vesicle always contains extracellular material or its equivalent–the contents of the cytocavitary network. When the process occurs in the reverse direction (reverse esotropy), the vesicle fuses with a membrane, bringing the vesicle contents into continuity with the extracellular space or with the space of the cytocavitary network. Examples of forward esotropy include phagocytosis, pinocytosis, elaboration of transitional vesicles from endoplasmic reticulum at the forming face of the Golgi apparatus, elaboration of secretory vesicles from the maturing face of the Golgi apparatus, and formation of microbodies. A model of esotropy is provided by treatment of normal red blood cells with the antimalarial compound primaquine (Fig. 2-21). Examples of reverse esotropy include fusion of secretory granules with the cell membrane, fusion of Golgi vesicles with phagosomes, and fusions between various secondary lysosomes.

Exotropy (*Greek:* "a turning out") refers to the opposite membrane movement, wherein the membrane turns out from the cytoplasm into the cytocavitary or extracellular space so that inner faces of the membrane face toward one another. An exotropic vesicle thus always contains cell sap. In reverse exotropy, fusion of an exotropic structure brings the two portions of cell sap into contact. Exotropy into the endoplasmic reticulum appears to be a common mechanism of autophagocytosis. Many viruses have appropriated this mechanism, acquiring their outer envelope by exotropy into the endoplasmic reticulum (Fig. 2-22) or into the space of the nuclear envelope, or by exotropic budding from the surface plasma membrane. At the extreme, mitotic division could be considered a gross example of exotropy. Examples of reverse exotropy include viral entry into cells, where the viral envelope fuses with the cell membrane, and, at the cell level, fusion of cells to produce syncytial giant cells. Fusions between exotropic and esotropic vesicles have not been reported.

Although much remains to be learned about the precise basis of these membrane movements, available evidence strongly indicates that they depend on high-energy compounds such as ATP, and are modified by cyclic AMP, possibly through mechanisms involving cell filaments and microtubules.

b. The lysosome

The term *lysosome* was originally used by de Duve and his associates (see review by de Duve and Wattiaux, 1966) to refer to a class of cytoplasmic particles

Figure 2-23. Rat proximal tubule, illustrating distribution of acid phosphatase. Note reaction products in secondary lysosomes (SL) and maturing face (arrows) of the Golgi apparatus (Go). TL, tubular lumen; BM, basement membrane; AV, autophagic vacuole. (Courtesy of Dr. Elizabeth M. McDowell)

a

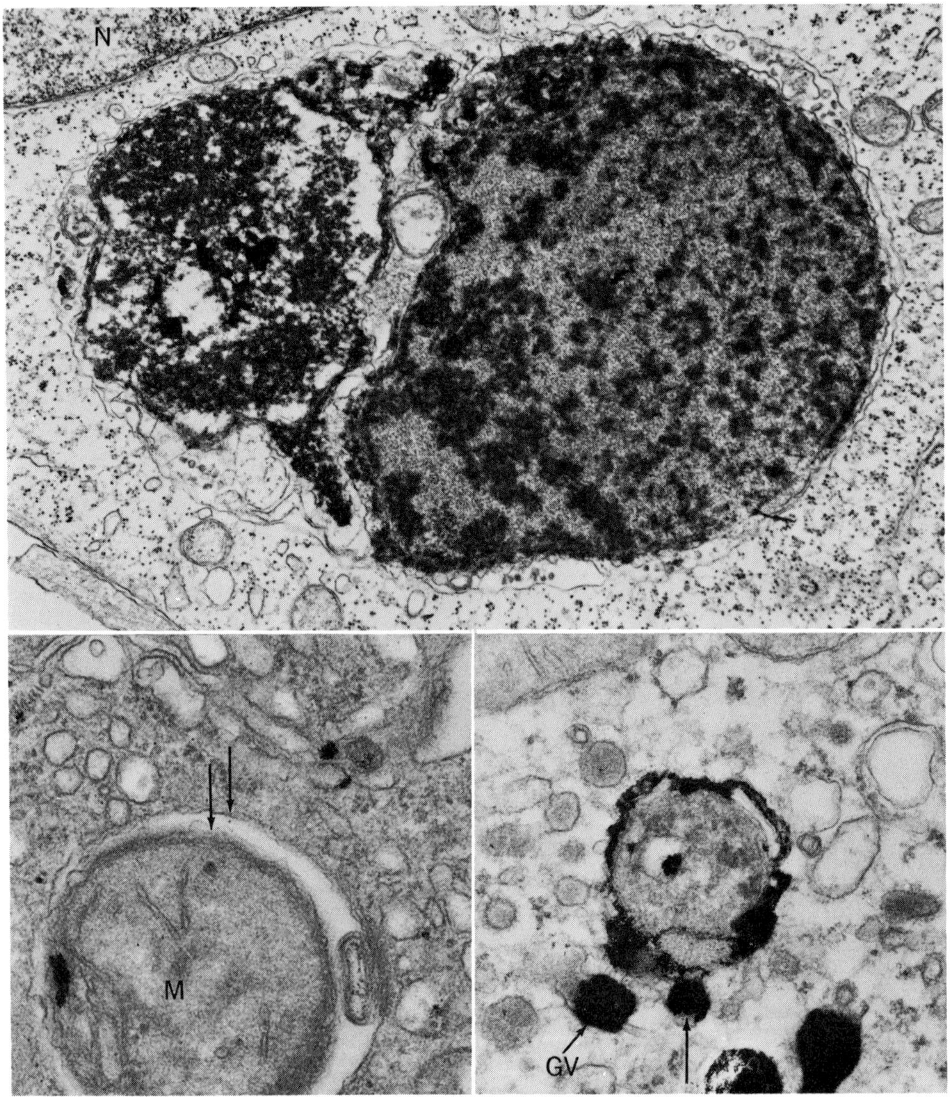

b c

Figure 2-24. **a.** Giant heterophagic vacuole in a HeLa cell 12 hours after infection with Herpes virus. The digestive vacuole contains debris from necrotic cells that have been phagocytosed. N, nucleus.

b. Newly formed autophagic vacuole in rat liver 1 hour after administration of glucagon. Note the double limiting membrane (arrows). The vacuole contains a mitochondrion (M) and a focus of acid phosphatase reaction product probably representing phagocytosed Golgi vesicles. Gomori lead phosphate technique.

c. Autophagic vacuole 1 hour after the administration of glucagon, showing apparent fusion of an acid phosphatase-containing vesicle (arrow) with the outer wall of an autophagic vacuole. Note the nearby Golgi vesicle (GV) with acid phosphatase activity.

limited by a membrane and containing hydrolytic enzymes, active at acid pH, and capable of rapidly digesting many components of the cell (see review edited by Dingle and Fell, 1969) (Fig. 2-23). The enzymes exhibit the property of structure-linked latency; when the particles are intact the substrate cannot gain access to the enzyme, and measured enzyme activities are low. If the membrane is damaged, substrate gains access to the enzyme and the enzyme activity can be measured (Fig. 2-10). If the damage is severe, the enzymes may escape completely from the lysosomes.

Although the concept of the lysosome as defined by its content of acid hydrolases is extremely useful, one should not lose sight of the fact that secretory and digestive vacuoles exist in a continuous spectrum from acid hydrolase-rich lysosomes to structures completely free of acid hydrolases, and indeed transform from the one type into the other. In the present chapter, therefore, the term lysosome is used to refer to that part of the cytocavitary network chiefly concerned with intracellular digestion, regardless of acid hydrolase content.

c. Heterophagocytosis

Heterophagocytosis refers to the esotropic uptake of particles such as macromolecules or macromolecular complexes from outside the cell or on the surface of the plasma membrane (Fig. 2-24a). Often this uptake is referred to as phagocytosis (cell eating) or pinocytosis (cell drinking), or collectively as endocytosis. The following case illustrates lysosomal storage of environmental materials taken in by heterophagocytosis.

CASE 4 A 38-year-old man had been employed in a titanium dioxide factory for ten years. During the past four years he had recurring episodes of a productive cough associated with fever. Dyspnea was aggravated by work, and the symptoms were considerably relieved by vacations. The patient was also a moderate-to-heavy smoker. Laboratory examination of the blood revealed no abnormalities. Tests of pulmonary function indicated severe loss. A chest x-ray showed many densities suggesting diffuse fibrosis of the lungs. A surgical biopsy was taken from the lateral aspect of the lingula.

Examinations of sections of lung under polarized light revealed abundant birefringent crystals within many cells, including alveolar epithelial cells. By electron microscopy the titanium particles could be readily demonstrated within the lysosomes of the alveolar epithelial cells and alveolar macrophages. Particles were also noted in reticuloendothelial cells within the draining lymph nodes. The intralysosomal particles could be characterized by their x-ray spectra. (Fig. 2-26a–c)

During heterophagocytosis the phagosome carries ingested particles into the cell, where it acquires digestive hydrolases by reverse esotropic fusion with pre-existing digestive vacuoles to form a new digestive vacuole. The material within

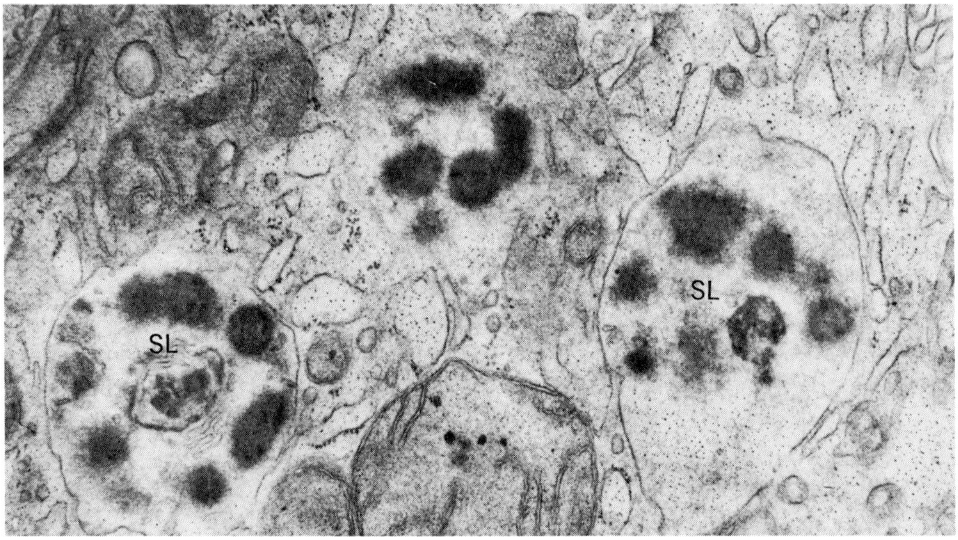

a

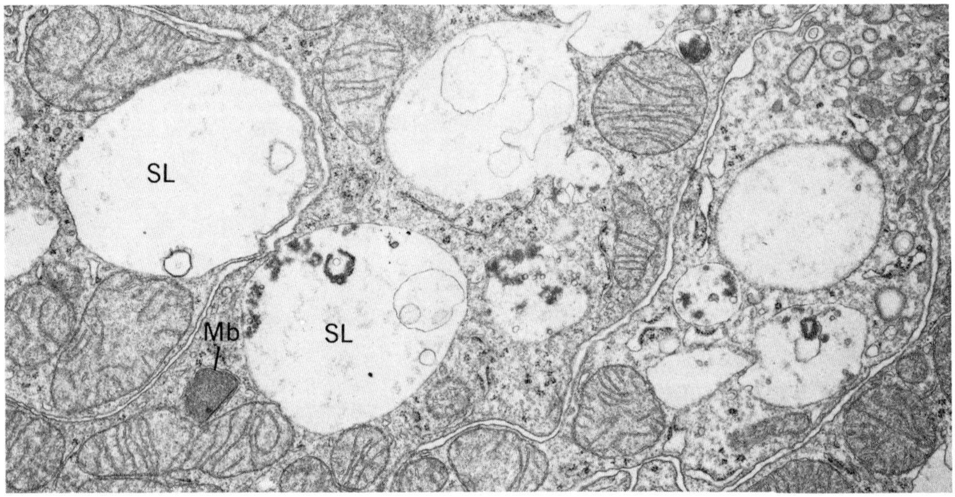

b

Figure 2-25. **a.** Kidney tubule cell from a child with glomerulonephritis. Reabsorbed proteins accumulate in the proximal tubule lysosomes (SL). By light microscopy hyaline droplets can be seen.

b. Proximal tubule from a human patient dying of shock and treated with mannitol. Secondary lysosomes (SL) are dilated because of the accumulation of mannitol and fluid in these bodies. Mb, Microbody may then be hydrolyzed either to indigestible debris or to soluble intermediates such as small dipeptides or amino acids, which can be reutilized or released from the cell.

Heterophagocytosis has critical implications in health and disease. The cells lining the proximal convoluted tubules of the kidney, for example, have well-developed systems for heterophagy (Fig. 2-25b) and are continually reabsorbing the protein that passes through the glomerulus into the filtrate (see review by Trump and Ericsson, 1965). When the glomerulus is diseased, as in glomerulonephritis, much more protein leaks through it and much more is reabsorbed and thus conserved by the tubules (Fig. 2-25a). Heterophagocytosis of microorganisms by leukocytes constitutes an important defense mechanism against infection (see Chapter 4). After phagocytosis the specific granules of the leukocyte fuse with the phagosomes, releasing digestive enzymes and other antibacterial substances into it. It has recently been suggested that antigen processing via heterophagocytosis by macrophages is an essential preliminary step in the stimulation of immunoglobulin synthesis by antibody-producing cells. More controversial is the possible role of heterophagic uptake in memory transfer and in the uptake of interferon. Certain endocrine secretory cells, such as thyroid epithelium, take up colloid via heterophagocytosis before processing and then releasing it into the bloodstream. Heterophagocytosis is apparently at work also in the newborn intestine during suckling to absorb maternal immunoglobulins present in milk. A general mechanism for removal of necrotic cells is heterophagocytosis by scavenging phagocytes.

In addition, although most material within digestive vacuoles is digested, some debris remains in all cells. Ordinarily this debris is largely lipid. It often becomes oxidized and forms pigmented autofluorescent materials termed *lipofuscin* or "aging pigment." The debris-filled bodies are called residual bodies. In some cells the residual bodies are known to fuse by reverse esotropy with the plasma membrane and to discharge their contained debris. In others, however, this probably cannot occur, and lipofuscin-filled residual bodies will tend to accumulate. The neuron is such a cell; neuronal lipofuscin increases in a linear fashion with age. Neurons become, as it were, filled with the debris of a lifetime.

Non-biological material is often retained within the digestive vacuoles of phagocytes. In tattooing, for instance, these pigments are retained for years in the digestive vacuoles of cutaneous macrophages, and in anthracosis inhaled carbon is retained for years in pulmonary phagocytes. Storage of certain types of material such as silica (Fig. 2-26d), asbestos, titanium dioxide pigments as in Case 4 (Fig. 2-26a-c), and perhaps other environmentally acquired materials in lysosomes may be of great importance in the pathogenesis of pulmonary disease.

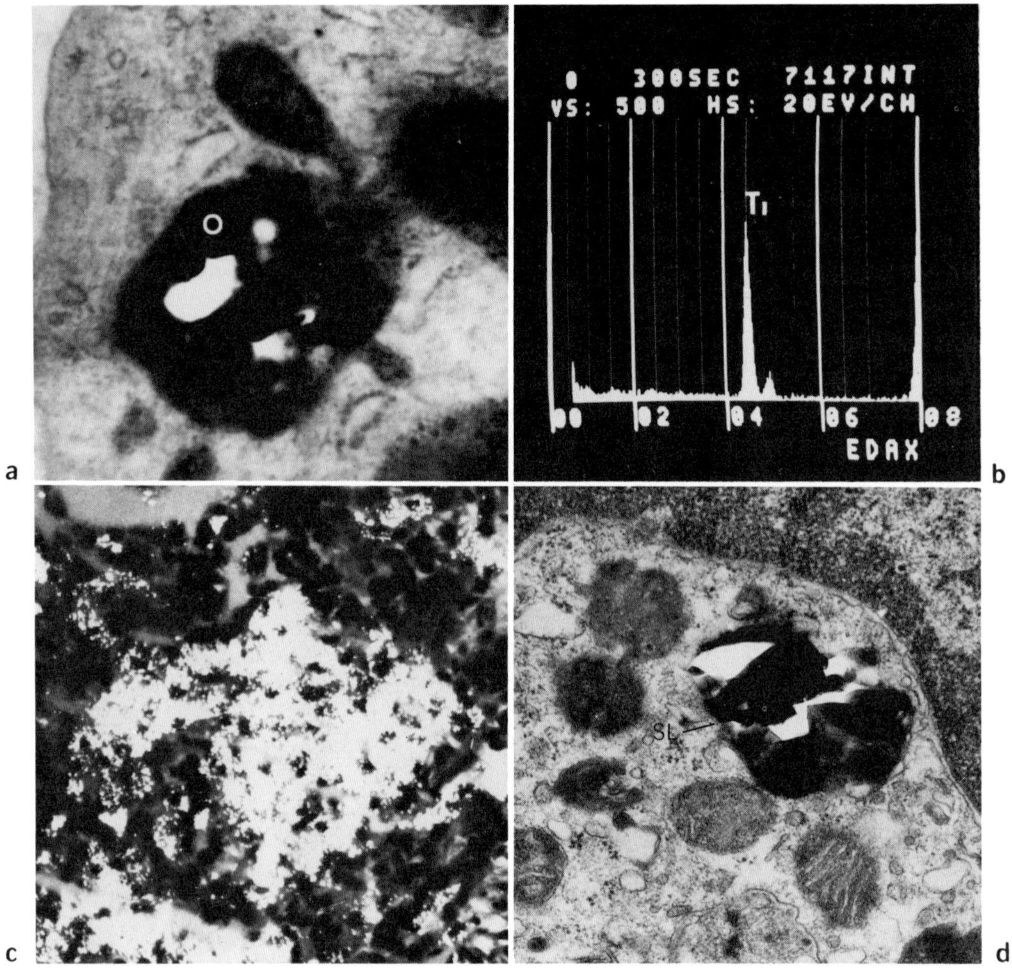

Figure 2-26. **a.** Electron micrograph of an alveolar macrophage from a titanium dioxide worker. Extremely electron-dense particles are in secondary lysosomes. O indicates the area of x-ray microprobe analysis.

b. X-ray spectrum from the area indicated, showing Ti to be present.

c. Polarized light shows the pigment to be birefringent. (Reproduced from R. Elo **et al.**, Arch. Pathol., **94**:417, 1972. Copyright 1972, American Medical Association)

d. Macrophage exposed to SiO_4 showing concentration of silica in a secondary lysosome (SL). (Courtesy of Dr. Moon L. Shin)

d. Autophagocytosis

Autophagocytosis is quite similar to heterophagocytosis (Fig. 2-24b, c), except that digestion of cells and organelles occurs within the vacuoles. Autophagic vacuoles appear to form by exotropy into a cisterna of endoplasmic reticulum or other portion of the cytocavitary network, resulting in the enclosure of a portion of cytoplasm, which may include organelles, such as a mitochondrion, in a double-walled sac. Enzyme is added by fusion of endosecretory vesicles or digestive vacuoles with the outer membrane of the sac in the double-walled stage. The inner membrane thickens to resemble the membrane of other digestive vacuoles, and debris-filled vacuoles often result (Fig. 2-24). Autophagocytosis thus provides an obvious means for organelle turnover. In the liver cell, for example, it is estimated that the rate of mitochondrial turnover (ten day half-life) could be accounted for by autophagocytosis, and at least some hepatic glycogen turnover occurs within autophagic vacuoles (Hers, 1965). Autophagocytosis may serve also as a nutritional mechanism under unfavorable conditions, such as general starvation or specific dietary deficiencies. Utilizing its own substances, the cell seems to accept a reduction in the number of organelles in order to maintain homeostasis.

Some of the most dramatic examples of increased autophagocytosis occur in association with involutionary processes, such as the atrophy of the mammary gland after lactation, the atrophy of the secondary sex organs in elderly persons, and the atrophy of functional units that accompanies progressive sub-lethal ischemia in organs such as the liver or kidney (see review edited by Dingle and Fell, 1969). In all such cases, organ remodeling is accompanied by the appearance of large autophagic vacuoles that ultimately become pigmented residual bodies.

Autophagocytosis may be important in differentiation and cell division as well. Phytohemagglutinin-stimulated lymphocytes exhibit numerous autophagic vacuoles. Large numbers of autophagic vacuoles are observed in the regenerating liver after hepatectomy. It has been suggested that autophagocytosis may have the function in cell division of destroying antimitotic materials.

e. Role of digestion in injured cells

In the following case several episodes of shock over three days led to the formation of numerous large residual bodies from autophagic vacuoles in the liver and kidney.

CASE 5 After being crushed between two tractors, a 48-year-old man was admitted to the hospital with a comminuted pelvic fracture, rupture of the mem-

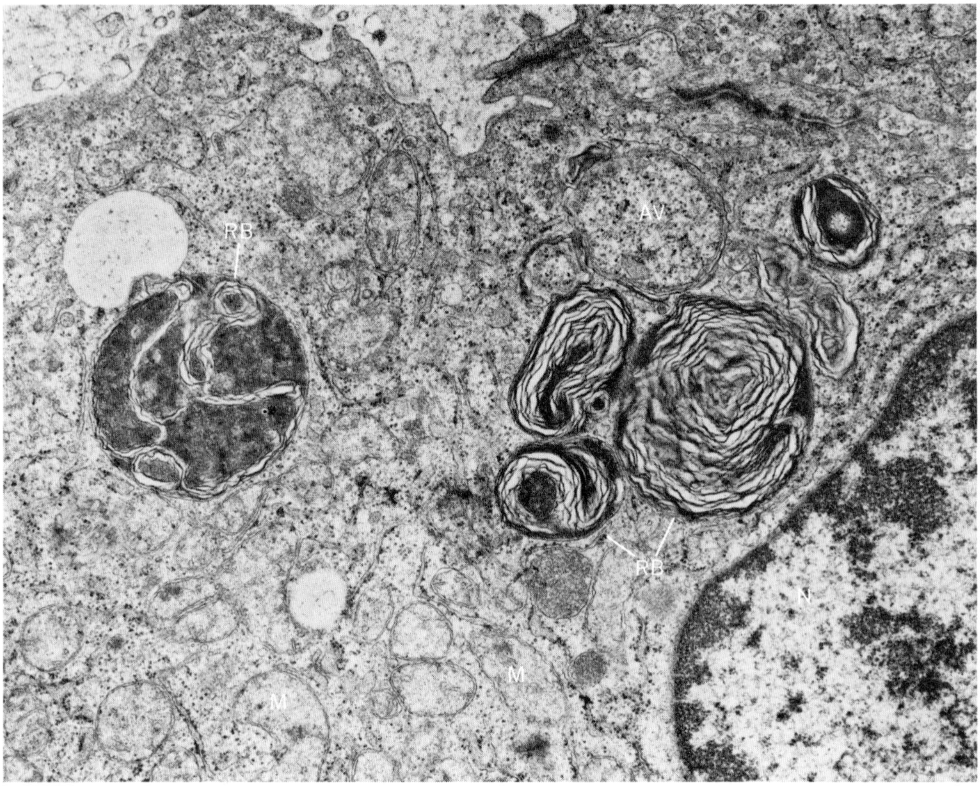

Figure 2-27. Hepatic parenchymal cell from patient (Case 5) who had suffered several episodes of shock. Several autophagic vacuoles (AV) are filled with lamellar debris formed from incomplete digestion material taken in by autophagy. N, nucleus; RB, residual bodies; M, mitochondria.

branous urethra, perforation of the extraperitoneal rectum, and transection of the left external iliac artery. These injuries were repaired at surgery. Blood pressure remained at 90/50 mm Hg over an 8-hour period but had risen to 160/120 within 18 hours after injury. The patient's pulse stabilized at 140. His urinary output dropped, however, and the blood urea nitrogen rose to 160 mg per dl.* He was placed on peritoneal dialysis but developed light stupor, which progressed to coma with absence of respiration and signs of injury to the brain stem. His blood pressure fell repeatedly to shock levels, and blood cultures were positive for Proteus species. He died three days after surgery.

The chief sub-lethal change in the renal tubular cells was an alteration of

* Normal value: 10–20 mg per dl.

lysosomal digestion that led to accumulation of large secondary lysosomes filled with debris. These autophagic vacuoles probably derived in large part from incomplete organelle digestion, the organelles entering the lysosome system by either heterophagy or autophagy. Considerable debris of a similar type—the product of cell lysis or normally occurring defecation of lysosomal contents—appeared also in the tubular lumen. Parallel alterations were found in the patient's liver cells (Fig. 2-27).

Increased formation of autophagic vacuoles is a common sub-lethal reaction to injury in the liver, kidney, and other organs. By light microscopy these autophagic vacuoles are often seen as large eosinophilic inclusions. As the vacuoles form and digestion occurs, debris accumulates—as in this case—often including lamellar myelin-like material. Ultimately, conversion to lipofuscin-type pigment occurs, and residual bodies filled with that pigment accumulate in the involved cell.

Several types of sub-lethal injuries result in the formation of increased numbers of autophagic vacuoles. Pathogenetic factors include damage to membranes in organelles, decreased nutrition, regeneration of cells, neoplasia, and damage by bacterial products. Damage to organelle membranes, which occurs as a nonspecific feature of many diseases, seems to be especially effective in promoting the formation of autophagic vacuoles. One known pathogenetic factor involved in membrane damage is the lipid peroxidation that occurs experimentally in animals deficient in antioxidants such as vitamin E. Numerous autophagic vacuoles result promptly from such deficiencies. Allison (1968) has proposed a hypothesis of carcinogenesis based on autophagic destruction or alteration of chromosomes to produce mutations; but this theory is yet to be confirmed. Some hormonal effects mediated by cyclic AMP are associated with the formation of autophagic vacuoles.

f. Changes in lysosomal enzymes

In some cells, stimulation of pinocytic uptake of digestible materials induces the synthesis of acid hydrolases. This apparently represents genetic induction, and can be blocked by inhibitors of RNA or protein synthesis.

In contrast to this increase in lysosomal enzymes, decreases may also occur. Since many enzymes are present in the digestive vacuoles, one could postulate a series of diseases with one of the enzymes deficient or absent in each (see chapter and review by Reisbois *et al.*, 1970). Many such diseases have been identified; they are characterized by accumulation of complex lipids or carbohydrates within digestive vacuoles in various cells throughout the body (Fig. 2-4b; Fig. 2-28c). Many of these so-called "storage diseases" exert their most serious effects on neu-

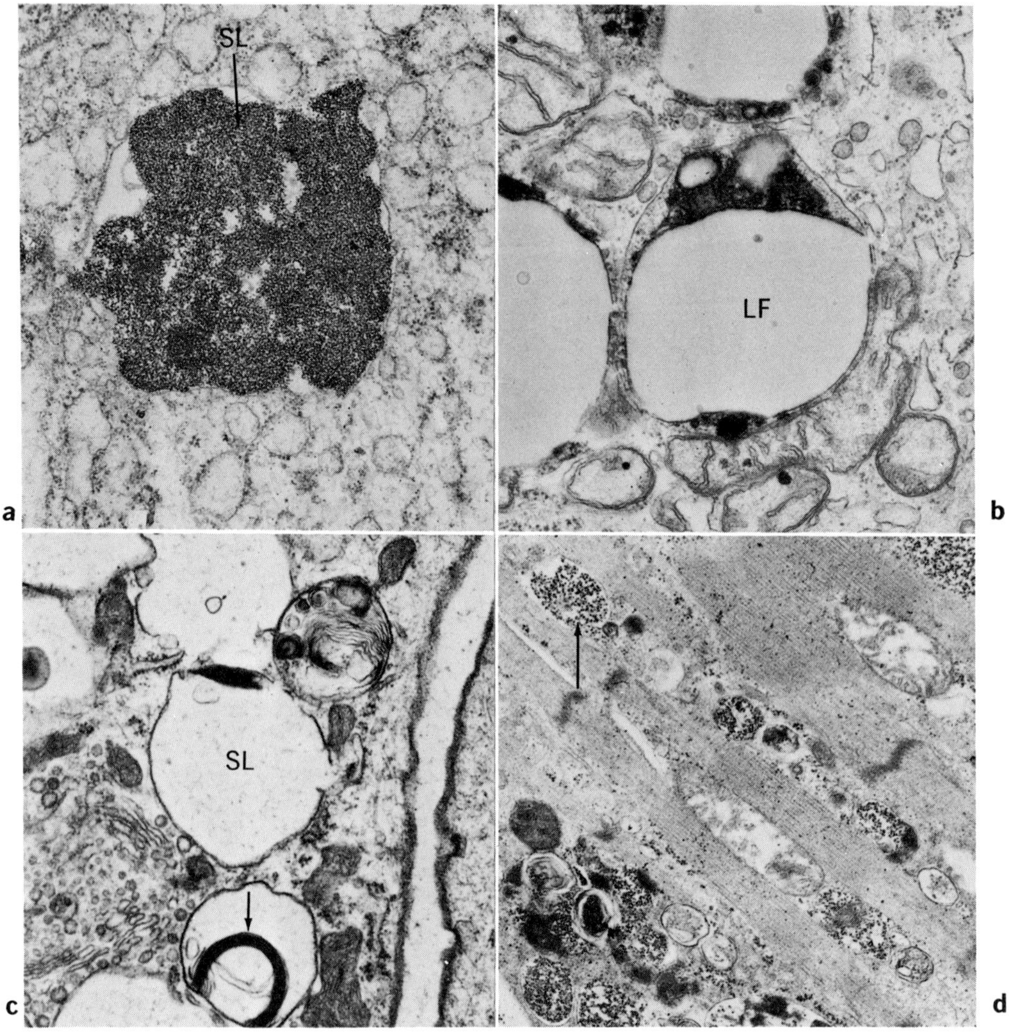

Figure 2-28. **a.** Hepatic cell from a patient with hemosiderosis. A large lysosome (SL) is almost filled with fine dense granules of ferritin and hemosiderin. Similar granules are scattered in the cell sap.

b. Kidney tubule cell from aging human patient. Large accumulations of lipofuscin (LF) are seen in several lysosomes.

c. Visceral epithelial cell of the glomerulus from a patient with neurovisceral lipidosis. Large lysosomes (SL) contain lipid debris forming myelin figures (arrow) and with acid mucopolysaccharides (which appear pale in these preparations).

d. Heart-muscle cell from a patient with Pompe's disease. Glycogen-filled lysosomes (arrows) are present in the sarcoplasm. (Courtesy of Dr. Doyle Graham) rons. These diseases may be susceptible to therapy by replacement of the missing enzyme in at least some organs, applying the principle that allows the mixing of contents between heterophagic and autophagic vacuoles.

The dramatic consequences of lysosomal deficiency are illustrated in the following case of Pompe's disease, or type II glycogenosis, in which lysosomal alpha-1-glucosidase is deficient.

> CASE 6 A 9-month-old baby boy was admitted to the hospital because of slowness of feeding, frequent choking, and constant drooling. Upon physical examination, the baby appeared weak, small, and poorly developed, and was found to have a large heart. Liver and muscle biopsies revealed large amounts of glycogen, much of which was within lysosomes. Assay of lysosomal acid hydrolases revealed normal or elevated levels, except for alpha-1-glucosidase, which was present in greatly diminished quantities.

This is only one of many types of glycogen-storage disease in which enzymes involved in glycogenolysis are deficient. It does, however, illustrate the serious consequences of abnormal lysosomal digestion. In Pompe's disease, glycogen accumulates in the lysosomes and ultimately in other compartments, including the cell sap as well (Fig. 2-28d). It is conceivable that the abnormal overloading and interference with lysosomal turnover cause severe cellular defects such as the myocardial failure seen in Pompe's disease.

g. Lysosomal storage

Under some conditions, lysosomes may act as reservoirs for certain biological materials. An example of increased transport of material to the lysosomes for storage is provided by ferritin and hemosiderin storage in the liver cell (see review by Kinney, 1973). Apoferritin is synthesized, in part, on the rough endoplasmic reticulum and transported through that system to the Golgi apparatus and then to the lysosomes, where storage and turnover occur. More apoferritin is synthesized on free polysomes and released into the cell sap. In conditions associated with increased levels of iron in the bloodstream, iron taken up by the liver cell may be added to the apoferritin in the cytocavitary network to form ferritin, which is relatively immune to attack by lysosomal enzymes and hence accumulates within all hepatic lysosomes. Iron is also added to apoferritin in the cell sap and enters lysosomes via autophagy. As this continues, the liver becomes loaded with iron, and much of the ferritin becomes converted to an insoluble, poorly characterized iron-containing protein called hemosiderin (Fig. 2-28a). In periods of iron depletion, iron is released from ferritin within the lysosomes and re-enters the bloodstream. In two disease states–hemochromatosis and hemosiderosis–abnormal amounts of both ferritin and hemosiderin are stored within hepatic lysosomes.

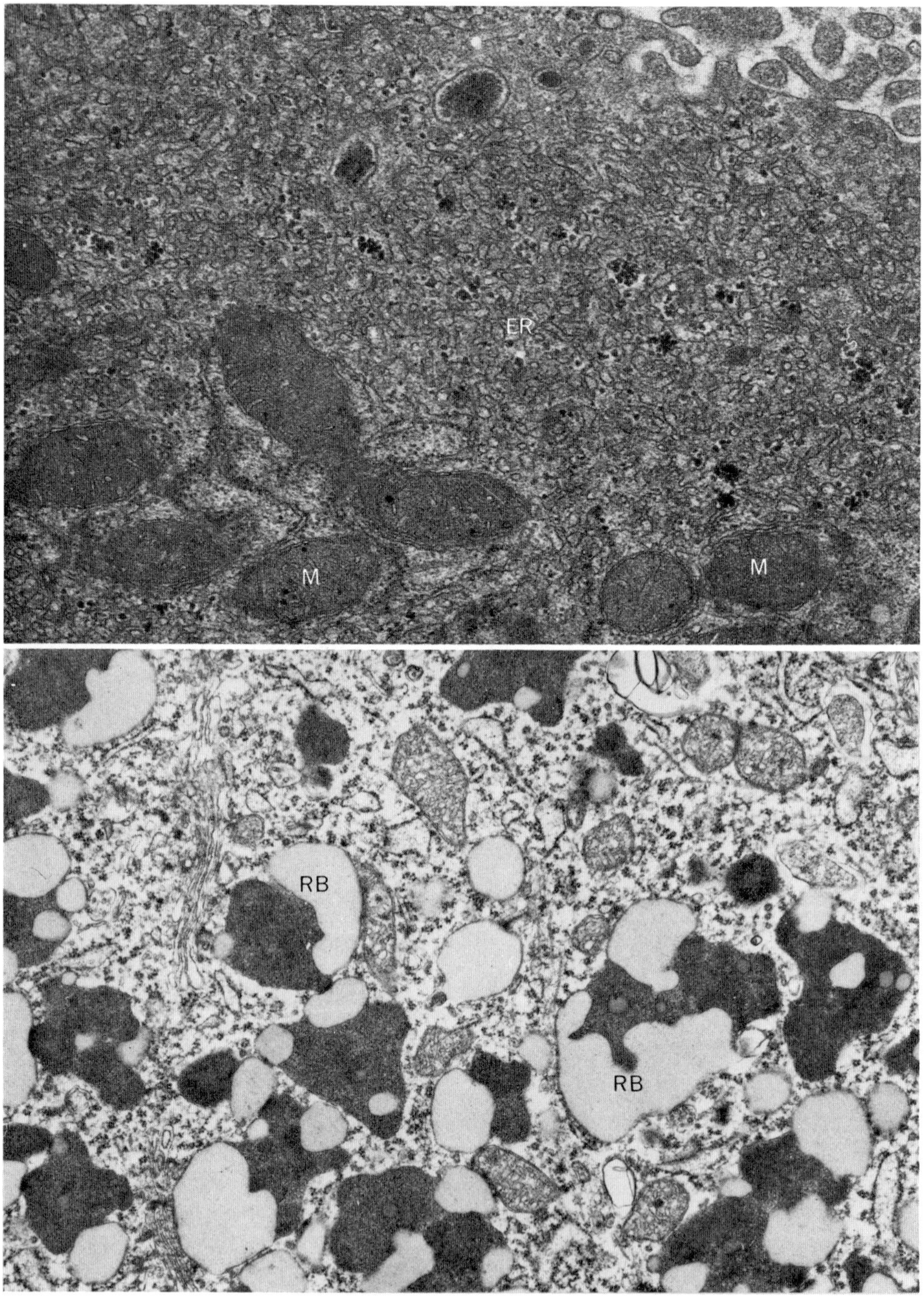

a

b

Since ATP is necessary for transport within the endoplasmic reticulum and through the Golgi system, ATP deficiency can result in defective transport of lysosomal enzymes and non-enzymatic components. This may result in their accumulation in the endoplasmic reticulum.

2. Cell growth, cell size, and aging

a. Hypertrophy

Cellular hypertrophy, an increase in the size of cells, results from an increase in the mass of their structural components. Ultrastructurally, it is often reflected by an increase in the size and number of organelles such as mitochondria, endoplasmic reticulum, and ribosomes; that is, hypertrophy of the cell may be caused by both hypertrophy and hyperplasia of organelles.

An interesting example of cellular hypertrophy occurs during the metabolism of certain drugs (Orrenius and Ernster, 1971). An important protective mechanism against these drugs is the mixed-function oxidase electron transport pathway, found in the endoplasmic reticulum of the liver and other organs. This enzymatic system catalyzes the metabolism of many exogenous compounds including drugs, carcinogenic hydrocarbons, insecticides, steroids, fatty acids, and other endogenous compounds.

Administration of such compounds will induce both protein and phospholipid synthesis and production of new membrane material—first in the rough and then in the smooth endoplasmic reticulum—associated with increased activity of the mixed-function oxidase system. This appears as masses of endoplasmic reticulum within the cell, and results in cellular hypertrophy and hypertrophy of the liver as a whole (Fig. 2-29a), as in the following case.

CASE 7 A 40-year-old woman was involved in a single car accident and suffered a severe closed head injury. Witnesses to the accident stated that the car was operated in an erratic manner suggestive of drunken driving; yet the blood alcohol level was only slightly elevated. Further examination of the blood demonstrated the presence of barbiturates. Upon questioning the next-of-kin, it was discovered that the patient had been taking phenobarbital and other "tranquilizing" drugs for anxiety, over a period of one year. The patient died from irreversible brain damage on the third hospital day.

Figure 2-29. a. Liver of a rat fed a polychlorinated biphenyl, showing proliferation of smooth endoplasmic reticulum (ER). M, mitochondria. **(courtesy of Dr. Lucy A. Barrett)**

b. Neuron from cerebral cortex of case No. 8, showing numerous residual bodies (RB) filled with lipofuscin pigment. **(courtesy of Dr. Julio H. Garcia)**

Examination of the liver tissue at autopsy revealed a massive increase in the amount of rough- and smooth-surfaced profiles of endoplasmic reticulum within the hepatocytes. Pieces of liver tissue assayed for hydroxylase and cytochrome P450 levels contained 2-to-3 times the normal amount.

The effects of stimulation of the microsomal system with phenobarbital and the subsequent hypertrophy of the endoplasmic reticulum are evident in this case. There is considerable cross-reactivity between drugs metabolized by this system; and once its activity is induced by one compound, it will frequently show increased metabolic activity with other compounds. This can be either protective or harmful to the cell, depending on the particular compound. For example, induction of the system with phenobarbital results in tolerance to dilantin. On the other hand, there is also increased metabolism of carbon tetrachloride to the toxic free radical, and thus relatively small amounts of carbon tetrachloride become toxic.

Hypertrophy has been well studied in muscle cells, where it represents a response to an increased work load. In hypertrophied muscle cells there is an increase in the amount of sarcoplasmic reticulum, ribosomes, and numbers of myofilaments, all of which increase the work capacity of the muscle cell.

b. Atrophy

This terms refers to a decrease in the size and activity of cells resulting from such factors as hypoxia, decreased work load, decreased nutrition, and decreased hormonal stimulation. The decrease in cell mass implies that turnover of cell components continues while replenishment decreases. Increased numbers of autophagic vacuoles are often found in cells undergoing atrophy. The debris within these vacuoles may be converted to residual bodies, resulting in granules of lipofuscin pigment (Fig. 2-28b); in the heart and liver this may impart a brown color to the organ, and this gives the process one of its names, *brown atrophy*. Atrophic changes in muscle include breakdown of myofilaments, fragmentation of the endoplasmic reticulum, and swelling and degeneration of mitochondria. A striking example of the effects of atrophy of the CNS is found in the following case.

CASE 8 A 50-year-old stevedore came to the emergency room repeatedly over a five-year period with lacerations, contusions, and abrasions he had received in numerous brawls. He was finally admitted to a psychiatric hospital, where he was found to have impaired judgment, dysgraphia, and visual agnosia. The electroencephalographic pattern showed diffuse bilateral slowing, and pneumoencephalography disclosed enlargement of the lateral ventricles. The diagnosis was presenile dementia. While on leave of absence from the hospital, the patient had another fight and suffered a fatal stab wound in the chest.

At autopsy severe cerebral atrophy was observed. This was reflected by the presence of many lipofuscin granules in both neurons and glial cells (Fig. 2-29b).

The cause of this atrophy affecting specifically the central nervous system is obscure, but the effects on cerebral function as reflected in judgment and personality are clear.

c. Abnormalities in organelle size and number

Certain cellular disorders are characterized by alterations in the size and number of organelles such as mitochondria. As methods for quantitating the number and size of organelles have been developed, more of these disorders have been found. Obviously there is some overlap between these changes and those discussed under hypertrophy and atrophy.

MITOCHONDRIA. Alterations in mitochondrial growth and replication often lead to the production of large, abnormally shaped mitochondria, sometimes called *megamitochondria* (mitochondrial giants) (Fig. 2-30a). These large mitochondria are to be distinguished from mitochondrial enlargement due to swelling, in which the increased size is caused chiefly by uptake of fluid. Megamitochondria can be observed in the liver cells of alcoholics, and by light microscopy may appear as large, round eosinophilic inclusions, sometimes larger than the cell nucleus. Other conditions associated with enlarged liver mitochondria include treatment with copper-chelating agents, essential fatty-acid deficiency, vitamin E-selenium deficiency, cirrhosis, and non-hemolytic jaundice. Mitochondrial enlargement is seen also in kidney proximal tubular epithelium, in tubular necrosis, in muscle cells in megaconial myopathy, and in tissue culture cells under abnormal growth conditions. The pathogenesis of the enlargement may involve fusion of mitochondria or failure of mitochondrial fission. Quantitative studies on mitochondrial mass in cells with megamitochondria indicate that the total mitochondrial volume may remain constant—which implies that there are fewer though larger mitochondria.

In addition to heterogeneity in size, mitochondria may show extreme pleomorphism, with scalloping of margins, protrusions of one mitochondrion into another, and formation of crystal-like patterns within the mitochondria. Pleomorphism has frequently been seen in neoplastic cells.

Variation of mitochondrial number can also be observed. Simple starvation of the rat produces within a few days a marked decrease in mitochondrial number in the liver cells. Following re-feeding, mitochondrial division and growth occur (Scarpelli *et al.,* 1971).

PEROXISOMES. At present little is known about the role of catalase-containing

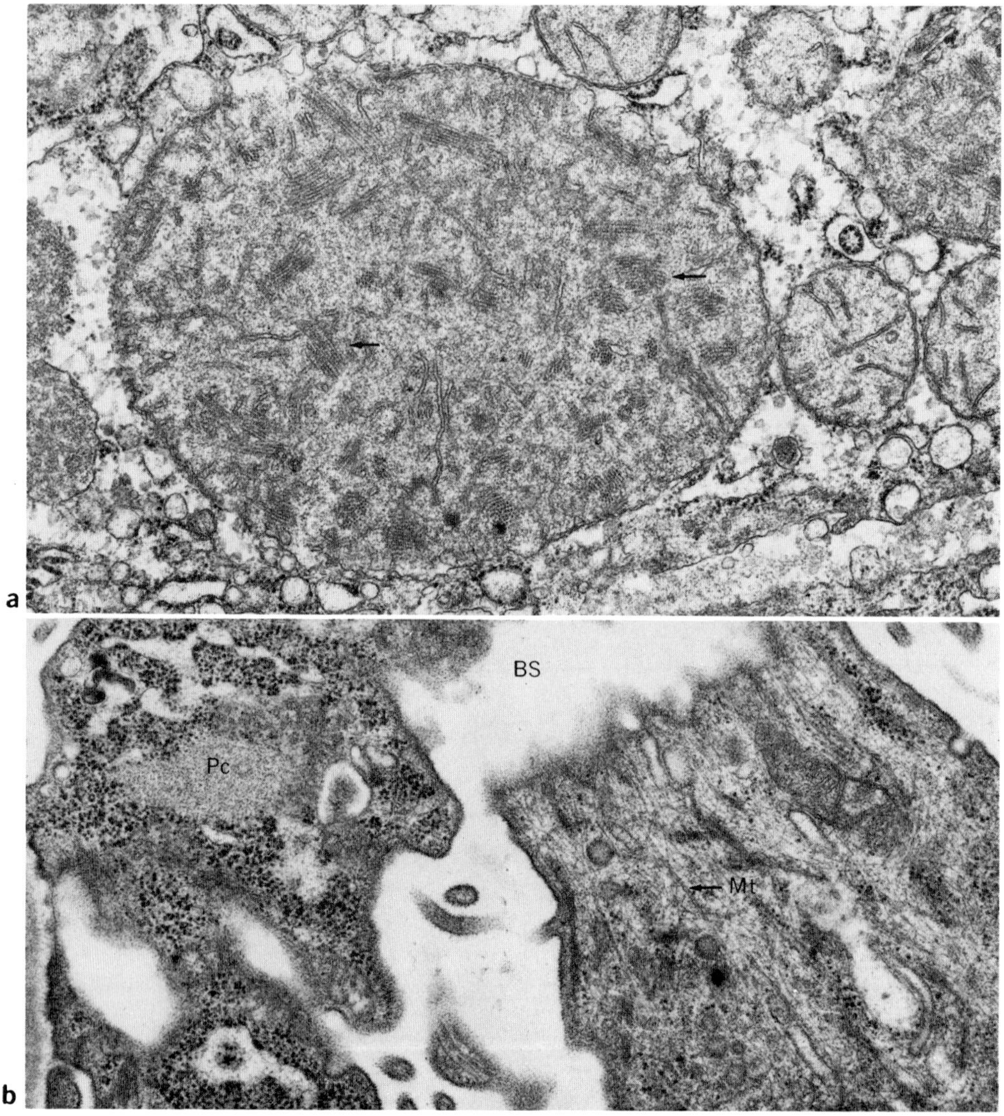
a
b
BS
Pc
Mt

peroxisomes in the pathogenesis of cellular injury (Hruban and Rechcigl, 1969; Svoboda and Reddy, in press). The number of hepatic microbodies is greatly increased following the administration of ethyl alpha chlorophenoxyisobutyrate (CPIB) and mefenopin, agents that produce hypolipidemia; this is associated with liver hypertrophy. An interesting hypothesis regarding a possible role of catalase in cellular injury was proposed by de Duve and Baudhuin, 1966, who suggested that this enzyme may form a safety device for oxidation of hydrogen peroxide in case of its accelerated production. Since free hydrogen peroxide is a potent inducer of lipid peroxidation, the excess of catalase within microbodies could thus serve as an inhibitor of intracellular lipid peroxidation.

d. Aging

Effects of aging on cells are undoubtedly complex, and no specific cellular features of aging have been identified. Still, in many cells, especially neurons, the accumulation of lipofuscin pigment exhibits a roughly linear increase with age (this has already been discussed). Other changes that may occur in aging are similar to those seen in atrophic cells, and the neurons in some types of presenile dementia (Case 8) are typical of them. Many theories of aging have been advanced, among them defective or altered immune recognition, thermal denaturation of cell proteins, free radical damage as by long-term action of cosmic irradiation, and accumulation of genetic errors; but definitive data have been difficult to obtain.

3. Changes in cell shape and motility; filaments and tubules

The cytoplasmic ground substance consists of a gel-like, protein-rich material in which are suspended such structures as microtubules, cytoplasmic filaments, glycogen deposits, free ribosomes, and lipid droplets. At times, abnormal accumulation of vesicles, filaments, and other puzzling structures occur. Cell shape, contractility, and movement, cytoplasmic viscosity, and intracellular movements in the cytoplasm, depend on or are influenced by these structures.

In particular, attention has recently been focused on cytoplasmic filaments and microtubules. The most common filaments are those present in masses in

Figure 2-30. **a.** Megamitochondrion from liver of a human alcoholic. Note the disordered cristae and paracrystalline inclusions (arrows). (courtesy of Dr. Kook Kim)

b. Glomerular visceral epithelial cells from a rat following administration of vinblastine. Note some normal-appearing microtubules (Mt) on the right, and a microtubule derived pericrystal (Pc) on the left. (Courtesy of Dr. Greta Tyson) muscle cells, both actin and myosin, which are responsible for cell contractility. Similar fibrils are also seen in smaller quantities in a number of othe cell types. The number and size of these filaments vary with atrophy and hypertrophy in muscle cells; and under the influence of some unusual drugs fragmentation, clumping, and dissolution–associated with changes in contractility and cell motility–may occur.

Microtubules appear to function in intracellular transport and movements, such as movements of the chromosomes during mitosis, and so-called "saltatory" movements of cell particles–the linear back-and-forth motion of mitochondria, lysosomes, and other organelles. When cells are treated with colchicine these tubules fragment (Fig. 2-30b), and both mitotic movements of chromosomes and saltatory movements are diminished.

a. Abnormal fibrillar inclusions

A striking accumulation of cytoplasmic filaments occurs in hepatocytes of alcoholics.

CASE 9 A 54-year-old man was admitted to the hospital with the chief complaint of jaundice. He had been passing large quantities of bloody stools, vomiting

Figure 2-31. **a.** Electron micrograph of alcoholic hyaline from a liver biopsy of a human alcoholic patient. **(courtesy of Dr. Kook Kim)**

b. Hepatic cell cytoplasm from a patient with alcoholic cirrhosis. An accumulation of alcoholic hyalin is present (AH). This deposit is formed by a tangle of fine filaments within the cytoplasm. See also Figure 2-3e. (Courtesy of Dr. Oscar A. Iseri)

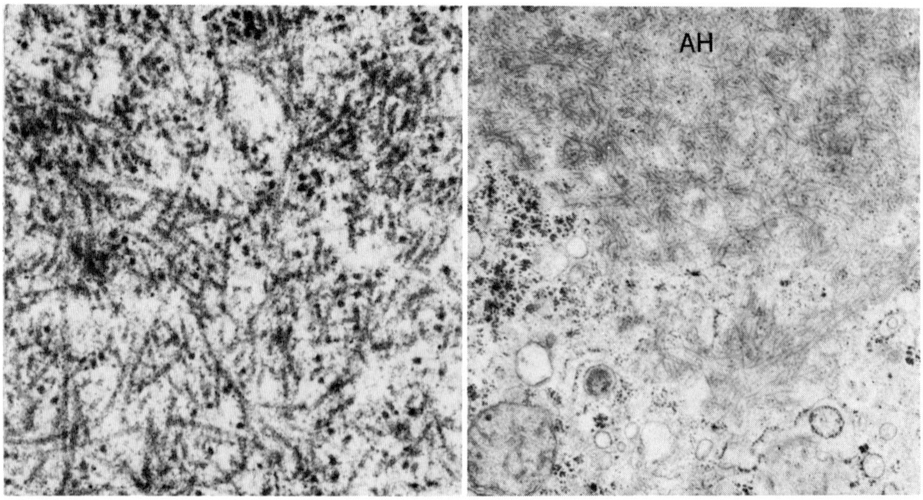

a b

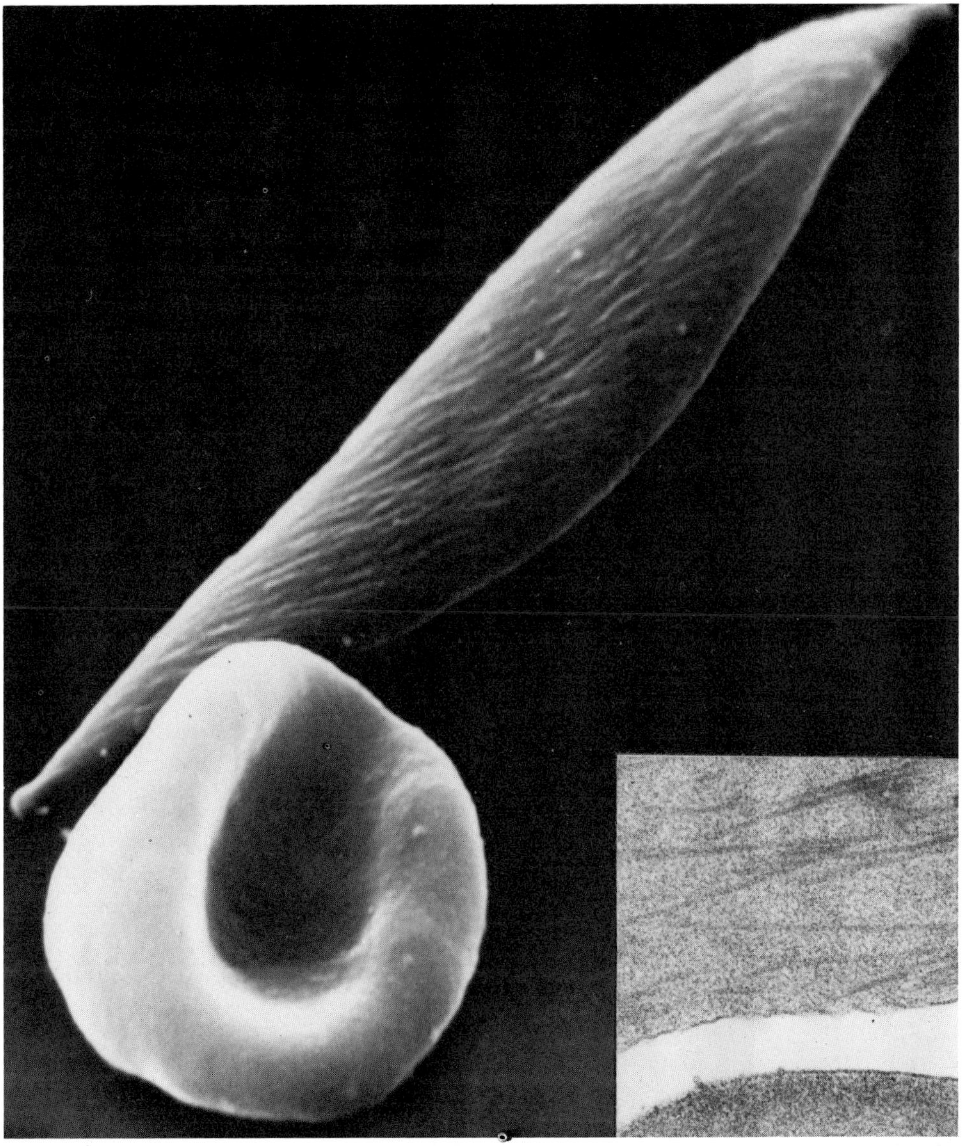

Figure 2-32. Scanning electron micrograph of a sickled human erythrocyte. A more normal erythrocyte is shown near the bottom. Inset shows a transmission micrograph of portions of two sickled human erythrocytes illustrating the microtubular forms in the cytoplasm, resulting from the stacked hemoglobin molecules. (Courtesy of Mr. Robert Pendergrass)

blood, and had a history of chronic alcoholism and poor eating habits. Physical examination revealed a chronically ill, deeply jaundiced man with a blood pressure of 80/60 mm Hg, pulse 100, and respirations 30. Blood tests showed severe anemia, leukopenia, and thrombocytopenia; LDH and SGOT levels were 207 and 165 milliunits per ml.* A firm, nodular, non-tender liver was palpable at the level of the umbilicus. On the second hospital day the patient began to go into coma, his urine output dropped and he had bloody stools. On the seventh hospital day his blood pressure fell to 60/40 mm Hg. He became unresponsive and died as a result of liver failure.

By light microscopy the liver cells showed necrosis, swelling, considerable fat, and masses of eosinophilic homogeneous material identified as alcoholic hyalin.

The term *alcoholic hyalin* designates a type of degeneration within hepatic cells, and was described originally by Mallory in patients with alcoholic cirrhosis. By light microscopy, alcoholic hyalin can be seen to consist of cytoplasmic clumps of eosinophilic hyaline material which form multiple droplets and irregular masses distributed predominantly in the perinuclear cytoplasm of hepatic cells. With the electron microscope it is found to be composed largely of a meshwork of fibrils approximately 80–100 Å thick (Fig. 2-31a), and it is associated with disarray, fragmentation, and disappearance of the rough endoplasmic reticulum. The pathogenesis of alcoholic hyalin is not clear. Somewhat similar in appearance, but probably unrelated, are aggregates of microfibrils that occur in the cytoplasm of aging neurons and other altered cells.

b. Cell sap proteins

Hemoglobin, the major cytoplasmic protein of mammalian erythrocytes, may exhibit several types of pathologic change. In certain types of hemolytic anemia, precipitates called Heinz bodies occur within the red blood cell. These precipitates consist of relatively insoluble products of hemoglobin denaturation, and they may form also during the normal process of red cell senescence, leading to red cell destruction. The initial morphologic lesion in Heinz body development is the formation of a dense structure that appears to grow by coalescence and condensation, finally coming to lie just beneath the cell membrane. These structures

* Normal values: LDH 30–110, SGOT 5–20 milliunits per ml.

Figure 2-33. a. Kidney tubule cell fixed with osmium tetroxide. Note the even distribution of the nuclear chromatin and interchromatin granules. N, nucleus; Nc, nucleolus.

b. A similar kidney tubule cell after fixation with glutaraldehyde followed by osmium. The chromatin is clumped along the nuclear envelope and around the nucleolus (Nc). N, nucleus.

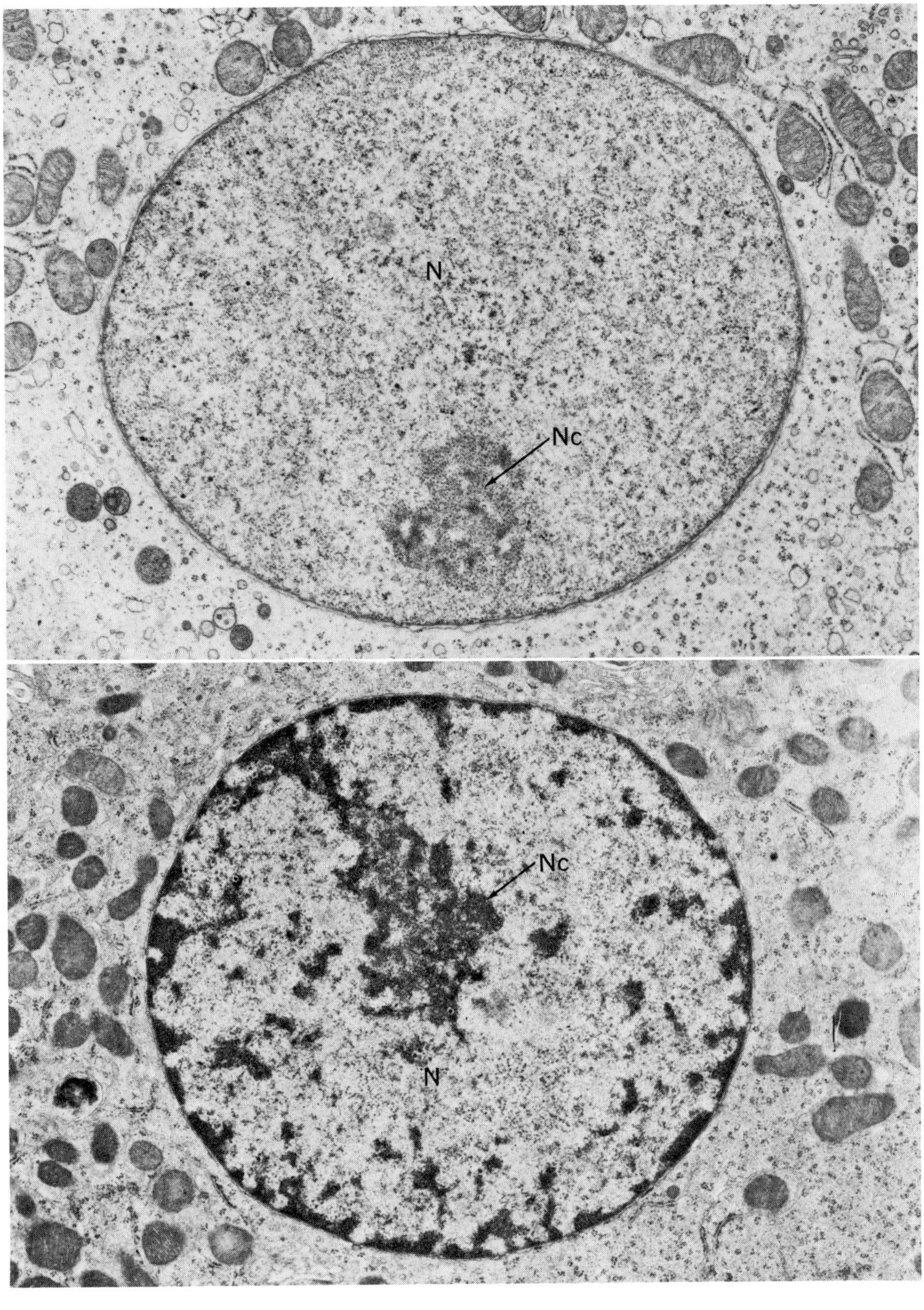

a

b

result in considerable distortion of cell shape and deformation of the plasma membrane, render the cells relatively rigid, and increase the chances of injury as cells pass through limited spaces such as the splenic cords. The resulting injury to the cell membrane presumably predisposes to hemolysis by accelerating erythrophagocytosis.

A striking conformational change in the red cell sap occurs in sickle cell anemia (Murayama, 1971), illustrated in the following case.

CASE 10 A 25-year-old black man was admitted to the hospital with fever and left-sided chest pain. Physical examination showed his pulse to be 92/min, and regular, blood pressure 120/60 mm Hg, respiratory rate 28/min, and temperature 101°F. Examination of the patient's chest demonstrated a decrease in expansion of the left side with dullness to percussion, decreased breath sounds, and crepitant rales. The heart was slightly enlarged. The liver was palpated two fingerbreadths below the costal margin and the sclerae of the eyes were yellow. The spleen could not be felt by physical examination. Laboratory examination of the blood revealed a white blood cell count of 20,000 per cu mm, a red blood cell count of 3.2 million per cu mm, and reticulocytes 16 per cent.* Target cells were seen in a blood film, along with nucleated red blood cells. A sickling test was positive, and hemoglobin SS was found by electrophoresis. The diagnosis was sickle cell anemia with lobar pneumonia. Despite treatment with antibiotics and packed cells, the patient developed congestive heart failure and died on the third hospital day.

The autopsy revealed multiple infarcts in the spleen, kidneys, lungs, and liver, with numerous capillary thromboses present. The right ventricle of the heart was massively hypertrophied. Sickled red cells could be seen in several tissues. The liver also contained large amounts of hemosiderin and ferritin within lysosomes.

In well oxygenated blood from patients with this disease, the red cells are morphologically very similar to normal erythrocytes. When the oxygen tension is reduced, the cells assume sickle or holly leaf shapes (Fig. 2-32). The only chemical difference between normal and sickle hemoglobin lies in the substitution of valine for glutamic acid at the sixth position in the two beta chains. This single amino acid substitution has two major effects: first, deoxygenated hemoglobin S is much less soluble than deoxygenated normal hemoglobin or either form of oxyhemoglobin; second, a new molecular conformation ensues which predisposes to neat molecular packing. Microscopic study reveals "microtubular" birefringent structures that, on further study, are found to represent hollow cables, each formed of six monofilaments of hemoglobin S.

* Normal values: WBC 4,800–10,800 per cu mm; RBC 4.6–6.2 million per cu mm; reticulocytes 0.2–1.5 per cent.

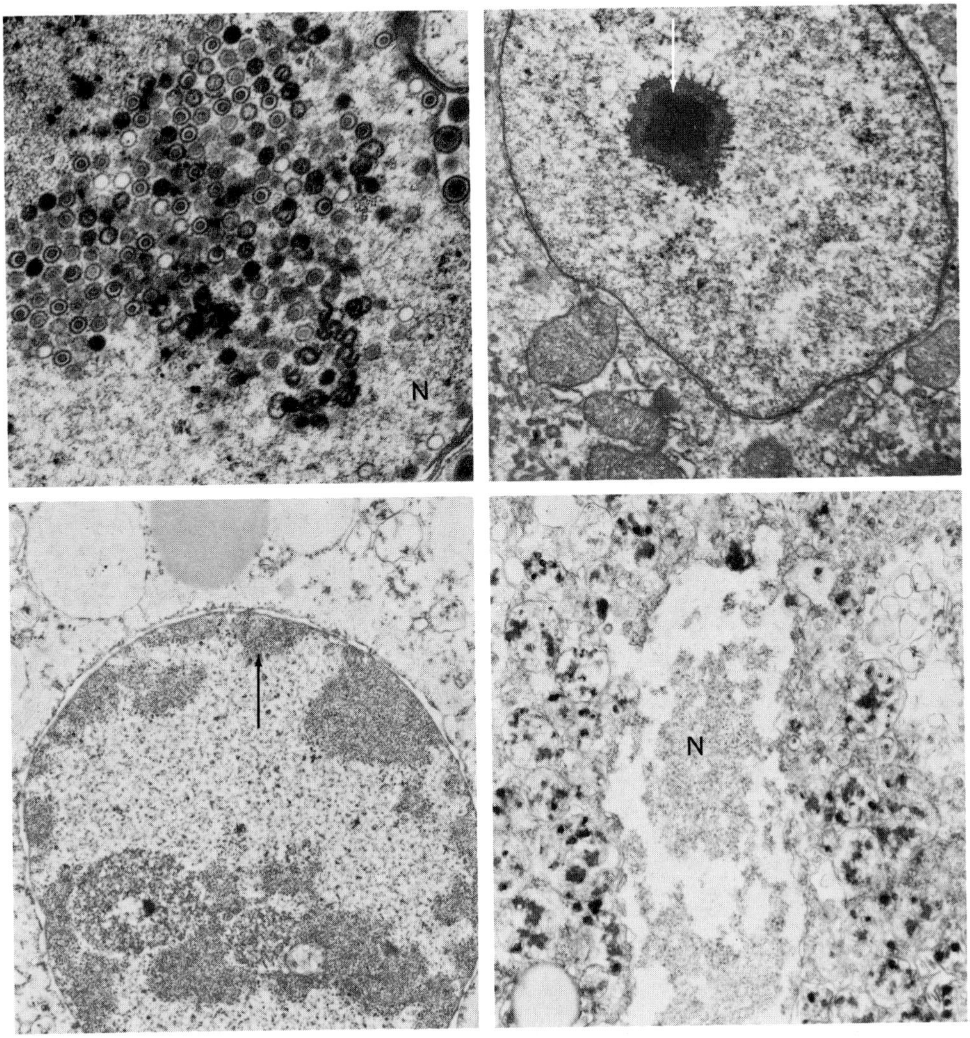

a b c d

Figure 2-34. a. Nuclear inclusion formed from packed Herpes virions in the nucleus (N) of a HeLa cell following infection with Herpes simplex virus. Note virions in the nuclear envelope as well. **(courtesy of Dr. Bernard B. Poeschel)**

b. Lead-induced nuclear inclusion (arrow) in a rat kidney tubule cell. (Courtesy of Dr. Robert Goyer)

c. Clumping of chromatin (arrow) and partial dissolution of the nucleolus in an Ehrlich ascites cell after treatment with mercuric chloride for 2 hours. (Courtesy of Dr. Kauno Laiho)

d. Karyolysis of the nucleus (N) in a kidney tubule cell 24 hours after administration of mercuric chloride. (Courtesy of Dr. Thomas Gritzka)

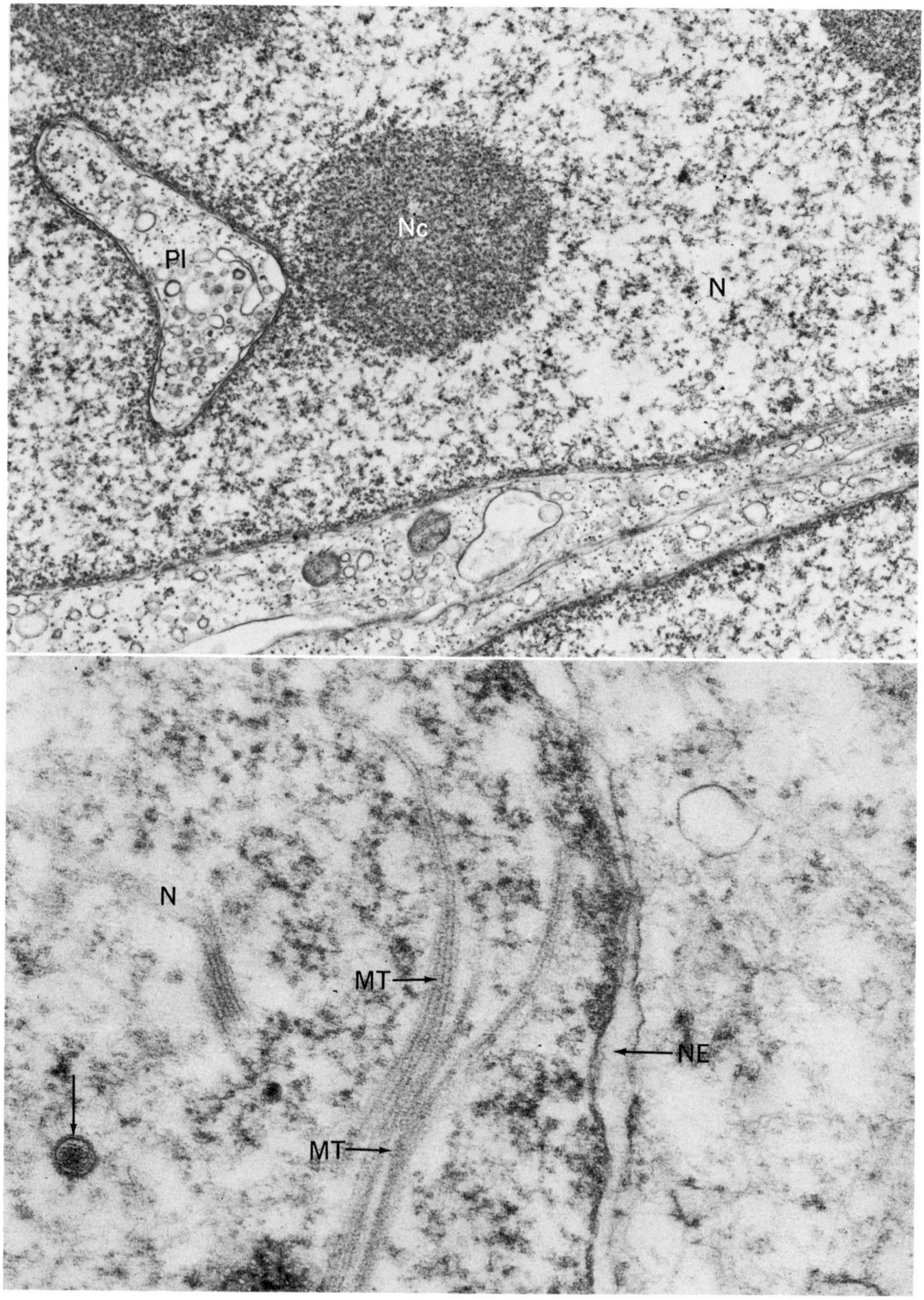

a

b

The manifold lesions, signs, and symptoms of this disease seem to be a direct result of the molecular alteration in hemoglobin and the gelling of the erythrocyte cytoplasm. This increases the rigidity of the erythrocytes and causes change in shape: the result is a shortened red cell life span. In addition, the altered red-cell shape and increased rigidity lead to increased blood viscosity, and this promotes multiple capillary thromboses with ischemic infarcts in many tissues. The entire sequence occurs more readily at reduced oxygen tensions, and affected individuals are at risk at high altitudes. They are even susceptible to flying in commercial aircraft normally pressurized to 5,000 ft. above sea level. Once set in motion, the sequence of sickling, thrombosis, infarcts, and red cell destruction can lead to a self-perpetuating cycle termed "sickle cell crisis." Recently urea has been used to treat this condition; it may act by destroying the hydrophobic bonds responsible for the abnormal hemoglobin polymerization.

4. Alterations in transcription and replication

There are marked variations in the structure and function of the nucleus during different phases of the mitotic cycle, and between cells of different types (Baserga and Wiebel, 1969)—which complicates the task of analyzing possible alterations in nuclei. In addition, differences in fixation are reflected in different morphologies (Fig. 2-33). Finally, the effects of nuclear alterations in cell injury depend on the stage of the cell cycle at the time of injury. In postmitotic cells, interference with nuclear function is not immediately lethal for the cell, and cannot explain the rapid progression to cell necrosis that occurs after such acute injuries as infarction. In some cells, in fact, the entire nucleus may be removed from a cell by microdissection without causing cessation of cytoplasmic function until several days have passed.

a. Nuclear inclusions (Figures 2-34a, b)

Various types of nuclear inclusions have been described in cells. Some structures that seem to be inclusions actually represent deep cytoplasmic indentions

Figure 2-35. a. HeLa cell showing pseudoinclusion (PI) of the nucleus (N). Note that the pseudoinclusion is surrounded by a typical double-layered nuclear envelope and contains cytoplasmic structures. Nucleolus (Nc).

b. Nuclear microtubules (MT) in cultured fibroblasts 36 hours after infection with Herpes simplex virus. Note a virion (arrow) within nucleoplasm. NE, nuclear envelope; N, nucleus. (Courtesy of Dr. William D. Bradford)

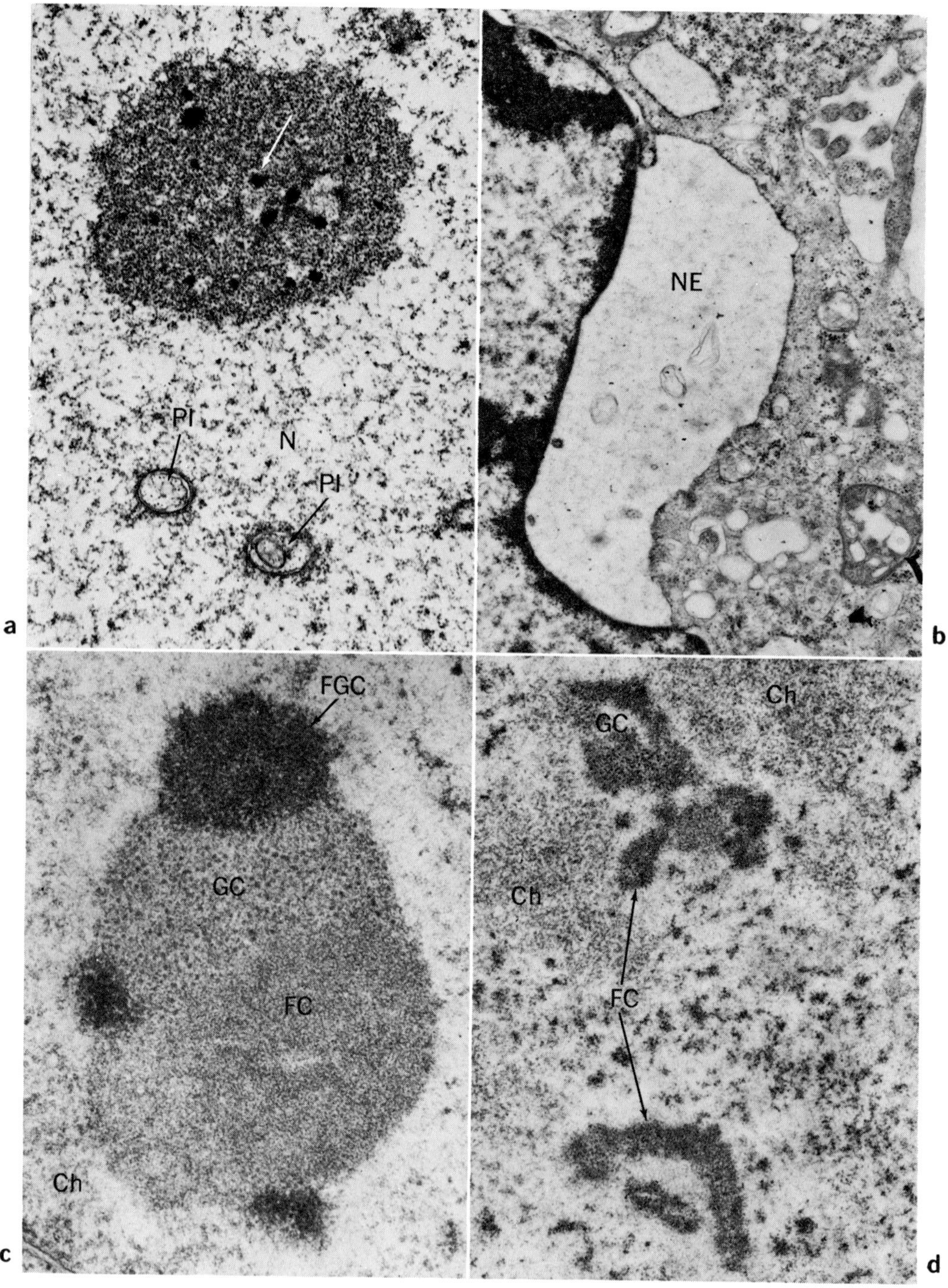

a
PI
N
PI
b
NE
FGC
GC
FC
Ch
c
GC
Ch
Ch
FC
d

into the nucleus, and, because the plane of section does not demonstrate continuity with the cytoplasm, such indentions appear to reside within the nucleoplasm. These pseudoinclusions can be identified easily by the nuclear pores in the envelope surrounding them. Pseudoinclusions are often observed in the nuclei of cells undergoing rapid turnover (Fig. 2-35a).

True inclusions are abnormal depositions or accumulations actually lying within the nucleoplasm. A variety of vesicles, glycogen, concentric lamellar bodies, fibrillar structures, vacuoles, and tubular or filamentous inclusions (Fig. 2-35b) have been described but are of unknown significance. More characteristic are inclusions formed by virus particles or virus-induced products that may be striking because of their crystalline array. Intranuclear inclusions may occur also in the nuclei of renal tubules in heavy-metal poisoning with bismuth or lead.

b. Nucleolus

Nucleoli in most cells have at least three intermingling components: (1) one contains dense ribosome-like particles 150–200 Å in diameter; (2) one contains filaments of 80–100 Å; and (3) one contains intranucleolar chromatin fibrils identical with the fibrils in the nucleoplasm (Busch and Smetana, 1970) (Fig. 2-36). The fibrils, arranged in an open skein-like structure somctimes termed the nucleolonema, contain the intranucleolar chromatin which, together with the condensed chromatin in the periphery of the nucleolus (nucleolus-associated chromatin), probably represent the nucleolar organizer. The ribosome-like particles and the 80–100 Å filaments both seem to represent RNA and protein and are part of the synthetic machinery responsible for ribosome synthesis.

Numerous carcinogenic and antimetabolic agents, including actinomycin D, lasiocarpine, aflatoxin, and ultraviolet irradiation, can cause segregation or stratification of the various nucleolar components into three distinct regions. This dis-

Figure 2-36. **a.** Nucleolar changes in a HeLa cell nucleus 12 hours after infection with Herpes simplex virus. The nucleolus has a spotty, moth-eaten appearance with highly condensed areas (arrows). Two pseudoinclusions (PI) are present at the left.

b. A perinuclear vacuole, caused by massive dilatation of the nuclear envelope (NE), appears in an Ehrlich ascites cell 2 hours after treatment with cyanide and iodacetic acid. The chromatin is densely clumped.

c. Segregation of the nucleolus of a rat liver cell after administration of actinomycin D. FGC, fibrillar granular component (plaque); GC, granular component; FC, fibrillar component; Ch, chromatin. (Courtesy of Dr. Peter J. Goldblatt)

d. Nucleclus of a rat liver cell 12 hours after administration of ethionine to a male rat. The various components are disintegrating. GC, granular component; FC, fibrillar component; Ch, chromatin. (Courtesy of Dr. Peter J. Goldblatt)

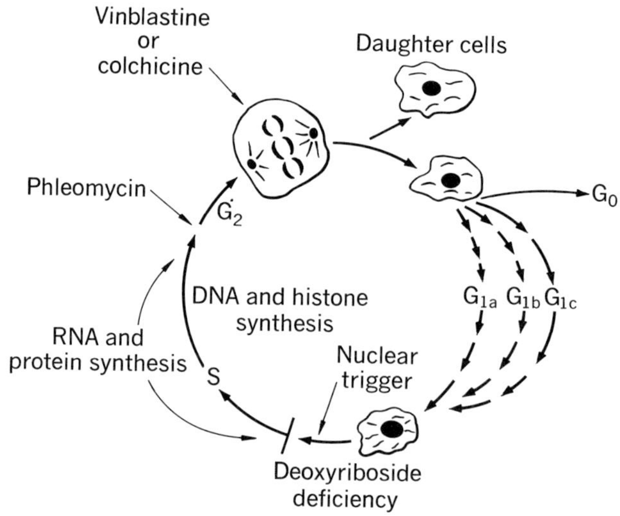

Figure 2-37. Concepts of the cell cycle in relation to cell injury. The replication of animal cells is a highly ordered sequence of molecular events requiring the expression of specific genetic information at certain steps in the cycle. S phase, an interval lasting 6-7 hours in many cells, is concerned with the synthesis of a complete complement of DNA and histones; progression through this interval requires the timely synthesis of RNA as well as DNA and proteins. The G_2 interval, mitosis, and cell division require approximately 2-3 hours and are concerned with the formation of newly synthesized chromatin into chromosome pairs and the distribution of the condensed chromosomes into the daughter cells. Progression into the G_2 interval requires the completion of DNA synthesis and the antecedent synthesis of RNA and protein. In HeLa cells phleomycin blocks the cell cycle near the end of the DNA synthesis period. Colchicine and other agents active against the microtubules—e.g., vinblastine—block the progression of cells through metaphase. Cells with different replication times vary mainly in the duration of the G_1 interval and are depicted in the diagram as G_{1a}, G_{1b}, G_{1c}, and G_O. During this interval the cell expresses the phenotypic character of its particular differentiated state. Depending on intracellular and extracellular factors, cells progress through G_1 and become triggered for nuclear replication and histone synthesis. (Modified from Mueller, Fed. Proc., **28**:1780, 1969)

tinct stratification is associated with marked interference with DNA-dependent synthesis of all classes of RNA (Fig. 2-36c).

Ethionine, which traps adenine in the form of *s*-adenosyl-ethionine, inhibits RNA and protein synthesis and causes fragmentation of nucleoli (Fig. 2-36d). The components of the nucleolus are widely dispersed but can be reaggregated when the effect is neutralized by the administration of adenine.

Through the use of synchronized cell cultures it has been possible to study variations in sensitivity to toxic agents throughout the division cycle (Baserga

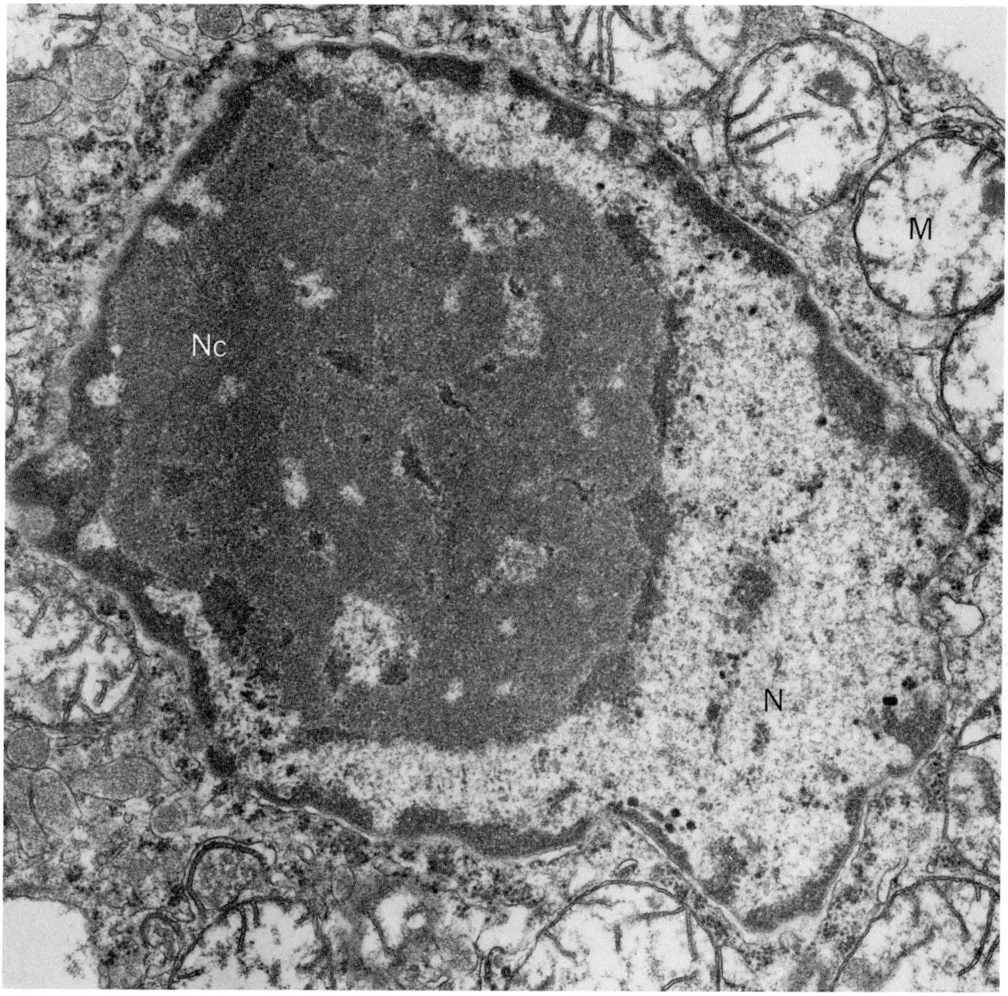

Figure 2-38. This cell from a human adenocarcinoma of the kidney has the characteristics of an undifferentiated cell. The nucleus (N) is large in comparison with the cytoplasm, and contains massive nucleoli (Nc). In the cytoplasm are numerous free ribosomes, scant endoplasmic reticulum, and mitochondria (M). (Courtesy of Irene K. Berezesky)

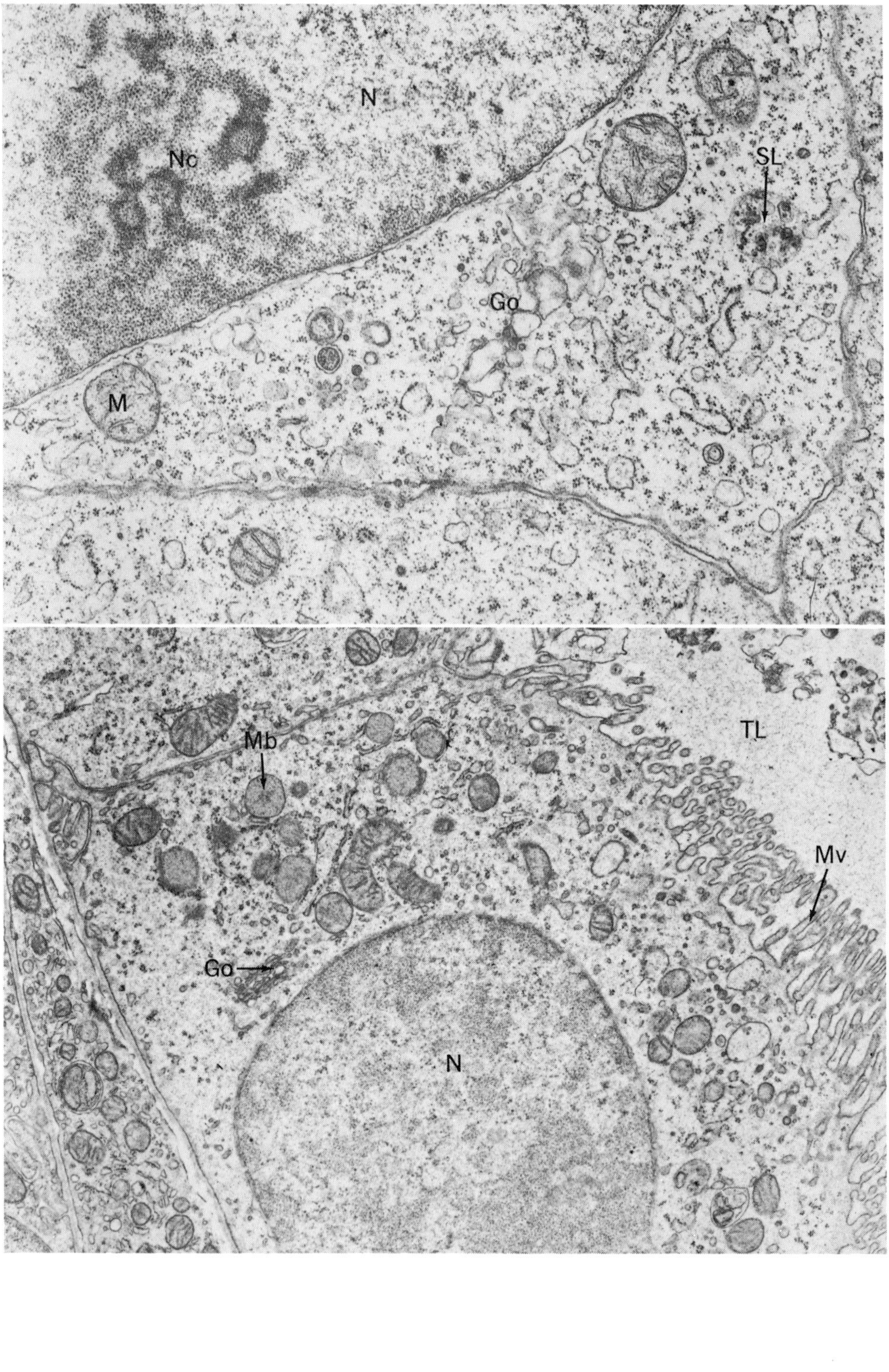

a

b

and Wiebel, 1969). This variability may be extremely important in clinical medicine inasmuch as it constitutes a possible basis of cancer chemotherapy and radiotherapy, and helps substantially to explain the undesirable side effects of these methods of treatment.

Variation in sensitivity to injury in different phases of the cell cycle (Fig. 2-37) is especially evident during therapy with ionizing radiation or radiomimetic agents such as the nitrogen mustards ("alkylating agents"). Cells in early G1 and G2 phases are the least sensitive, and cells in M, late G1, or early S phase are the most sensitive. Thus, in cancer therapy, it becomes desirable to treat cells that are not in G1 or G2. Characteristic changes are observed in the nucleus during cell division in the irradiated cell, including chromosome breaks, bridge formation between chromosomes at anaphase, and chromosomal fragmentation. In contrast, some cells such as lymphocytes and spermatogonia apparently undergo an immediate, cytolytic type of death after irradiation.

Changes in the nucleus caused by acute lethal injury such as chromatin clumping (Fig. 2-34c), dilatation of nuclear envelope (Fig. 2-36b), and karyolysis (2-34d) have already been mentioned.

c. The undifferentiated cell

Undifferentiated cells, which occur in embryonic tissue, regenerating epithelia or mesenchyma, many types of hyperplasia, elements of the hematopoietic system, and neoplasia (Haguenau, 1969), have structural and functional characteristics that are distinctive and differ little from one cell to another. Even the cells of highly malignant neoplasms share some or all of these features.

Undifferentiated cells are usually rounded, have only a few irregular cytoplasmic processes, and usually do not show complex membrane specializations of differentiated cells such as microvilli or cilia. Their shape depends on their environment and on the adjacent structures. They are characterized by a high ratio of

Figure 2-39. Stages of regeneration of rat kidney tubule cells after the administration of mercuric chloride.

a. Regenerating cell after 2 days. There is a large nuclear cytoplasmic ratio and a prominent nucleolus (Nc) containing many ribosome precursors. Many ribosomes are lying free in the cell sap. Mitochondria are scarce, as is endoplasmic reticulum. SL, secondary lysosome; Go, Golgi apparatus; M, mitochondrion.

b. After 7 days the cell is differentiating. Mitochondria are elongated and much more numerous. A regular brush border of microvilli (Mv) is forming at the luminal surface, the Golgi apparatus (Go) is more closely organized, and microbodies (Mb) are appearing. TL, tubular lumen; N, nucleus.

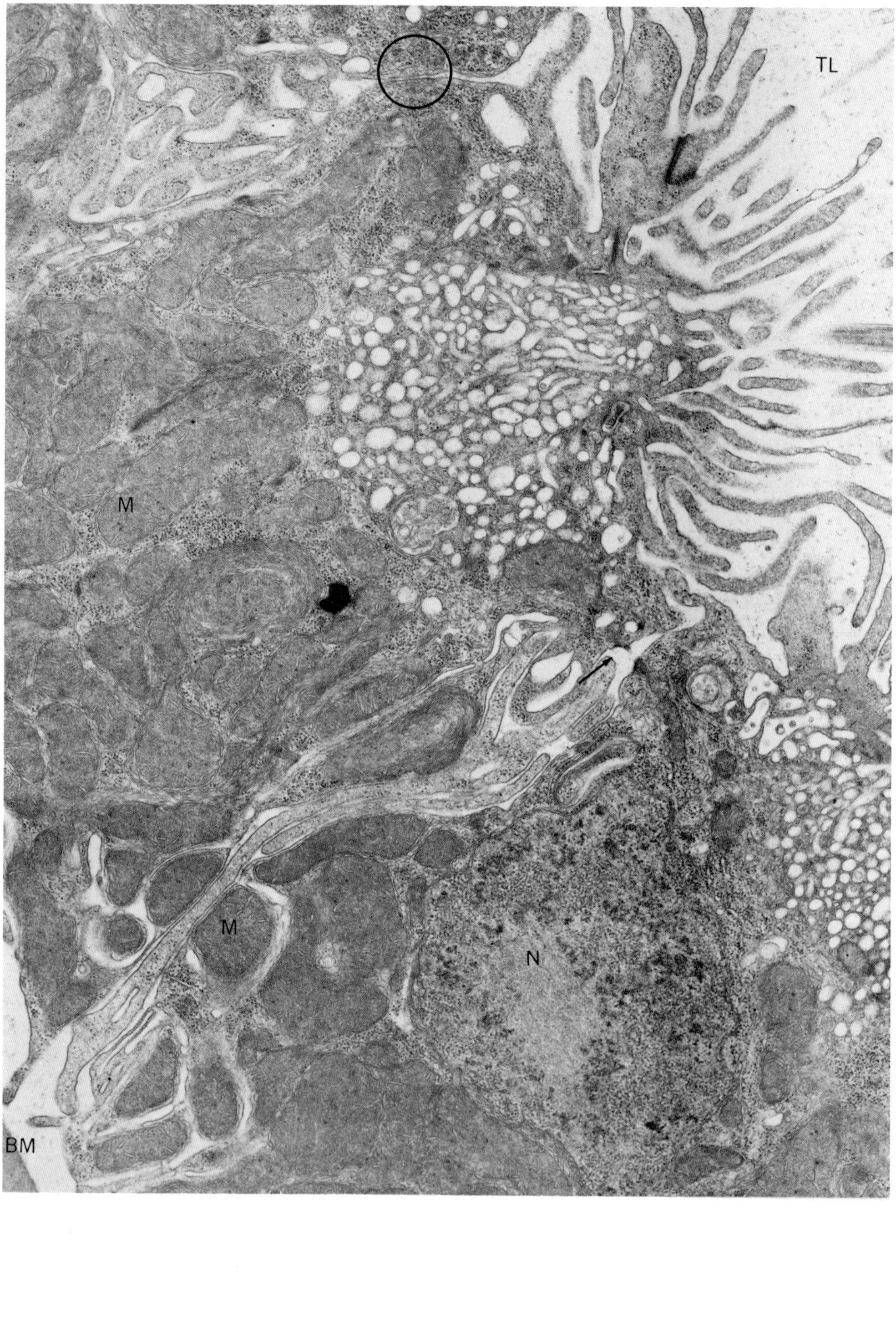
TL
M
M
N
BM

nuclear to cytoplasmic volume, and the cytoplasm is quite basophilic and pyroninophilic, due to the high concentration of RNA in the form of numerous polysomes that lie predominantly free in the cell sap. Relatively few profiles of rough endoplasmic reticulum are present. The mitochondria are inconspicuous, a characteristic probably related to the fact that these cells usually have well-developed systems for aerobic and anaerobic glycolysis. Digestive vacuoles or lysosomes are usually not prominent, although large autophagic vacuoles often occur early in regeneration in some organs such as the liver and kidney. The nuclei are large–often because they are polyploid; and various abnormalities of mitotic division may occur. Nucleoli are numerous, large, and full of particles representing ribosome precursors and perhaps other forms of RNA (Fig. 2-38).

These features of undifferentiated cells probably reflect the fact that the transcription and translation systems are primarily directed away from differentiation and toward the task of division. One example is the regeneration of renal tubular epithelium that occurs after acute tubular necrosis (Fig. 2-39a,b) (see Case 3); approximately one to two weeks is required for complete regeneration. During this time the differentiated function of the tubular epithelium is deficient, reabsorption is marginal, and there is a saline diuresis because the undifferentiated cells lack the ability for proper sodium reabsorption. When regeneration is complete, differentiation continues, and normal tubular function is restored.

d. Virus-cell interactions

These interactions are discussed in Chapters 4 and 6. It is sufficient here to point out that, although many viruses cause rapidly lethal responses in cells, other viruses have achieved variable degrees of adaptation. Latent infections, slow virus infection, and malignant transformation of cells are examples of such adaptation. Depending on the type of virus and the type of infection, structural abnormalities in the infected cells may accompany these functional changes. In many infections with DNA viruses, large nuclear inclusions–often containing crystalline aggregates of virions–are typically seen (Fig. 2-34a). In RNA virus infection, inclusions representing sites of virus production may be seen in the cytoplasm. In both cases membrane changes in the cell may be numerous, including virus-specified

Figure 2-40. Isolated flounder kidney tubule after incubation in solutions devoid of calcium. Note the separation of the cells and pulling apart of desmosome (arrow). Note also that at the top all junctions, including tight junctions, have separated (circle). M, mitochondria; N, nucleus. Note also the irregular contours of the microvilli and the clustering of apical vesicles and vacuoles. The tubular lumen (TL) is at the upper right, and basement membrane (BM) at the lower left. (courtesy of Dr. Ruth E. Bulger) changes in plasma membrane composition in the case of influenza virus, extensive fusion and redundancy of the nuclear envelope in Herpes virus infection, proliferations of endoplasmic reticulum in vaccinia virus replication, and large filamentous cytoplasmic inclusions due to measles virus. Virions may be found also within lysosomes–this perhaps resulting from fusions with virion-containing cisternae or vacuoles, or as a result of direct exotropy of virions from the cell sap into the lysosome (Fig. 2-22).

5. Disorders of cell-cell interactions

A number of cellular reactions to injury affect the relations between cells, reflecting alteration of either the cell surface or the specialized cell junctions. Since the effective surface of the cell is the glycocalyx, much attention has been directed recently to this extremely complex "sugar coat" in trying to explain these disorders. Nonetheless, precise identification of specific alterations resulting in defective cell-cell interactions has not been achieved.

In the nervous system, junctions between endothelial cells form part of the "blood-brain barrier," which limits the transfer of materials from the endothelial lumens to the brain parenchyma. These junctions are modified by the swelling and shrinking of the endothelial cells, as occur in a variety of injuries. These changes in the blood-brain barrier allow increased freedom of diffusion into the brain substance.

In some way, onset of mitosis and rate of cell growth are controlled by cell surface properties. In malignant transformation, for example, loss of control over cell growth and division is associated with several specific alterations of membranes. Changes in antigenic determinants on the membrane surface are important reflections of malignant transformation. Released into the blood stream, these tumor antigens can be measured (though still imperfectly) in an effort to determine the type and amount of tumor in the body. Changes at the cell junctions also occur in malignant transformation, with impairment of cell-to-cell communication. The junctions are more than cell attachment sites, since important molecular transfers between cells occur normally through some of them. In the absence of calcium, cell junctions of all types lose their integrity (Fig. 2-40).

The synapses in the nervous system are specialized cell junctions for neural transmission. Organic phosphates, several animal toxins derived from toads and other amphibians, and a variety of other toxins exert their effects on these junctions. Alterations of synaptic vesicles in CNS boutons occur quite early in ischemia.

In the inflammatory process, modification of cell junction integrity makes possible the migration of leukocytes from the capillaries (see Chapter 3). Changes in cell adhesion properties are critical factors in platelet aggregation and attachment to the endothelial cells in thrombosis, as well as in margination of leukocytes.

The formation of multinucleated giant cells is relatively common in pathologic processes and reflects a change in cell-cell interactions, sometimes involving contact, dissolution, and fusion of cell plasma membranes. This produces polynucleated or polykaryocytic cells. Among the stimuli to cell fusion that have been studied are viruses such as Herpes virus, measles virus, and Sendai virus, which bind to the glycocalyx and fasten several cells together. The Sendai virus has been of special interest because it can be used to produce fusion between cells from different species.

Polykaryocytic cells also occur commonly in granulomatous inflammation caused by infection with tuberculosis bacteria and fungi. Tuberculous giant cells may be formed partially by nuclear division without cytokinesis.

The number of nuclei, their location in the cell, and other morphologic features vary somewhat from cell to cell, depending on the agent; knowledge of these patterns may enable the pathologist to make specific diagnostic inferences when the etiologic agent is not known.

a. Alterations in membrane transport and transduction

Some changes in injured cells are best considered as alterations of plasma membrane transport and transduction. Some of these were mentioned in the section on acute lethal injury, since severe changes in permeability and in the sodium-potassium transport systems of the cell membrane can quickly lead to cell death. Many alterations in cellular transport systems are not lethal to the cell in question but may have important secondary consequences for the body as a whole. A striking example of this is the group of disorders known as amino-acidurias, in which defects of membrane-associated transport enzymes of renal tubular epithelial cells result in defective amino acid reabsorption, causing a characteristic series of signs and symptoms. Many such specific transport defects have been described, and it is beyond the scope of this chapter to consider them.

b. Alterations in myelin

Myelin sheaths are multilayered structures derived from plasma membranes of Schwann cells in peripheral nerves and from oligodendroglia in the central nervous system. Changes in myelin, usually involving degeneration (demyelination), are seen as part of the response to virtually any lesion in the nervous system involving tissue destruction. They are seen also in specific diseases of the central and peripheral nervous system such as multiple sclerosis and experimental

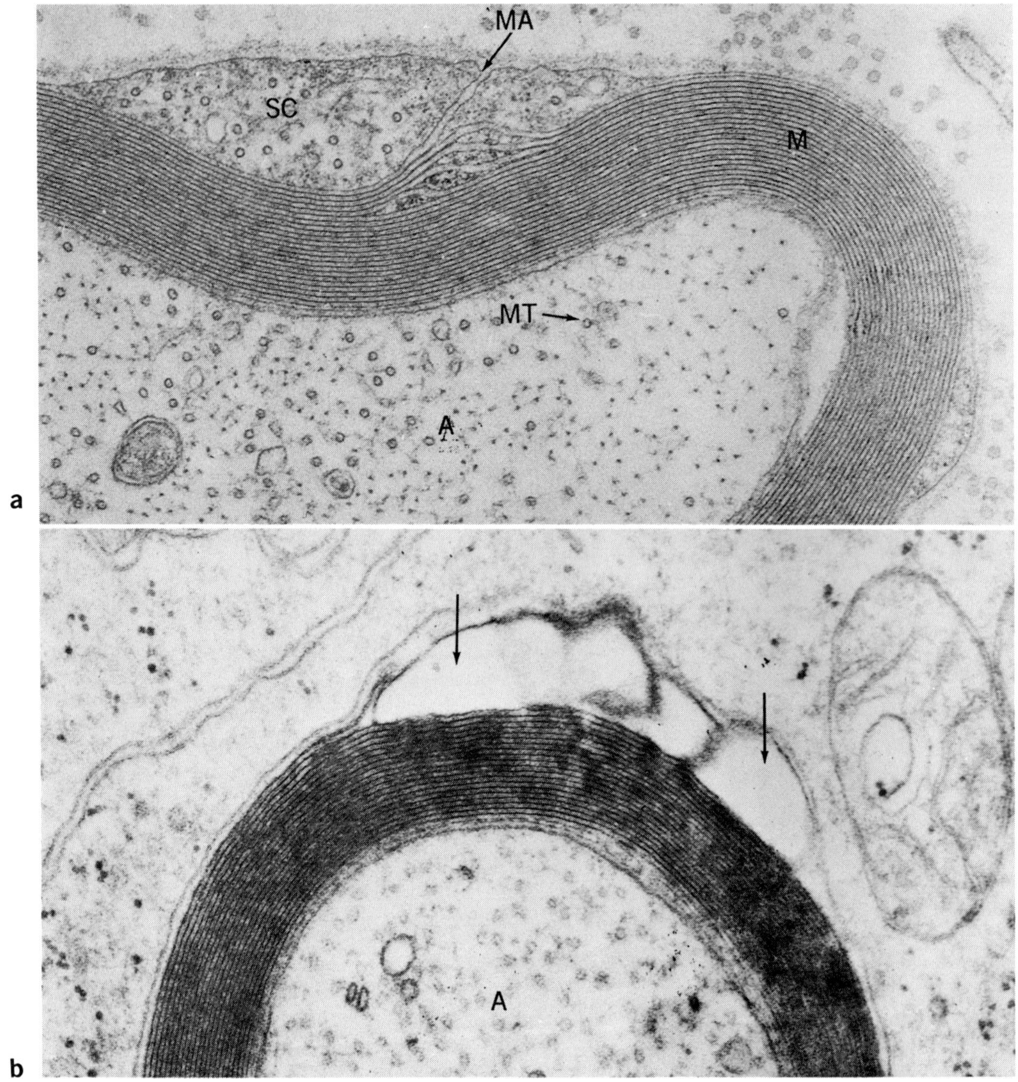

Figure 2-41. **a.** Normal peripheral nerve showing axon (A) with microtubules (MT), myelin (M), and Schwann cell (SC). MA, mesaxon. (Courtesy of Dr. Peter W. Lampert)

b. Peripheral nerve from an animal with experimental allergic neuritis. The central axon (A) is surrounded by myelin sheath consisting of regular, closely packed membranes. The arrows indicate blebs (bubbly degeneration) between myelin lamellae, an early sign of demyelination. (Courtesy of Dr. Peter W. Lampert) allergic encephalomyelitis (Fig. 2-41), and in the axonal reaction appearing after interruption of axons.

Demyelination occurring in multiple sclerosis and other central demyelinating diseases is presumably the result of primary injury to the oligodendrocyte, or Schwann, cell. The myelin lamellae are transformed into granular debris, and many undergo vesiculation.

Another type of change in myelin, consisting of separation of myelin lamellae with splitting of both minor and major dense lines, can occur in cases of cerebral edema due to vascular injury or the administration of certain chemical poisons. In these cases large amounts of fluid accumulate and form large vacuoles (spongy encephalopathy) easily visible with the light microscope. This is not the only cause of brain swelling, which may result also from swelling of astrocytic or other glial processes, from distended extracellular spaces, and from swollen axons.

6. Alterations of intracellular transport and compartmentation

Because of its roles in intracellular transport and compartmentation of material, the cytocavitary network is inevitably involved in alterations of these functions. Various rate-limiting steps of transport occur within the network. Although some of these steps are ATP-requiring–such as the transport from the endoplasmic reticulum to the proximal side of the Golgi apparatus–the controls over movement of materials within most of the system are not understood.

One result of alteration in transport and compartmentation is the accumulation of material within the reticulum in the form of inclusions (Goldblatt, 1972). A prominent example is the Russell body of plasma cells, in which large amounts of protein, much of it immunoglobulin, distend the cisternae of the rough-surfaced endoplasmic reticulum, producing large eosinophilic inclusions (Fig. 2-42c).

Accumulation of lipid within the cell cytoplasm is a common sub-lethal reaction to injury and may also reflect an alteration in transport and compartmentation. Although their appearance is greatly changed, cells containing large amounts of triglyceride can exist for long periods of time without appreciable impairment of function. The fatty liver of the alcoholic is an example.

Lipids reach the liver for the most part as alimentary chylomicrons or fatty acids from adipose tissue and are either utilized within the liver or secreted as lipoproteins (Fig. 2-43). The small triglyceride droplets that appear within the endoplasmic reticulum and the Golgi complex reflect the formation of lipoprotein particles (Lombardi, 1965) (Fig. 2-42a). There is good evidence that any

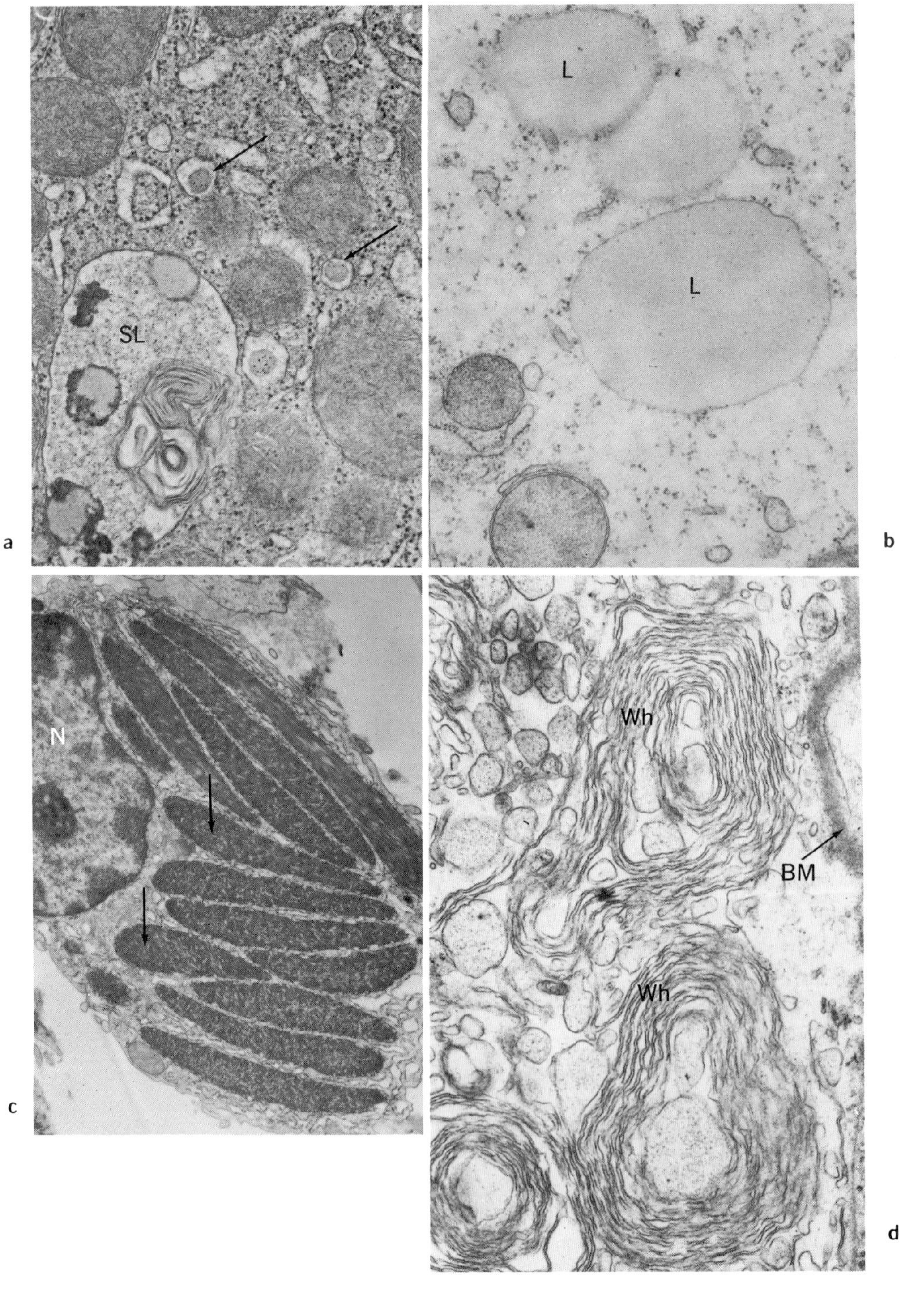
a
SL
L
L
b
N
c
Wh
Wh
BM
d

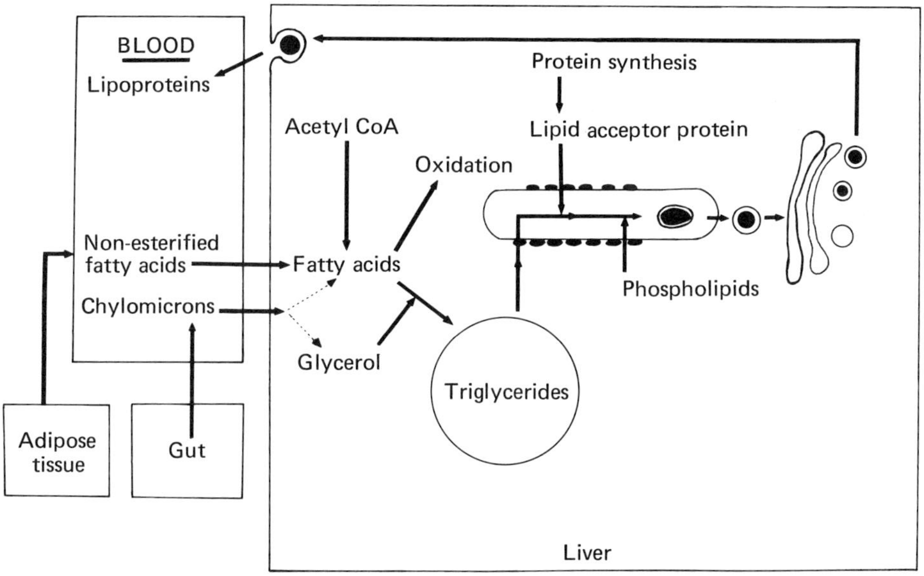

Figure 2-43. Diagram illustrating basic pathogenetic mechanisms involved in the formation of fatty liver.

imbalance between supply, utilization, and secretion of lipid by the liver cell can result in a fatty liver. For example, interference with phospholipid metabolism (as in choline deficiency) or interference with protein synthesis (as in the presence of many hepatotoxins) results in imperfect lipoproteins and consequent accumulation of triglycerides within the liver (Fig. 2-43). If the delivery of lipid to the liver is greatly increased–in adipose tissue mobilization, for example–the metabolic capacity of the liver may be exceeded, and triglyceride will accumulate. It has also been suspected that interference with mitochondrial fatty acid oxidation will increase the fatty acid pool and result in lipid accumulation.

Figure 2-42. a. Cytoplasm of a liver cell from a female rat after the administration of ethionine, which reduces ATP levels by approximately 80 per cent. A large lysosome (SL) is present; triglyceride droplets (arrows) accumulate within the cisternae of the endoplasmic reticulum as a result of the lack of ATP.

b. Large lipid droplets (L) in the cytoplasm of a choline-deficient rat.

c. Plasma cell showing a Russell body, consisting of accumulation of paracrystalline material (arrows) within ER cisternae. (Courtesy of Dr. William O. Dobbins, III)

d. Base of kidney tubule 24 hours after administration of mercuric chloride, showing characteristic whorls (Wh) derived from basilar cell membrane. BM, basement membrane.

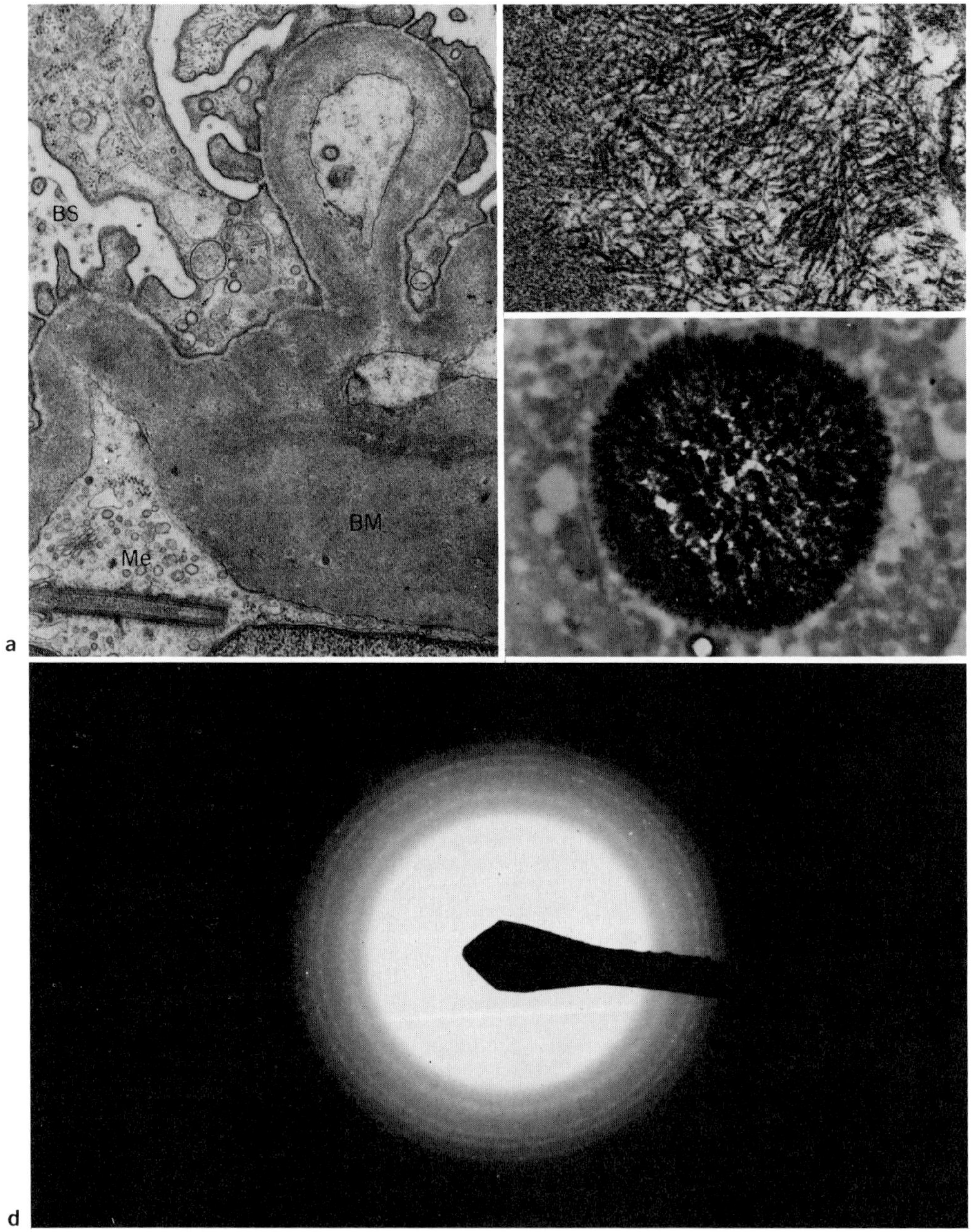
BS
BM
Me
a
b
c
d

In most conditions resulting in fatty liver, the stored lipid is in the form of triglycerides that exist as droplets of moderate density within the cell sap (Fig. 2-42b). Their precise relation to cytoplasmic structures has not been identified; but in view of the high surface energy of lipid droplets, it seems rather unlikely that they exist in a free state within the cell sap. They may be surrounded by a monolayer of phospholipid, with the hydrophilic ends directed toward the cell sap.

Another, and very different, type of fatty accumulation in cells occurs in lethally injured cells, where phospholipid released from damaged membranes reforms into lamellar, myelin-like bodies (Fig. 2-42d).

7. Abnormal cell products and extracellular phenomena

Excessive production of cell-secretory substances is a cellular reaction that occurs in many disease processes. Among the important secretory products of some cells is basement membrane material, a mixture of a variety of glycosylated proteins including collagen. When cells such as glomerular epithelial or mesangial cells are stimulated by various injuries, they produce much more basement membrane material, and this accumulates and ultimately may interfere with function. In diabetes mellitus, for example, massive accumulations of basement membrane material in both glomerular (Fig. 2-44a) and other capillary basement membranes can result in significant alterations of vascular function.

The protein amyloid is another abnormal cell-secretory product. In many instances, amyloid consists largely of altered antibody light-chain peptides. This protein accumulates along vessels and in parenchyma as a characteristic fibrillar structure and can seriously interfere with both vascular and parenchymal function (Fig. 2-44b).

Calcification of material within the extracellular space commonly occurs in

Figure 2-44. **a.** Portion of glomerular capillary wall from an individual with arteriolar nephrosclerosis. Note the marked thickening and irregularity of the basement membrane (BM). BS, blood space; Me, mesangial cell.

b. Electron micrograph of amyloid from the glomerulus of a patient with systemic amyloidosis. Note the characteristic appearance of the closely packed amyloid fibrils. (Courtesy of Dr. Ray Jones)

c. Extracellular calcification from human aortic valve in an individual with calcific aortic stenosis. Note the dense crystals of mineral which represent hydroxy apatite.

d. Electron diffraction pattern from **c.** illustrating characteristic rings of hydroxy apatite. (**c** and **d** courtesy of Dr. Kook Kim)

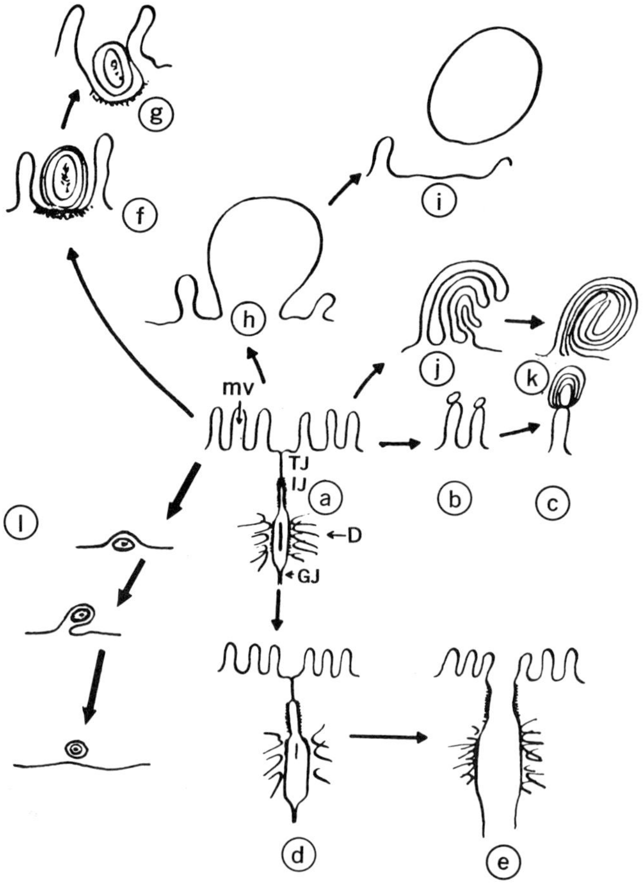

Figure 2-45. Conformational changes in the cell membrane after cell injury.

a. A typical normal membrane with microvilli (MV) and components of junctional complex, including tight junction (TJ), intermediate junction (IJ), desmosome (D), and gap junction (GJ).

b & **c.** Myelin forms produced by elaboration of bimolecular leaflets representing extracted phospholipid.

d & **e.** Stages of separation of junctional complexes occurring as a result of removal of calcium or treatment with chelating agents such as EDTA.

f & **g.** Stages in phagocytosis of bacteria in small intestine showing induced formation of spine-like coatings on cytoplasmic surface of membrane adjacent to the ingested organism.

h & **i.** Stages in elaboration of an exotropic bleb from the membrane surface.

j & **k.** Elaboration of tubular forms with formation of concentric arrangements when these protrude into a constrained space such as a kidney tubule or a bile canaliculus.

l. Stages in budding of virus.

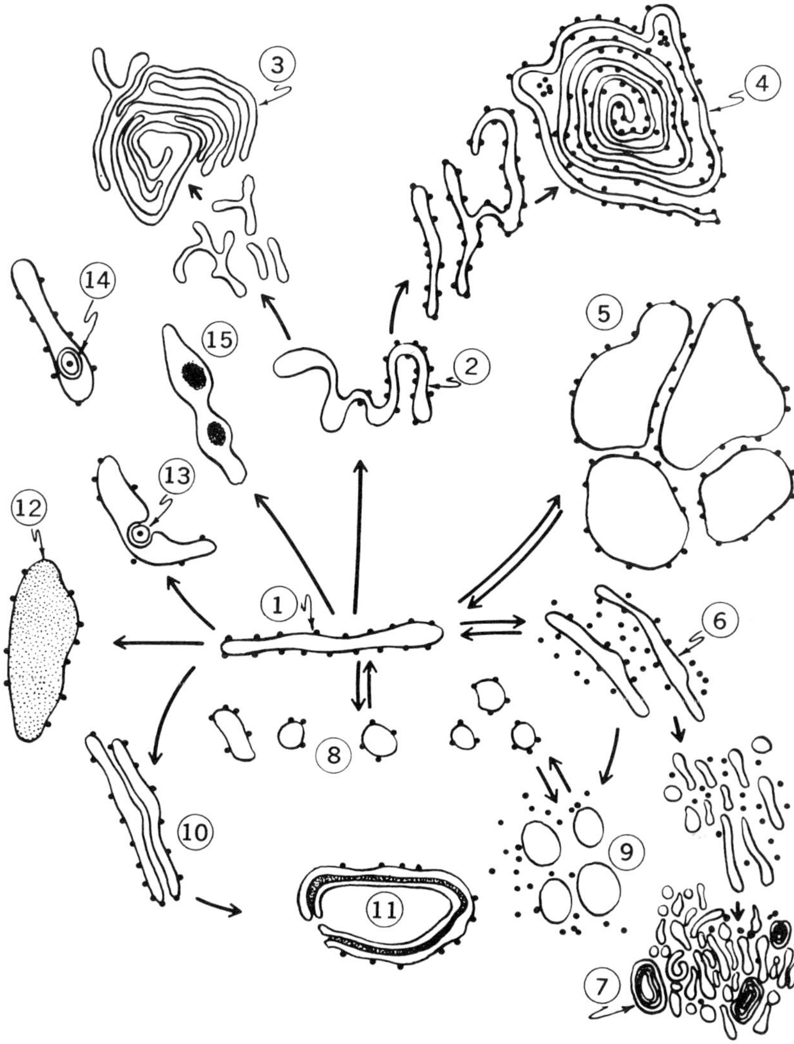

Figure 2-46. Conformational changes in endoplasmic reticulum.
(1) Normal conformation. (2) Stimulated synthesis of rough and smooth ER membranes results in (3) Proliferation of masses of smooth ER, as after administration of phenobarbital, and (4) complex proliferations of rough endoplasmic reticulum. (5) Dilatation of endoplasmic cisternae is caused by mild injuries that result in changes in ion and water movements. (6) Degranulation (loss of polysomes from the endoplasmic reticulum) is a common response to injury. (7) Peroxidation leads to changes of membrane conformation and accumulation of dense deposits. (8) & (9) Progressive fragmentation of ER results in smooth vesicles and detached polysomes. (10) & (11) Paired cisternae are formed after treatment with certain hormones including cortisone. (12) Materials such as glycoproteins may accumulate within ER cisternae. (13) & (14) Exotropy of naked virions into the endoplasmic reticulum cisternae results in an enveloped virus within ER. (15) Lipoproteins may accumulate in ER.

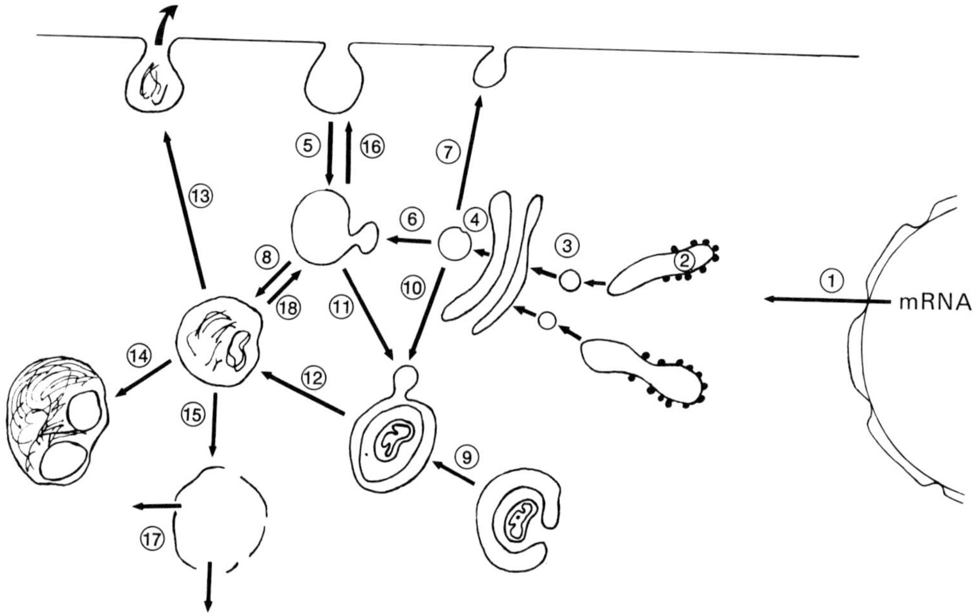

Figure 2-47. Basic reactions to cell injury of the lysosome system.
(1) Messenger RNA for synthesis of acid hydrolases moves from nucleus to cytoplasm. If genetic defects exist, as in Pompe's disease, enzyme deficiencies will occur. (2) Acid hydrolases, presumably synthesized on membrane-bound ribosomes, are injected into the lumen of the endoplasmic reticulum and transported to the Golgi region. An obstacle to release from the ER, as in ATP deficient states, may result in accumulation within the ER. (3) Transitional vesicles carry acid hydrolases and other materials from the ER to the forming face of the Golgi apparatus. This step has been shown to be ATP dependent. In the Golgi apparatus formation of secretion products occurs, including addition of glycosyl moieties to form glycoproteins. (4) The hydrolases are released at the maturing face, to form primary lysosomes. Primary lysosomes may exist not as vesicles but as tube-like extensions from the maturing face. (5) Phagocytic vacuoles or phagosomes pinch from the cell surface and enter the cytoplasm, fusing with either primary lysosomes (6) or secondary lysosomes (18). (7) In some cases, primary lysosomes are discharged directly to the surface. This same process occurs in secretion of hormones. (9) Autophagic vacuoles are formed by exotropy, creating a double-walled sac, the outer membrane of which may fuse with either primary (10) or secondary (11) lysosomes. (12) Conversion of the double-walled stage to a residual body or secondary lysosome occurs. (13) In some cells there is defecation of residual body contents to the cell surface. (14) Formation of increased amounts of residual bodies appears to be an event occurring in aging, especially in neurons and muscle cells; it can result also from increased autophagic and/or heterophagic events in many cell types after injury. (15) Lysosomes in necrotic cells deteriorate, the membrane leaks, and enzymes escape to the cell sap (17). (16) Secondary lysosomes or enzyme-containing phagosomes may fuse with the cell surface, leaking enzymes into the extracellular space.

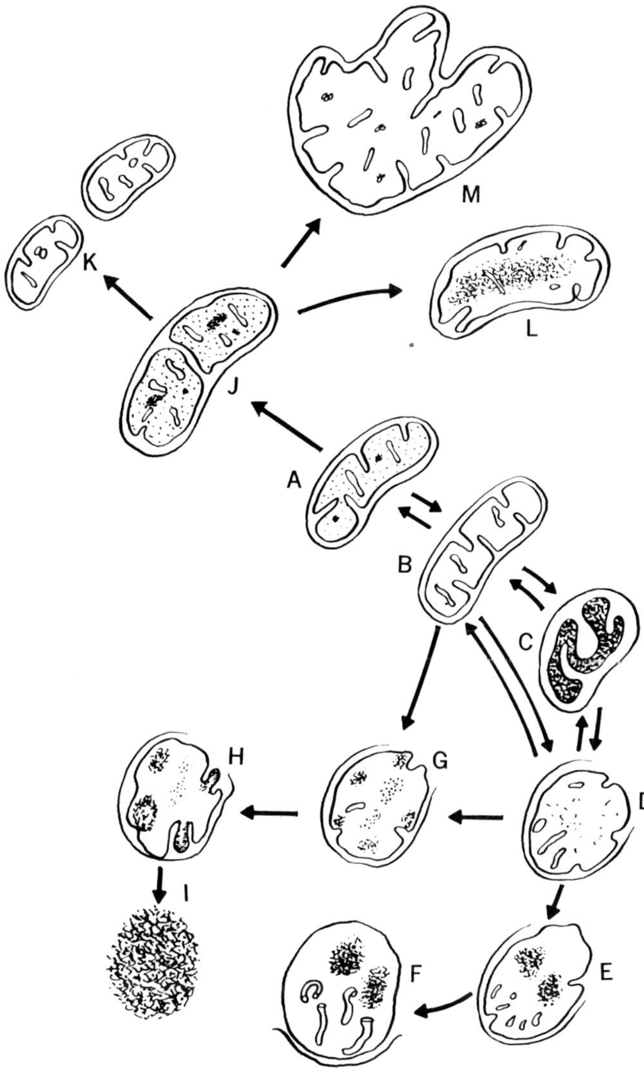

Figure 2-48. Progressive mitochondrial changes in cell injury.
A. Typical normal mitochondrion. B. The mitochondrial granules are lost, concomitantly with a decrease in ATP. C. Condensed mitochondrion in which the matrix is contracted, possibly the result of condensation of matrix proteins following changes in ADP/ATP ratio. Increased levels of ADP often produce contraction. D. High-amplitude swelling follows ion and water movements into the mitochondrion, with rupture of the outer membrane. E. Fluffy deposits that probably represent aggregations of denatured proteins are seen; at this stage mitochondria are severely damaged, and P/O ratios approach zero. F. Tubular forms have arisen from the inner membrane. G. Deposits of apatites occur

chronic cell injuries. This calcification often has the form of hydroxyapatite crystals that may begin as colloidal calcium phosphate precipitates on nuclei of uncertain nature, though both glycosaminoglycans and phospholipids have been suggested as representing the original nidus. These calcification sites commonly enlarge by deposition of concentric rings of crystals and represent—in contrast to the mitochondrial calcification described above—an energy-independent form of dystrophic calcification (Fig. 2-44c,d).

E. Classification of Reactions by Organelle

Reactions to injury have been presented in this chapter in a unified manner, organized as *patterns* of response at the cellular level. It is possible to categorize these reactions according to those that are characteristic of each organelle, subjected to a variety of injuries. Figures 2-45–48 present such a classification for the convenience of the student, who can thus review cellular pathophysiology from a different point of view. The most characteristic reactions of each organelle or subcellular system to cell injury are presented in diagrammatic fashion.

---

following calcium and phosphate accumulation by mitochondria. H. The calcium deposits are in annular patterns adjacent to the inner membrane. I. The entire mitochondrion has calcified. J. Beginning mitochondrial division with a septum separating the inner compartment into two phases, each of which contains clumped mitochondrial DNA in the matrix. K. The division is completed. L. A paracrystalline aggregate in the mitochondrial matrix, as seen in human livers. M. A megamitochondrion that may arise from defective mitochondrial division or from fusion. N. Mitochondrion with hemosiderin stored in matrix, from an erythropoietic cell in a case of sideroblastic anemia. O. Mitochondria with closely packed zigzag cristae, as is seen in non-thyrotoxic hypermetabolism states.

References

Allison, A. (1968), The role of lysosomes in the action of drugs and hormones, Adv. in Chemotherapy, *3*:253.

Baserga, R., and Wiebel, F. (1969), The cell cycle of mammalian cells, *in* Int. Rev. of Exp. Path., vol. 7, pp. 1–20, G. W. Richter and M. A. Epstein, Eds., Academic Press, New York.

Busch, H., and Smetana, K. (1970), The Nucleolus, Academic Press, New York.

de Duve, C., and Baudhuin, P. (1966), Peroxisomes (Microbodies and related particles), Physiol. Rev., *46*:323.

de Duve, C., and Wattiaux, R. (1966), Functions of lysosomes, Ann. Rev. Physiol., *28*:435.

Dingle, J. T., and Fell, H. B., Eds., (1969), Lysosomes in Biology and Pathology, Parts I and II, North-Holland Publishing Co., Amsterdam.

Goldblatt, P. J. (1972), Molecular pathology of the endoplasmic reticulum, Subcell. Biochem., *1*:147.

Haguenau, F. (1969), Ultrastructure of the cancer cell, *in* Biological Basis of Medicine, vol. 5, pp. 433–86, E. E. Bittar and N. Bittar, Eds., Academic Press, New York and London.

Hruban, Z., and Rechcigl, M. (1969), Microbodies and related particles, *in* Int. Rev. Cytology, Suppl. 1, pp. 1–251, G. H. Bourne and J. F. Danielli, Eds., Academic Press, New York.

Kinney, T. D., Ed. (1973), President's Symposium: Iron Overload, Am. J. Path., *72*:263.

Lombardi, B. (1965), Considerations on the pathogenesis of fatty liver, *in* Biochemical Pathology, pp. 1–15, E. Farber, and P. N. Magee, Eds., Proc. 1st Int. Symp. in Biochemical Path. (Seven Springs, Champion, Pa.), Williams & Wilkins Co., Baltimore.

Majno, G., LaGattuta, M., and Thompson, T. E. (1960), Cellular death and necrosis; chemical, physical and morphologic changes in rat liver, Virchows Arch. Path. Anat., *333*:421.

Murayama, M. (1971), Molecular mechanisms of human red cell (with HbS) sickling, *in* Molecular Aspects of Sickle Cell Hemoglobin: Clinical Applications, pp. 3–19, R. M. Nalbandian, Ed., Charles C Thomas Co., Springfield, Ill.

Novikoff, A. B., and Holtzman, E. (1970), Cells and Organelles, Holt, Rinehart and Winston, New York.

Orrenius, S., and Ernster, L. (1971), Enzymatic properties of membrane-associated cell fractions as related to drug metabolism, *in* Cell Membranes: Biological and Pathological Aspects, pp. 38–53, G. W. Richter and D. G. Scarpelli, Eds., Williams & Wilkins Co., Baltimore.

Parsons, D. F. (1965), Recent advances correlating structure and function in mitochondria, Adv. Exp. Path., *5*:1.

Resibois, A., Tondeur, M., Mockel, S., and Dustin, P. (1970), Lysosomes and storage diseases, Int. Rev. of Exp. Path., *9*:93.

Scarpelli, D. G., Chiga, M., and Haynes, E. (1971), Experimental modification of mitochondrial biogenesis in rat liver cells, *in* Cell Membranes: Biological and Pathological Aspects, pp. 151–74, G. W. Richter and D. G. Scarpelli, Eds.

Scarpelli, D. G., and Trump, B. F. (1971), Cell Injury (Prepared for Universities Associated for Research and Education in Pathology, Inc.), Upjohn Co., Kalamazoo, Mich.

Svoboda, D. V., and Reddy, J. K. (1974; in press), Some biological properties of microbodies (peroxisomes), *in Pathobiology* Annual, vol. 4, H. L. Ioachim, Ed., Appleton-Century-Crofts, New York.

Tosteson, D. C. (1963), Regulation of cell volume by sodium and potassium transplant, *in* The Cellular Functions of Membrane Transport, pp. 3–22, J. F. Hoffmann, Ed., Prentice-Hall, Englewood Cliffs, N.J.

Trump, B. F., Croker, B. P., and Mergner, W. J. (1971), The role of energy metabolism, ion, and water shifts in the pathogenesis of cell injury, *in* Cell Membranes: Biological and Pathological Aspects, pp. 84–128, G. W. Richter and D. G. Scarpelli, Eds.

3

INFLAMMATION

Peter A. Ward, M.D.

A. General Description

As one of the most common and visible responses of the vertebrate body to injury, the inflammatory process has occupied the attention of physicians since the time of the early Greeks. It was recognized many years ago that without the inflammatory process a microbe would be free to enter a wound or mucosal surface, establish residence in the warm, well-nourished environment, proliferate, spread, and eventually kill the host. In quite another way, the benefits derived from the body's ability to marshal an inflammatory response have been evident in wound healing, since not only are microbial agents kept in check and infection thus prevented, but concomitantly events of the inflammatory response set into motion a complex series of reactions that result in healing and repair of the damaged tissue. Without inflammatory responses, then, we would go through life bearing all the open wounds of the past, a body unable to heal itself, quite like a machine that functions until a part wears out or breaks.

In all these respects, because it swiftly and dramatically copes with sudden changes in the body, the inflammatory response is important to the maintenance of life. But inflammation itself may also be destructive. The loss of homeostatic control in the inflammatory response can lead to self-mutilation or even death. The many hundreds of thousands of victims of rheumatoid arthritis, the thousands of patients dying yearly with glomerulonephritis, the increasing numbers of patients threatened by rejection of a vital homograft, all give testimony to the serious consequences of the inflammatory process that goes, for whatever reason, unchecked.

The constitutional signs and symptoms of an inflammatory process are well known. Who has not experienced the lassitude, the weakness, and the fever that are so prominent when an inflammatory response is in progress, as in the throat, the middle ear, the lungs, or anywhere else in the body? Precisely why a localized process should lead to such profound systemic changes is far from clear. Do substances released from the local area lead to an effect elsewhere in the body, and, if so, how is the inflammatory process involved in the mechanism? Perhaps the best answers to these questions come from the work of many groups who have defined a mechanism of fever that depends upon the role of granulocytes.

It is now well known that a substance termed *endogenous pyrogen* is elaborated from granulocytes as a result of contact of these cells with antigen-antibody complexes, bacterial endotoxin, or soluble substances present in inflammatory foci. Endogenous pyrogen is also elaborated during the phagocytic process of granulocytes. The pyrogen apparently has an action on the central nervous system, where the thermal regulatory mechanism is upset and the body's "thermostat" is set higher. In view of the variety of mechanisms for releasing endogenous pyrogen, it is not difficult to see why fever develops once granulocytes have accumulated in an inflammatory focus.

The classical local signs of inflammation–namely, heat, redness, swelling, and pain–are the result of functional changes in the vasculature of tissue in response to an injurious agent or altered state. Water, electrolytes and macromolecules, and cells, especially leukocytes, escape from the usual intravascular confines. When these substances appear outside the walls of vessels, provided this is not due to a simple physical destruction of the vessel wall, the inflammatory process is, by definition, present. Without intact blood vessels and without circulating elements within them, the inflammatory process cannot occur; but once the functional integrity of the blood vessels is lost, these substances quickly begin their exodus from the bloodstream. The redness caused by the inflammatory process is attributable to dilatation of vessels; the heat is due to the increased blood flow to the area; the swelling is due to the escape of liquids and cells into the extravascular spaces; and the pain is due to the pressure on nerve endings and/or the action of mediators such as bradykinin (see below) on these structures. Such changes usually lead to healing, but on occasion they may seriously interfere with the function of the involved organ; this is well represented in post-streptococcal glomerulonephritis, rheumatic carditis, or pneumococcal pneumonia, where the inflammatory process itself leads to a condition that is more life-threatening than the initial insult to the tissue.

B. Histology of the Inflammatory Response

The inflammatory response can be classified according to the types of cells that predominate in the inflamed tissue.

Acute inflammation is the common type that one might see when a wood splinter has penetrated the skin. Within hours redness appears, heralding the vascular dilatation and the accelerated blood flow through the area. Fluid (edema) accumulates in the tissues. Shortly thereafter, neutrophilic granulocytes can be seen clustering along the endothelial margins of blood vessels, the phenomenon of *margination* or peripheralization; and soon these leukocytes can be seen making their way into the adjacent connective tissue. These events accelerate over the period of several hours so that soon the entire area contains vast numbers of extravascular granulocytes that effectively wall off the foreign body. Much the same sort of response is seen whenever any acute injury to tissue occurs, such as a burn, a mechanical injury like an abrasion, or an infection.

Precisely what accounts for these changes in the functional behavior of the blood vessels is quite unclear. Many years ago Lewis (1927) emphasized the role of the autonomic nervous system in bringing about changes in the caliber of blood vessels. He emphasized that this occurs autonomously, in the nature of a reflex: that is to say, peripheral nerves are involved, the higher center of the central nervous system being by-passed. Why the granulocytes accumulate along the endothelial surfaces just prior to their movement out of the blood vessel has been a point of great controversy. It has been suggested that the endothelium has been modified, becoming "sticky" for leukocytes; but there is no convincing evidence for this conclusion. This does not, however, exclude a chemical or physical basis for the adherence of these leukocytes to endothelial surfaces.

Precisely why granulocytes would move beyond the confines of the vessel at this point could be explained by the role of chemotactic factors–that is, attractants that are present in the surrounding area and cause the unidirectional movement of leukocytes toward a concentration gradient or attractant. In the acute inflammatory response very few lymphocytes or monocytes accumulate in the extravascular sites. Possible reasons for this could be either a lack of specific mediators such as chemotactic agents causing extravascular migration of monocytes and lymphocytes, or the much slower responsiveness of lymphocytes and monocytes to stimuli such as chemotactic factors.

Ordinarily within one to three days the character of the cells in the acute inflammatory process has changed: this altered morphology defines the *subacute inflammatory response*. In the place of neutrophilic granulocytes, lymphocytes and monocytes can be seen scattered in the extravascular area. The most striking manifestation of the subacute inflammatory response, however, is the appearance of lush sprouts of very actively growing, tiny, fragile blood vessels and connective tissue cells. This angioblastic and fibroblastic proliferation, in aggregate referred to as *granulation tissue*, indicates that a stimulus to cell growth has occurred. It is because of the profusion of vascular sprouts and fibroblasts beginning to lay down collagen that the stage is set for the formation of a scar.

If the inflammatory process does not subside—particularly if the agent responsible for inducing the inflammatory process remains—the granulation tissue will continue to form, and dense collagenous connective tissue may be found. In addition, the population of leukocytes begins to change, almost exclusively, to lymphocytes, monocytes, and plasma cells. The persistence of these cells in areas where they ordinarily exist in small numbers (if at all), the continued laying-down of ever-increasing amounts of dense collagenous connective tissue, the continued influx of cells from the circulation and the accelerating disintegration of leukocytes (and also cells native to the area of injury) lead to a *chronic inflammatory process* that may present serious problems to the functional capacity of tissue, particularly if a critical area such as a heart valve or the myocardium is involved.

As just indicated, the staging of the inflammatory process is usually based upon histologic criteria—that is, the nature of the inflammatory cells (leukocytes) present. While the type of leukocyte in the inflammatory response can usually be predicted according to duration of the process, the clinical terms *acute* or *chronic inflammation* may also be based solely upon temporal considerations. Accordingly, acute inflammation usually implies a process of fairly short duration (days). It is usually characterized by an exudate of neutrophils, although in some cases—for instance, viral hepatitis—mononuclear cells predominate. On the other hand, persistent osteomyelitis would be termed a *chronic* inflammatory process because of its long duration, although histologically the inflammatory cells might consist almost exclusively of neutrophilic leukocytes. In this chapter the terms *acute, subacute,* and *chronic* are used according to established histologic criteria.

C. Phases of the Acute Inflammatory Response

In order to understand these very complex events, it is important to examine the various phases of the inflammatory process. It is possible to consider separately the permeability changes and the accumulation of leukocytes; these are independent events that may occur simultaneously or in sequence.

1. Permeability changes

Wilhelm and Mason (1960) and subsequently several other workers have now shown that the acute inflammatory process, which can conveniently be induced by thermal injury in rat skin, is characterized by two phases of altered per-

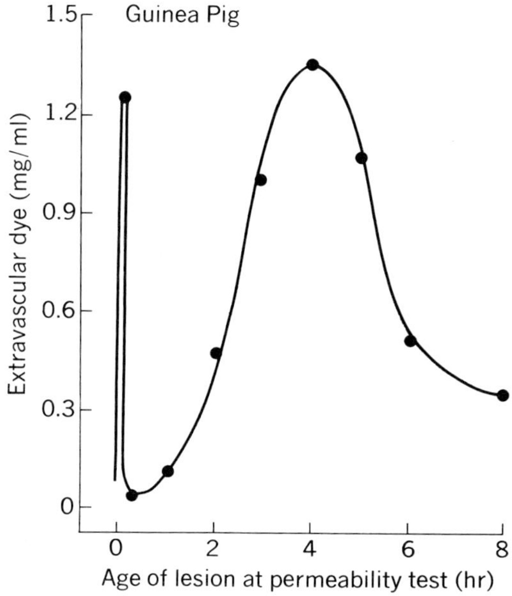

Figure 3-1. The two phases of capillary permeability (in rat skin) induced by thermal injury. The initial phase is transient and histamine dependent, whereas the secondary (delayed) or prolonged phase is independent of histamine. Extravascular leukocyte accumulation in tissue occurs during the secondary phase of permeability. (Courtesy of Wilhelm and Mason, 1960)

meability (Fig. 3-1) (see review of Wilhelm, 1962). The first phase appears to be mediated by histamine, since suitable chemical antagonists of histamine will completely ablate the change in permeability. As several groups have pointed out, this histamine-dependent phase is transient, lasting little more than a few minutes. Within 2-to-4 hours a prolonged and quite different phase occurs. In contrast to the histamine-dependent phase, the secondary phase is prolonged, lasting over the next 3-to-4 hours. It is during this period that leukocytes begin to migrate out of blood vessels (Hurley, 1964). The mediator of this secondary phase has not been identified, but it clearly is not histamine or serotonin.

Both the histamine-dependent and the histamine-independent phases of permeability are associated with the migration of fluids, not through endothelial cells, but between endothelial cells—that is, a percolation of proteins, electrolytes, and water through the junctional zones between endothelial cells, through the basement membrane of the vessel, and into the area around the blood vessel (Fig. 3-2).

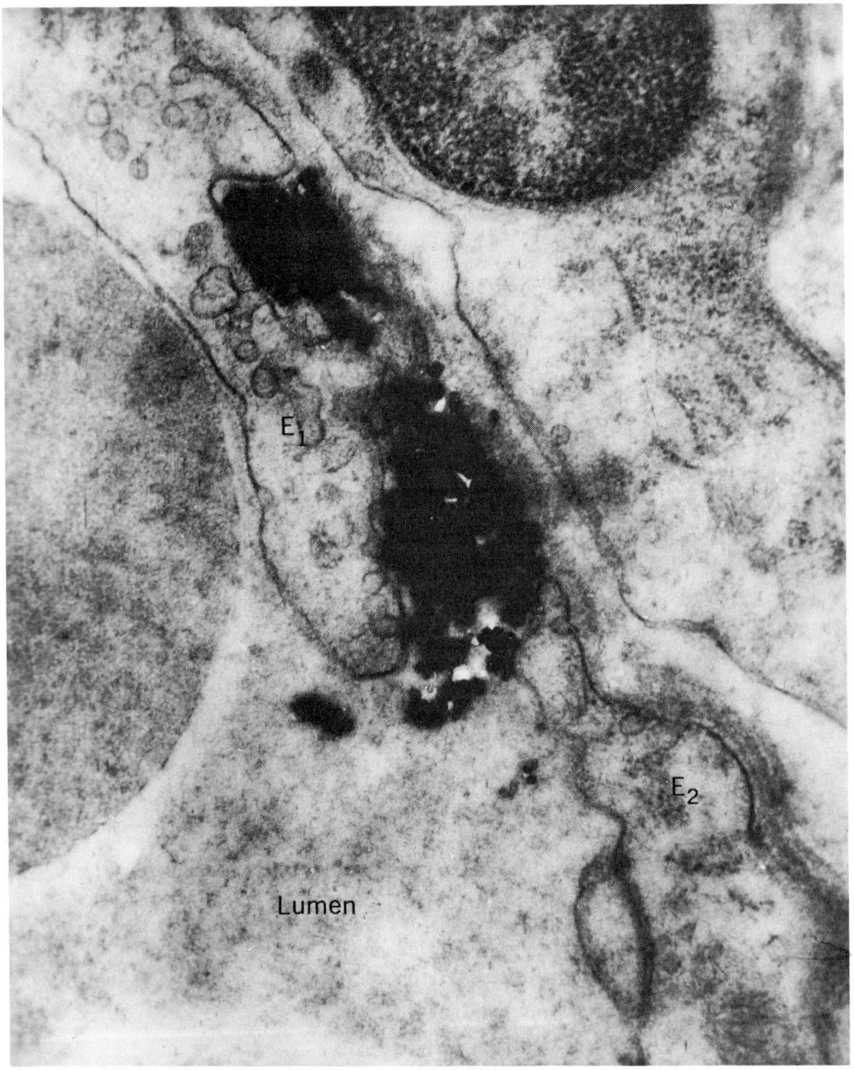

Figure 3-2. Movement of carbon particles through an interendothelial junction (between endothelial cells E1 and E2). The capillary lumen is indicated, with a red blood cell adjacent to the endothelial surface. (Courtesy of Marchesi, 1962)

Several classes of mediators affecting permeability of blood vessels have been described, and most appear to be an effect either on capillaries or on the postcapillary venules. The mechanism by which permeability agents accomplish their biological effect is not known, if in fact a common mechanism pertains. The suggestion that permeability changes are due to increases in hydrostatic pressure in the capillary, caused by contraction of postcapillary venules, has not been substantiated. Recently Majno and his associates have advanced the intriguing suggestion that permeability agents cause contraction of periendothelial cells, which surround capillaries. Since these cells seem to be structurally attached to endothelial cells, their contraction could result in a pulling apart of endothelial cells at their junctional zones, allowing escape of fluids with resultant permeability increases. Majno has shown electron-microscopic evidence of contractile-like events in periendothelial cells and has provided provisional evidence (by immunofluorescence) of the presence within these cells of antigenic material reactive with antibody to smooth-muscle antigen. This theory of permeability changes caused by contractile events of special cells awaits further study.

Table 3-1 Permeability Factors

FACTOR	SPECIAL CHARACTERISTICS
Vasoactive amines	Histamine, serotonin, stored in special cells in preformed state
Kinins	Generated by plasma kallikrein acting on α_2 globulin substrate in plasma
PF/dil	Present as inactive plasma enzyme, active product not defined; probably a fragment of Hageman Factor
Leukokinins	Generated by enzyme(s) derived from leukocytes (and other tissues), acting on substrate in serum
Anaphylatoxins (C3a, C5a)	Cleavage products from the third and fifth components of complement
SRS-A	Non-peptide but unknown structure; production somehow related to neutrophils in some situations
Prostaglandins (PG)	Derivatives of fatty acids, produced in many tissues, consisting of subclasses A, B, E, and F, of which E class appears to be most active biologically
Basic peptides from neutrophils	Preformed, highly basic peptides in lysosomal granules of neutrophils, released during phagocytosis

Listed in Table 3-1 are the permeability factors found in a variety of species of mammals, including man. *Vasoactive amines* consist of histamine and serotonin, which ordinarily do not exist free in the circulation but are stored in cells such as basophils, mast cells, and platelets. Intricate mechanisms account for the release of these amines; and when they are released in the vicinity of endothelium, permeability changes in the vessels occur. The natural antagonists to these permeability factors, including the catecholamines such as epinephrine and norepinephrine (Spector and Willoughby, 1964), do not exist in local stores but must be released from secretory granules in cells at a distant site (in the adrenal medulla), and then make their way via the circulation to the site of altered permeability.

Histamine is probably the more important amine in many of the allergic responses in man, especially in the case of hayfever, in which the symptoms of increased vascular permeability in the naso-pharynx can be dramatically reversed by therapeutic application of histamine antagonists (anti-histaminic drugs). Vasoactive amines may play a key role in the initial localization of immune complexes present in the circulation, the outcome of which is a severe glomerulonephritis with consequent structural and functional damage.

The *kinins* constitute a series of peptides derived from α_2 globulin in the plasma. The scheme of the kinin-generating system is described in Table 3-2.

Table 3-2 Scheme of Kinin-generating System

Activation by contact with glass surfaces or other agents	
Pre-Hageman Factor	Hageman Factor (active fragment also known as PF/dil)
Pre-Kallikrein (Pro-Kininogenase)	Kallikrein (Kininogenase)
Kininogen (Substrate)	Kinin
Kininase in Plasma*	Inactive Kinin

* Carboxypeptidase B

The complex series of reaction steps, featuring sequential activation (probably by cleavage) of proteins, results in the formation of several enzymes, each of which acts sequentially on the next protein, and so on down the pathway. The final result is the formation of at least one of three kinin peptides: bradykinin (a 9 amino acid-containing peptide), lysylbradykinin, and/or methionyl-lysylbradykinin. These peptides are known for their abilities to increase vascular permeability, contract smooth muscle, and produce pain in man when applied to the base of a blister. The kinins are rapidly inactivated by the presence in plasma of a potent carboxypeptidase B type enzyme that cleaves the C terminal arginine from the respective kinin. As will be pointed out later, this same enzyme inactivates the C3a anaphylatoxin, suggesting it is an important regulator of the inflammatory system. The kinin system has been the subject of an excellent recent review (Kellermeyer and Graham, 1968).

The *leukokinins* are kinin-like peptides, basic in charge, and, being somewhat larger molecules (mol. wt. around 2,500) than the classical kinins described above, are derived from the action of an enzyme(s) (leukokinin-forming enzyme) that exists in lysosomal granules of leukocytes. This enzyme is present also in a variety of other cells, including tumor cells. Leukokinins are potent permeability agents and are generated by the action of the enzyme(s) on a plasma substrate. The enzyme, the plasma substrate, and the leukokinin(s) are each structurally different from their counterparts in the kallikrein system. The leukokinin-forming proteins have been found in ascitic fluids of animals and humans with malignant neoplasms, suggesting that these permeability factors may be important in the causation of the tumor-associated exudate.

The *anaphylatoxins* constitute a completely separate class of vasoactive peptides and are derived from the third or the fifth component of complement (reviewed by Müller-Eberhard, 1968). Each of these peptides has an approximate molecular weight of 10,000, and apparently alters vessel permeability indirectly by causing the release of histamine from tissue mast cells. In addition, the anaphylatoxins contract smooth muscle, and this contraction may, in critical areas, lead to increased hydrostatic pressure and subsequent increased permeability. When injected into humans, in nanogram amounts, the C3a anaphylatoxin has been shown to cause potent permeability changes in the skin. It is likely that the C3a and C5a molecules will induce increases in vascular permeability as well as chemotactic attraction of neutrophils.

The substance *PF/dil* (*permeability factor in diluted serum*), described by Miles (1961), appears to be a plasma enzyme that can act on a plasma substrate to produce a material that increases vascular permeability. The nature of this biogenic agent is not known. There is now evidence that PF/dil is not directly a permeability agent but is, in fact, a fragment of the Hageman factor that can directly activate prekallikrein.

A substance termed *lymph node permeability factor* has been extracted from lymph nodes of animals exhibiting delayed hypersensitivity to various antigens. This material appears after sensitization and induces increased vascular permeability following intradermal injection. It has not been characterized, but Willoughby and Spector (1964) suggest a role for this factor in chronic inflammatory processes where immunologic mechanisms come into play. A substance termed *slow-reacting substance* (*SRS-A*) is released when sensitized lung tissue is perfused with antigen (Brocklehurst, 1960). SRS-A, which under some circumstances requires neutrophils for its elaboration and may be a product of them (Orange, Valentine, and Austen, 1968), induces increased vascular permeability as well as a characteristic contraction of smooth muscle, and may be important in certain allergic reactions where vascular permeability changes are prominent. There are also some suggestions that this factor may be responsible for the bronchoconstriction in asthmatic states, but direct evidence is lacking.

The *prostaglandins* (PG's) represent a new class of fatty acid derivatives with controversial biological functions. Certain PG's induce increases in the intracellular levels of cyclic AMP, which may result in a great change in the functional status of cells. For instance, significant metabolic shifts have been found in lipocytes, while the secretory activity of mast cells is markedly depressed. Certain of the PG's induce an increase in permeability when injected into the skin. Whatever, the true role of PG's in inflammation remains to be determined. Because certain non-steroidal anti-inflammatory drugs block PG synthesis, it has been concluded that this supports the role of PG's in inflammation. Much more study of the PG's is obviously necessary.

The last of the permeability factors listed in Table 3-1 are the *basic peptides from neutrophils,* present in preformed state in lysosomal granules of neutrophilic granulocytes. These peptides have potent, direct permeability activity on vessels. It is to be expected that each time the release of lysosomal contents occurs from neutrophils there will be delivery of these permeability agents with resultant intensification of the inflammatory response.

2. Transmigration of leukocytes

It is quite clear that a permeability change in vessels leading to the escape of proteins is not synonymous with the escape of granulocytes. Indeed, change in permeability may very well occur in the virtual absence of leukocyte emigration (as in urticarial or "hives" reactions), and vice versa. The transmigration of cells across vascular barriers is of central importance in inflammation.

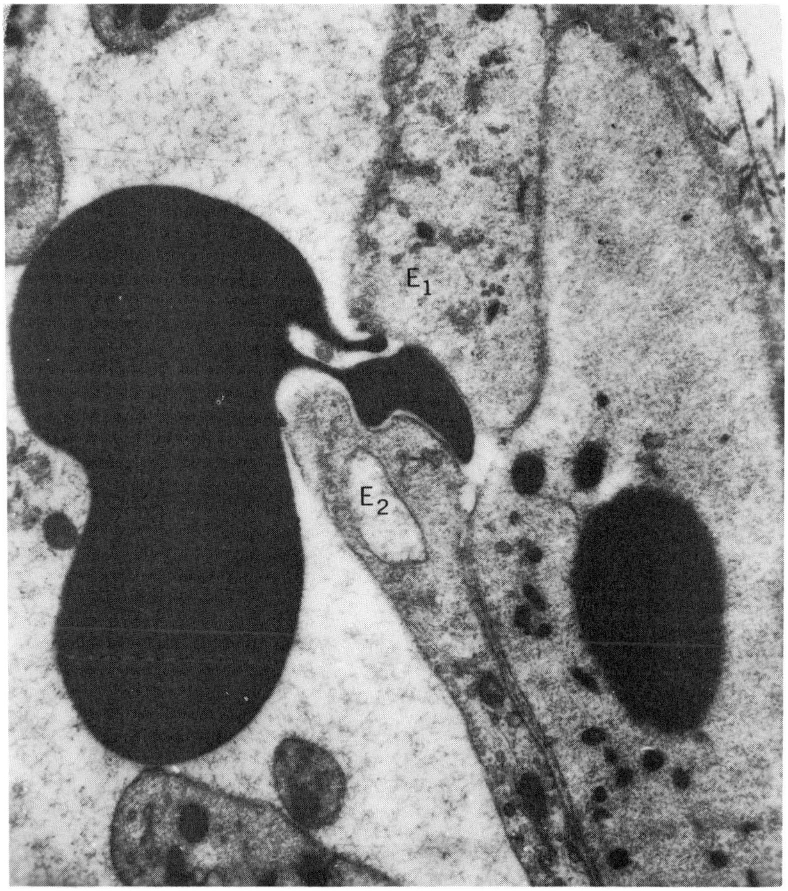

Figure 3-3. Movement of a red blood cell through an interendothelial junction, similar to the escape of carbon particles during inflammation. Plasticity of the red cell is evident. (Courtesy of Marchesi, 1964)

There is no evidence that red blood cells escape by other than passive means. Their exodus is via transit through interendothelial cell junctions (Fig. 3-3). Unless initial injury to the blood vessels results in physical disruption of blood vessels, the extravasation of red cells appears to be a late event in the inflammatory process and is often related to damage of vessels induced by the inflammatory process itself (to be discussed later). When it occurs, red cell escape (hemorrhage) usually reflects grave injury to the wall of the blood vessel. Hemorrhage should not be considered an integral part of the inflammatory process, even though a "hemorrhagic exudate" is sometimes described.

Granulocytes escape from the vessel in a manner that is anatomically similar to that for red cells. The very elegant electron-microscopic observations of Marchesi and Florey (1960) have defined morphologically the process of granulocyte emigration. These authors describe how granulocytes approximate the endothelial surface of the vessel and protrude pseudopods into the interdothelial junction, following which the pseudopod then squeezes along and arrives at the base (outer aspect) of the endothelial cell (Figs. 3-4, 3-5). Once there, the rest of the cell

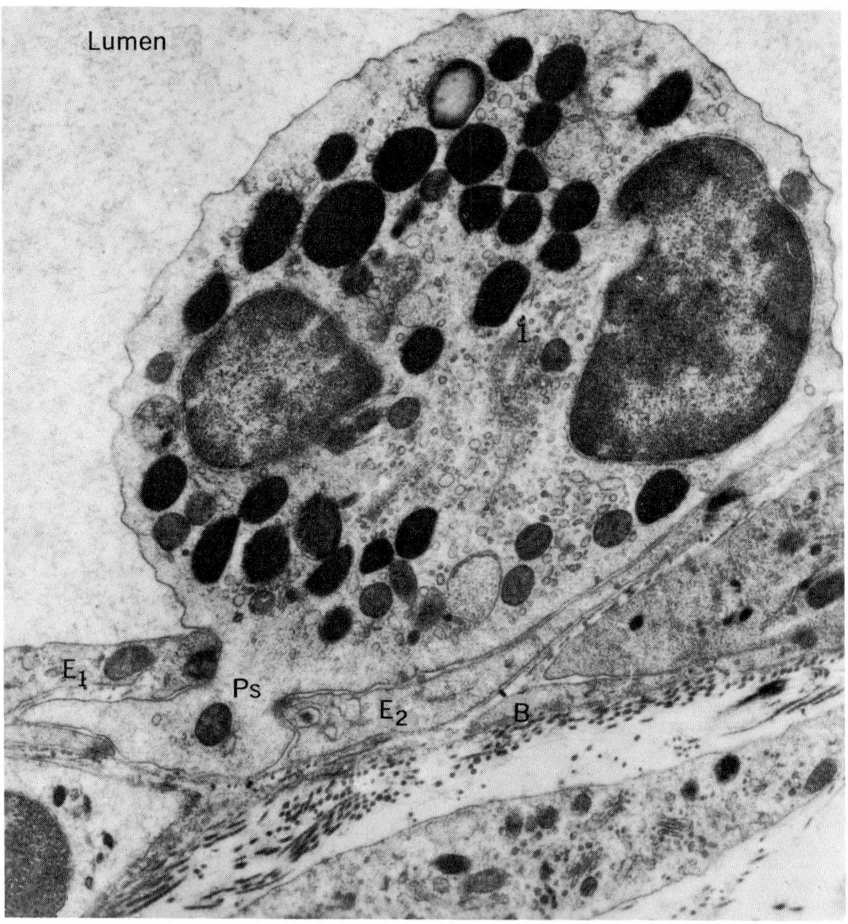

Figure 3-4. Intrusion of a pseudopod (Ps) from a neutrophil (1) through an interendothelial junction (defined by cytoplasmic processes of endothelial cells E_1 and E_2) as the cell moves through the capillary wall. (B represents basement membrane). Collagen fibers are in evidence outside the vessel wall. (Courtesy of Marchesi, 1961)

squeezes along this channel and is soon outside the endothelial cell, where it moves through the basement membrane of the vessel and into the extravascular connective tissue space.

The movement of leukocytes from the bloodstream into areas beyond the endothelial barrier has been explained at least in part by chemotactic mechanisms. For years it has been known that leukocytes on surfaces of glass slides will move toward certain substances, such as bacterial clusters; and time-lapse photography has revealed that this is unidirectional, linear movement rather than an aimless random migration (Harris, 1960). The possibility that such mechanisms apply

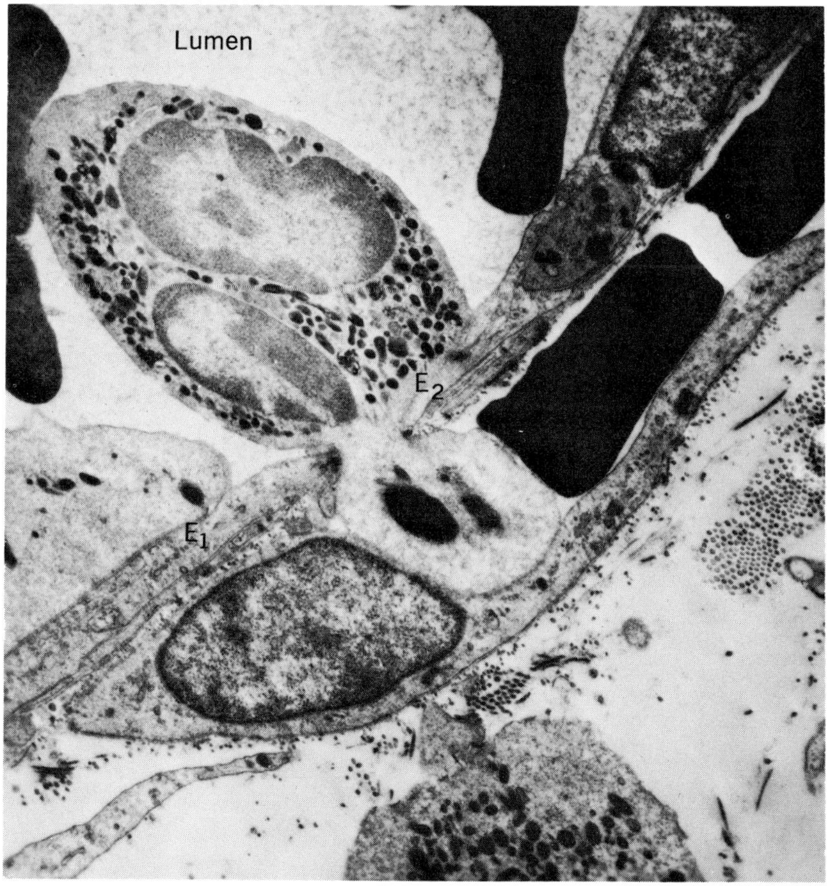

Figure 3-5. Movement of a neutrophil through a venular wall with intrusion of a pseudopod into the periendothelial space. Several red cells have escaped beyond the point through the same channel. (Courtesy of Marchesi and Florey, 1960)

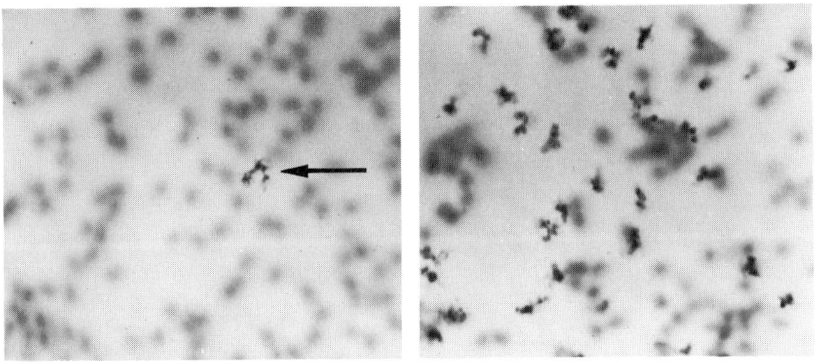

Figure 3-6. Chemotaxis of neutrophilic leukocytes, micropore filter technique. Micropore filters are from two chemotaxis chambers. The left frame from negative control chamber contains a single cell (arrow) that has migrated into the filter, while the right frame shows numerous neutrophils that have moved into channels of the filter in response to a complement-dependent chemotactic stimulus. (Courtesy of Ward, Cochrane, and Muller-Eberhard, 1965)

in vivo has appealed to many investigators, although direct confirmation has been difficult to come by. Nevertheless, it has been possible to demonstrate that neutrophilic granulocytes respond chemotactically to specific factors *in vitro*.

The latest era in the study of chemotaxis began in 1962, when Stephen Boyden popularized a new method for studying leukocyte chemotaxis–namely, by the use of a micropore filter that would separate leukocytes on the one side from the chemotactic substance on the other side of the membrane. It has now been rather convincingly shown that granulocytes will migrate only if the chemotactic factor is present at a distance from the cell (i.e., in the opposite compartment). When various concentrations of the chemotactic factor on the two sides of the membrane were used, it was found that the cells were responding to a gradient of concentration of the factor (Fig. 3-6) (Ward, Cochrane, and Müller-Eberhard, 1965, 1966; Keller and Sorkin, 1968). With this system it became possible to obtain precise quantitative data for leukocyte responsiveness, and the micropore filter technique has now become the most popular method for studying chemotaxis.

Neutrophilic granulocytes respond over a short interval of time–which is reminiscent of the behavior of leukocytes *in vivo*. Specifically, these cells require only 90 minutes to complete their response in the chemotactic chamber, in sharp contrast with the time course of response for mononuclear cells (Fig. 3-7). Several different factors that are chemotactic for neutrophils have been isolated. Curiously, many of these are derived from the nine-component complement system either as products of complement generated by enzymes extrinsic to or intrinsic to the complement system (Table 3-3). Sequential interaction of the complement

Table 3-3 Products of Complement System with Chemotactic Activity for Neutrophils

CHEMOTACTIC FACTOR	METHOD OF GENERATION
C567	Sequential interaction of first seven components of complement
	Trypsin
Low molecular factors C3 fragment	Complement enzymes (from classical pathway $C4\overline{2}$ or C3 convertase; from "alternate pathway," the C3 activator)
	Trypsin
	Thrombin
	Plasmin
	Tissue protease
C5 fragment	Sequential interaction of first five components of complement system
	Activation of the alternate complement pathway
	Trypsin
	Neutral protease in lysosomal granules of the neutrophil
	Protease in macrophages

system results in the activation of the macromolecular complex consisting of the fifth, sixth, and seventh components of complement. This factor, with a relatively high molecular weight, thereupon acquires chemotactic activity. It is possible also to activate the $C\overline{567}$ complex by trypsin, suggesting that protein cleavage is the important change that biologically activates the complex.

Chemotactic activity is present also in the two cleavage products of the third (C3) and the fifth components (C5) of complement. Each of the peptides has a molecular weight varying from 7,500 to 15,000. The C3 fragment can be produced by a series of enzymes, including the enzyme intrinsic to the "classical complement pathway" (C42, or C3 convertase), the enzyme of the "alternate path-

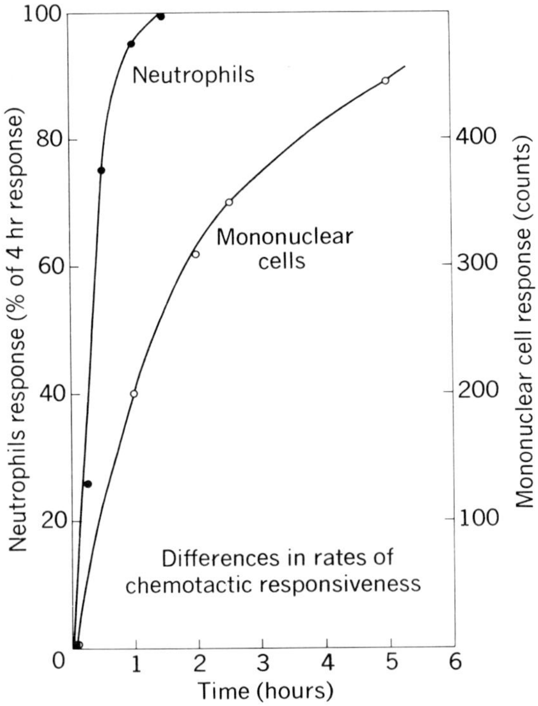

Figure 3-7. Differences in rates of responsiveness of neutrophilic and mononuclear leukocytes as measured by chemotactic migration. Neutrophils respond rapidly within 90 minutes, whereas mononuclear cells respond much more slowly. (Drawn from data of Ward and Becker, 1967; Ward, 1968)

way" (the C3 activator), and other non-complement-related enzymes such as trypsin, thrombin, plasmin, and a "C3 cleaving enzyme" that is present in most normal tissues and is active at neutral pH. The C5 fragment is highly chemotactic for both neutrophils and monocytes. It can be produced by an enzyme generated from the classical complement pathway (C423), and by an enzyme (as yet unidentified) from activation of the alternate complement pathway, as well as by trypsin, a neutral protease present in lysosomal granules of neutrophils, and a protease derived from macrophages.

In addition to all these chemotactic factors, there are other, non-complement-derived factors. For instance, in addition to causing the liberation of chemotactic fragments through enzymatic cleavage of C3 and C5, bacteria produce endogenous, highly leukotactic factors of low molecular weight (*circa* 20,000). It has also been reported that kallikrein is itself chemotactic for neutrophils. Breakdown products of collagen also are reported to have this biological activity (see review by Ward, 1970). Thus, while there appear to be many chemotactic factors, there is nevertheless a restriction in the number of factors. Proteolytic degradation of most serum proteins fails to give rise to chemotactic peptides. Structural information may eventually reveal a common or similar basis for these biological activities.

It is tempting to conclude that the production of chemotactic factors by bacteria in tissues accounts for the ability of most of these microorganisms to induce an acute inflammatory response characterized by the massive accumulation of granulocytes. The fact that the complement system appears to be closely involved in the generation of chemotactic factors suggests that it consists of a series of substrates involved in the production of mediators capable of initiating the acute inflammatory response. It should be pointed out that in addition to the chemotactic factors, the anaphylatoxins are generated also by sequential interaction of the complement system or by direct action of enzymes on C3 or C5 (see above). These factors increase the permeability of blood vessels. Thus, it is now well substantiated that many bioactive products can be derived from the complement system; one set of factors causes the soluble contents of plasma to leak out through permeability changes while the other brings about chemotactic emigration of leukocytes. Taken altogether, the stage is set for the acute inflammatory response. Precisely which factors are involved in a given inflammatory reaction is a very difficult question because of the very short life span of these mediators. As pointed out earlier, there is good evidence that in thermal or chemical injury not one, but several, permeability factors are operative. It seems quite possible that in the case of leukotactic mediators a similar story will be found to pertain.

Some information is available concerning the nature of the interaction of one of the complement-derived chemotactic factors with the neutrophil. It is now recognized that at least two different enzymes in the neutrophil are necessary if the cell is to respond to the chemotactic factor of high molecular weight. One of these enzymes exists as an inert precursor that is converted to an active enzyme upon contact of the cell with the chemotactic factor (Ward and Becker, 1967). This enzyme (esterase) has some features suggestive of chymotrypsin (Ward and Becker, 1968). The second exists naturally in the granulocyte in an active form and appears to be similar to an acetylase (Becker and Ward, 1967). Undoubtedly, a large series of enzymes is involved in the interaction of chemotactic factor with the leukocyte. The net result is that the cell eventually begins to move in a specific and unidirectional manner, probably by an expenditure of energy through glycolytic pathways. It will be important to understand these biochemical events if novel non-empirical approaches to anti-inflammatory therapy are to be developed. There is also recent evidence suggesting that microtubules within the neutro-

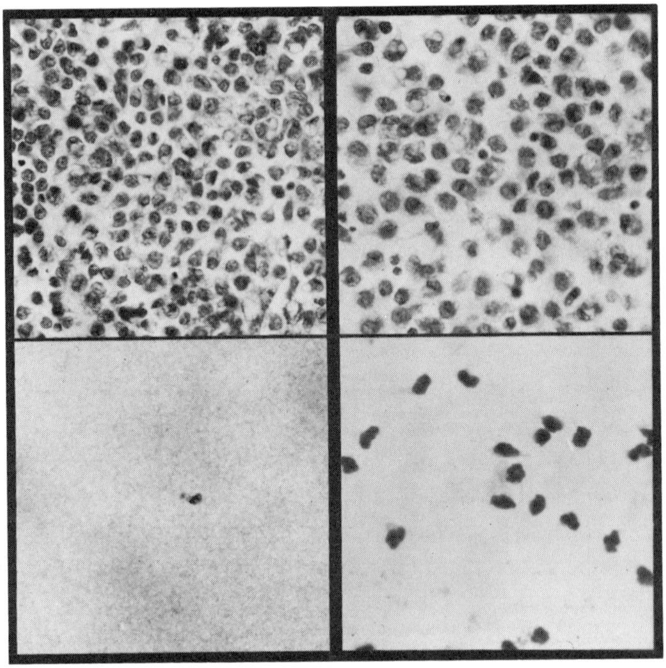

Figure 3-8. Chemotactic response of mononuclear cells. Two micropore filters are included showing non-responding cells (upper frames) and those which have moved completely through the filter to the opposite side (lower frames). In the lower right frame, cells have responded to a chemotactic stimulus, whereas the negative control (with a single migrated cell) is seen in the left lower frame. (From Ward, 1968)

phil are necessary for chemotactic responsiveness of neutrophils. Since this conclusion comes from studies employing drugs that disrupt certain anatomical structures, more direct approaches will be needed to verify the conclusions.

Mononuclear cells respond to chemotactic stimuli in a much more sluggish manner than those of neutrophils; the migrational response requires up to five hours, whereas neutrophils are able to complete their migration within a 90-minute period (Fig. 3-7). Such differences might account for the fact that in the first few hours mononuclear cells are rarely seen in inflammatory exudates but appear in significant numbers by the fifth or sixth hour. Chemotactic behavior of mononuclear cells can be studied also by the micropore filter technique (Fig. 3-8). Mononuclear cells respond to the following chemotactic factors: a factor generated in serum by interaction with antigen-antibody complexes (which is apparently not related to the complement system); fragmentation products of the third and fifth components of complement; soluble bacterial factors; a factor produced by the interaction of sensitized lymphocytes with specific antigen; and a factor present in lysates of neutrophils (Ward, 1968; Ward, Remold, and David, 1969; Ward, unpublished observations). It is obvious that both complement-associated and complement-independent systems are important in the generation of factors that are chemotactic for mononuclear cells. The fact that upon contact with antigen, sensitized lymphoid cells produce a chemotactic factor for mononuclear cells could explain the presence of these cells in reactions of delayed hypersensitivity. The neutrophil-contained factor that is chemotactic for mononuclear cells could explain the commonly observed sequential appearance of mononuclear cells after the arrival of neutrophils in an exudate. Perhaps relevantly, it has been shown in cyclic neutropenia of human beings that monocytes do not appear in inflammatory exudates unless there is an adequate supply of circulating neutrophils (Page and Good, 1958).

Concerning enzyme mechanisms involved in the chemotactic response of mononuclear cells, all that can be said is that mononuclear cells contain at least one enzyme, a serine esterase, which is required for the chemotactic response of the cell but which is distinct from either of the two enzymes required for the chemotactic response of the neutrophil (Ward, 1968).

How *lymphocytes* traverse blood vessels has been a mystery for a long time. It has been assumed for many years that lymphocytes are relatively slow moving, but this may not be an accurate assessment. Until recently there has not been much convincing evidence for the chemotactic responsiveness of lymphocytes to chemotactic factors. There is now some indication that lymphocytes can respond chemotactically to a factor produced by antigen-stimulated lymphocytes. Thus, in reactions of delayed-type hypersensitivity, this could explain why the bulk of accumulated lymphocytes are non-specific in terms of immunologic responsiveness.

Marchesi and Gowans (1964) and subsequently others have provided evidence that lymphocytes migrate out of blood vessels by at least one mechanism totally different from the emigration of neutrophils and mononuclear cells. By the process of *emperipolesis,* lymphocytes in contact with endothelial cell surfaces become surrounded and engulfed by the cytoplasmic processes of the endothelial cells (Figs. 3-9 to 3-11). The lymphocytes are then transported intact across the endothelial cell to be deposited on the basement membrane side. At this point the lymphocytes are effectively outside the blood vessel. The phenomenon of emperipolesis has been observed in postcapillary venules of lymph nodes, in choroidal vessels of the eye, and in vessels of nerves involved with experimental allergic neuritis. The fact that the emigration of lymphocytes from blood vessels involves an interaction (which may be passive on the part of the lymphocyte) with endothelial cells implies a mechanism of migration totally different from that for granulocytic leukocytes.

The concept of emperipolesis has been recently challenged as an artifact due to sectioning of tissue blocks for electron microscopic studies. The matter obviously merits further study. It should be pointed out that if the transendothelial

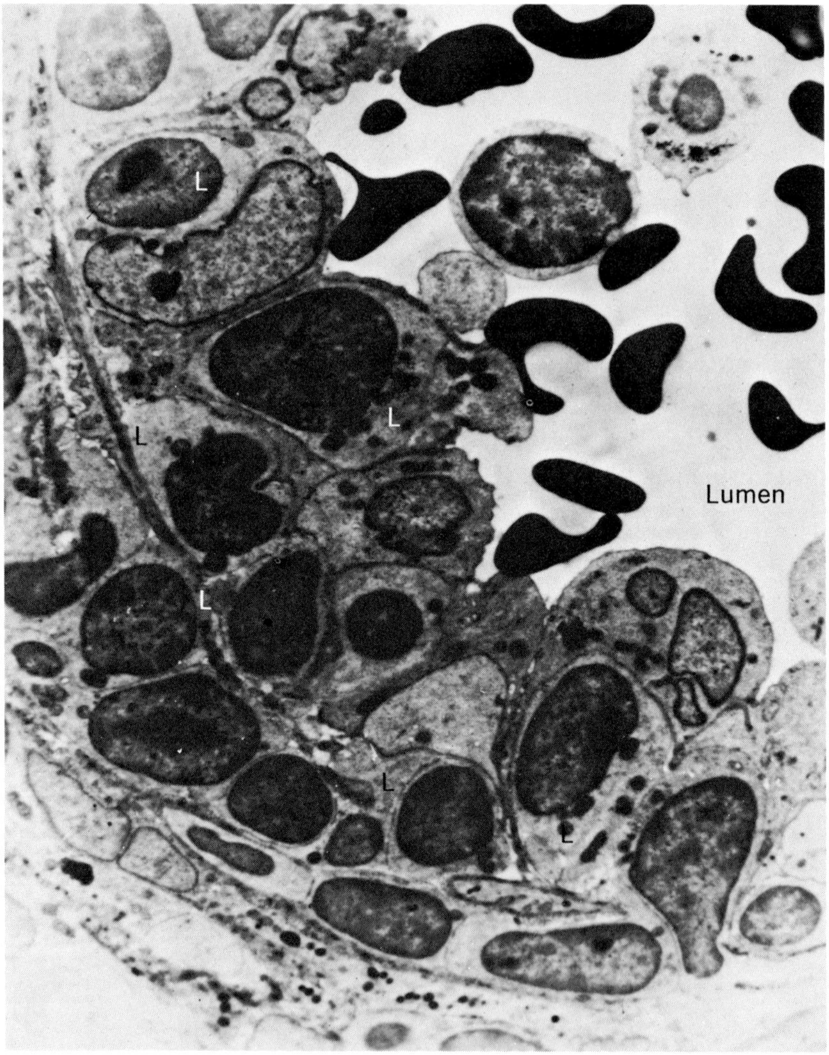

Figure 3-9. Postcapillary venule in a lymph node of a normal rat. Red blood cells are present in the lumen. Endothelial cells contain lymphocytes (L) characterized by their electron-dense nuclei. (Courtesy of Marchesi and Gowans, 1964)

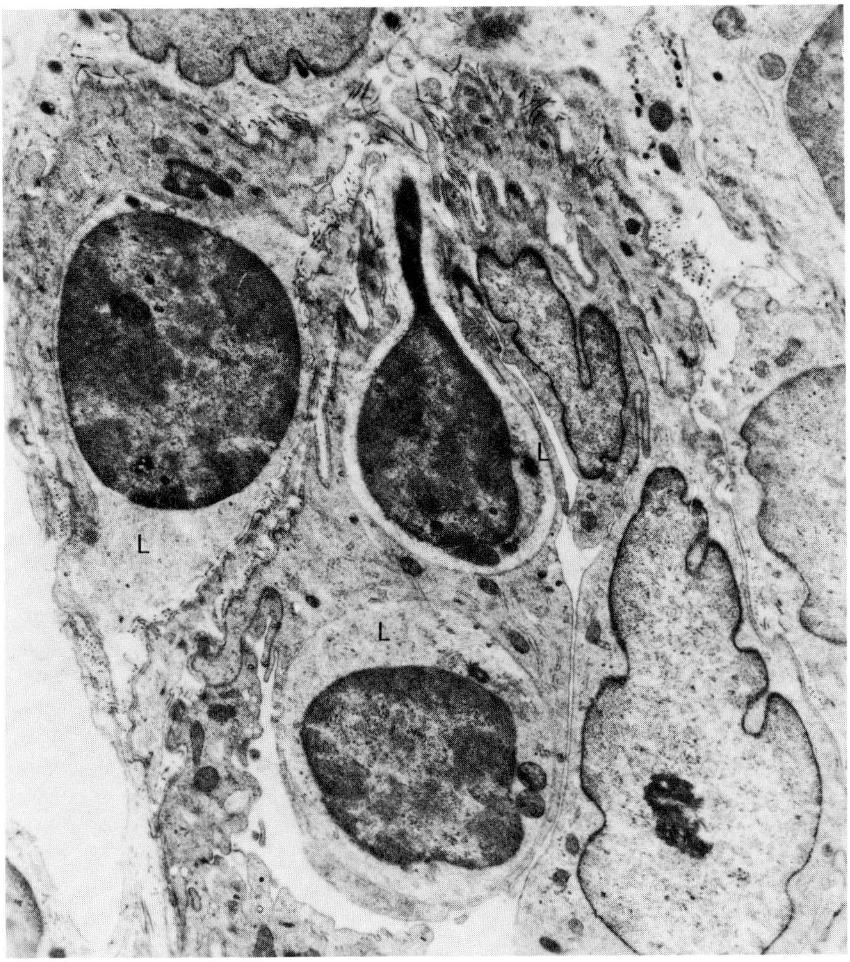

Figure 3-10. From the same vessel as Fig. 3-9. Three lymphocytes (L) with electron-dense nuclei are enclosed within endothelial cells. One lymphocyte has a pseudopod extending through an interendothelial junction. (Courtesy of Marchesi and Gowans, 1964)

passage of lymphocytes really exists, there also is a significant passage of lymphocytes through junctional zones of endothelial cells, as with all other types of leukocytes.

D. Reticuloendothelial System

At an inflamed site, phagocytic uptake and metabolic degradation of foreign material is readily accomplished by the macrophages (derived from blood monocytes or already resident in the tissue) and granulocytes that have arrived from

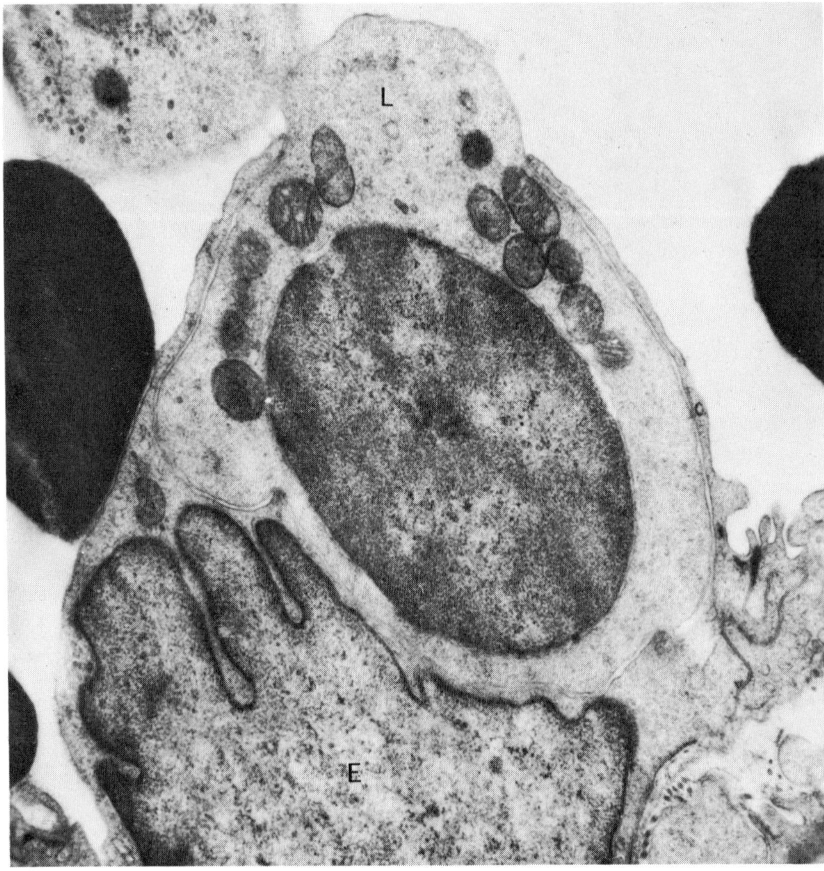

Figure 3-11. Additional area of the vessel pictured in Fig. 3-9, showing the intimate relationship between a lymphocyte (L) and an endothelial cell (E). Cytoplasmic processes of the endothelial cell almost completely enclose the lymphocyte. (Courtesy of Marchesi and Gowans, 1964)

the circulation. If the injurious agent is quickly contained, these phagocytic cells are adequate to deal with the clean-up task. Even so, there exists also an auxiliary system of phagocytosis that has as its main purpose the clearance of foreign matter from blood or lymphatic channels. The material being phagocytosed may be particulate, as in the case of a microbe or protozoan, or soluble, as in the case of an aggregated protein (autologous, homologous, or heterologous) or an antigen-antibody complex. All these substances will disappear from the circulation within hours.

The clearance mechanism can be ascribed to the fact that the body has a highly specialized system, termed the *reticuloendothelial system* (RES), that acts as an effective back-up system of phagocytosis for the inflammatory cells. In some instances the RES may be the sole means for phagocytic removal of foreign material, as in the case of erythrocytes that become coated with antibodies rendering them "foreign." The actively phagocytic cells of the RES lie along vascular channels of the liver and spleen. There are occasional, scattered cells in vascular channels of various other organs, and, under the proper stimulus, they also can engage in phagocytic function. The lymphatic channels and especially the peripheral sinuses of the lymph nodes contain macrophages that are very avidly phagocytic. These cells may completely remove microbes that have escaped from a wound site and have begun to percolate into the interior of the body. According to some definitions, the RES includes even phagocytic cells (histiocytes) that are scattered throughout the connective tissue of the body. In a special sense the RES is the reserve system that takes over protective, phagocytic functions when leukocytes that have been mobilized during an inflammatory response have failed in their efforts to contain an invading microbial agent.

It should be pointed out that there is some consideration now to change the term RES to the *mononuclear-phagocytic system.* This term is desirable because of the mounting evidence that all fixed as well as mobile macrophages are derived from precursor monocytes in the bone marrow. It would also remove the artificial division of macrophages based on anatomical locations. There may, of course, turn out to be exceptions to this classification. If, for instance, phagocytic (glial) cells of the central nervous system are non-bone marrow-derived, they will represent a special and unique population of phagocytes. But in general the phagocytic system throughout the body would appear to be distinguished by its similarity rather than by its diversity.

E. Fate of Inflammatory Cells

Because both mononuclear cells and neutrophils carry stores of enzymes potentially destructive for tissue proteins, the function and the fate of these cells once outside blood vessels is of considerable importance. Both types of leukocytes are actively phagocytic and possess numerous lysosomal enzymes such as lysozyme, which is ideally suited for destruction of bacteria by hydrolysis of sugar groups in the cell wall.

The engulfment and ingestion by the neutrophil of particulate material, such as bacteria, has been expertly documented by Hirsch (1962) and many others. The discharge of lysosomal contents into phagocytic vacuoles formed in the cytoplasm of the leukocyte is a necessary step in the destruction (by digestion) of phagocytosed particles and is a well-known phenomenon. Following phagocytosis, there is increased oxygen consumption, oxidation of glucose via the hexose monophosphate shunt, and formation of hydrogen peroxide (see review of Karnovsky, 1962). As will be seen in Chapter 4, when these mechanisms fail, bacterial invaders remain viable within the neutrophil and can cause serious disease. Much less is known about mononuclear cells–except that, while their enzyme content differs from that of neutrophils, the mechanism for phagocytosis is probably similar to that of the neutrophil.

The fate of neutrophils and mononuclear cells once outside the blood vessel is not clear. Neutrophils have little proliferative potential and have a life span of probably only a few days. If their accumulation is rapid, and emigration from the area fails to occur, they may begin to break down, as occurs in an *abscess* (see Fig. 4-1), with the discharge of enzymes potentially destructive to the surrounding tissue of the host. Neutrophils contain a variety of agents that can directly damage tissue or intensify the inflammatory process. Table 3-4 provides a partial listing of some of these agents. The listing emphasizes the potential that neutro-

Table 3-4 Enzymes and Other Substances Associated with Lysosomes*

Acid phosphatase	Hyaluronidase
Acid ribonuclease	Lysozyme
Acid deoxyribonuclease	Collagenase
Cathepsins B, C, D, E	Aryl sulfatases A and B
Phosphoprotein phosphatase	Phospholipase
Phosphatidic acid phosphatase	Acid lipase
Organophosphate-resistant esterases	Phagocytin and related bactericidal proteins
β-Glucuronidase	Endogenous pyrogen
β-Galactosidase	Plasminogen activator (? urokinase)
β-N-acetylglucosaminidase	Hemolysin(s)
α-L-fucosidase	Mucopolysaccharides and glycoproteins
α-1,4-glucosidase	Basic proteins: (a) Mast-cell-active; (b) Permeability-inducing, independent of mast cells
α-mannosidase	Kininase
α-N-acetylglucosaminidase	Elastase
Kininogenase	
Collagenase	

*Adapted from Cochrane (1968)

Table 3-5 Factors in the Neutrophil with Phlogistic Potential

1. Permeability factors
   a) leukokinin-forming enzyme
   b) basic peptides
2. Leukotactic factors
   a) C5-cleaving enzyme
   b) basic peptides (chemotactic for monocytes)
3. Tissue-damaging enzymes
   a) hydrolases for: elastin
      basement membrane
      collagen
      other structural proteins

phils have for intensifying the inflammatory response and/or for inducing tissue damage. The phlogistic factors of the neutrophil fall into three categories: permeability factors, chemotactic factors, and tissue-damaging enzymes (Table 3-5). The permeability factors or related factors are referred to above and include the preformed lysosome-associated basic peptides, as well as the leukokinin-forming enzyme that is active at an acid pH. The leukotactic factors or related factors associated with the neutrophil include the C5-cleaving enzyme (which produces the highly active C5 fragment) and the preformed basic peptides (in lysosomal granules) that have chemotactic activity for monocytes. These peptides are identical with the permeability-active basic peptides referred to above.

All the basic peptides have permeability-inducing activity; only a few are chemotactically active. The most obvious neutrophil-contained factors that are inimical for tissues are the enzymes that can degrade structural proteins. It is possible to cite enzymes that specifically degrade elastin, basement membrane, and collagen, while there almost surely exist several other tissue substrates that can be degraded by the battery of neutral and acidic (cathepsins) proteases contained within the lysosomal granules of the neutrophil. Very little comparable information can be cited for the monocyte and/or macrophage, but there is every reason to believe that these cells have an equally destructive battery of phlogistic-promoting and tissue-damaging factors.

Mononuclear cells apparently contain many enzymes similar to those in neutrophils, as indicated above, but these cells behave differently from neutrophil cells in the bone marrow and can be produced by rapid division of the precursor cells (Volkman and Gowans, 1965). Thus, large numbers of monocytes can be quickly delivered to the blood stream from the bone marrow. It appears possible

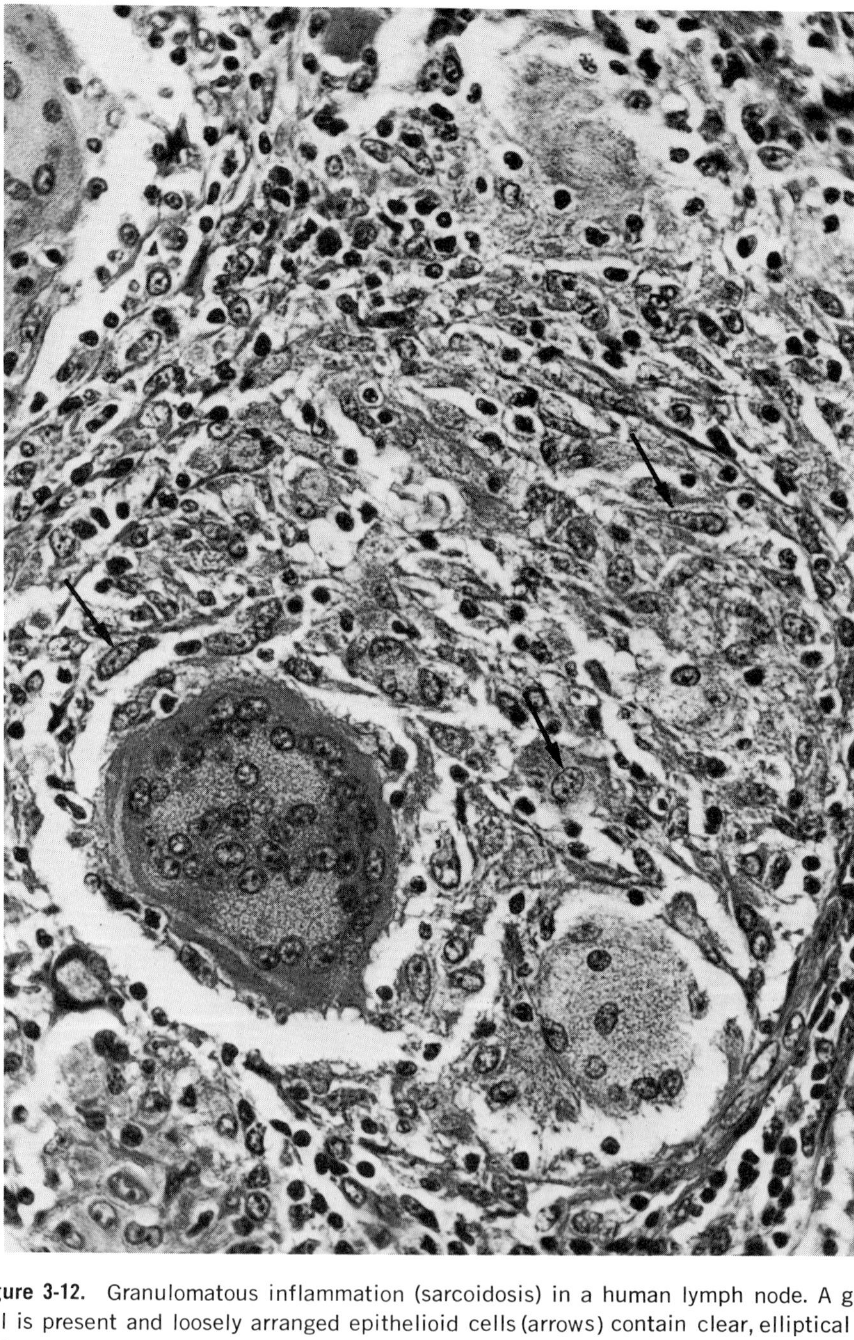

Figure 3-12. Granulomatous inflammation (sarcoidosis) in a human lymph node. A giant cell is present and loosely arranged epithelioid cells (arrows) contain clear, elliptical nuclei and abundant cytoplasm.

that mononuclear cells may continue to proliferate once in the extravascular site—accounting in part for a rapid increase in numbers of these cells in exudates.

Under certain influences mononuclear cells merge one with the other to acquire a common cytoplasm, while at the same time maintaining their distinct nuclei, forming the so-called *giant-cells* (Fig. 3-12). Often the giant cell appears when a vigorous attempt by the mononuclear cells to remove foreign material by phagocytosis has failed. Tuberculous inflammation, as well as the reactions to fungal infections, a wood splinter, or silk suture are such examples in which giant cells are commonly seen. The merging of monocytes into giant cells has been of great interest, since this represents a phenomenon of membrane fusion. It is known that the SV40 virus can cause cell fusion of dissimilar cells. That giant cells are seen frequently in measles (rubeola) and other infections suggests that many viruses capable of producing disease in man can induce cell fusion. In the case of giant cells formed by monocytes in tuberculous inflammation, the stimulus and mechanism for this cell fusion is not known.

The fate of lymphocytes in exudates is slightly clearer. These cells carry immunologic memory (see Chapter 5); and if they come into contact with the appropriate antigen, they may undergo a curious *transformation* process. Nucleic acid metabolism (both RNA and DNA) increases, the nucleus enlarges, the cytoplasm acquires new lysosomal structures, and the cells soon undergo mitotic division. In transformation many soluble substances (termed *lymphokines*) are produced, including the so-called migration inhibitory factor that causes cessation of random movement of mononuclear cells, a factor chemotactic for mononuclear cells as well as one chemotactic for lymphocytes, a substance cytotoxic for virtually any cell type (referred to as *lymphotoxin*), and a broad spectrum anti-viral agent (*interferon*). In addition, several serum proteins are synthesized (see review of David, 1973). Thus, the arrival at extravascular sites of specifically sensitized lymphocytes which then come into contact with the appropriate antigen can lead to the production of mediators that will lead directly or indirectly to tissue damage. As pointed out above, the bulk of lymphocytes making up a chronic inflammatory exudate are probably not specifically sensitized to an antigen present at the site of inflammation. It has been shown in skin reactions of delayed hypersensitivity that more than 90 per cent of the lymphoid cells are not specifically sensitized (Hamilton and Chase, 1967; Turk, 1962; McCluskey *et al.,* 1963). The diverse list of lymphokines may contain one or more factors responsible for tissue damage in a given reaction. It could well be, however, that the accompanying monocytes are really the cells responsible for tissue damage in chronic inflammation. It should be noted in passing that no one has yet described a function for lymphocytes unrelated to an immunologic mechanism.

The fact that lymphocytes continually recirculate in a shuttle between the bloodstream and lymphoid tissues is firmly documented by the studies of Gowans (1959). This phenomenon allows for a conservation of immunocompetent cells in the body, while providing a mechanism for the return of lymphocytes to lymphoid tissues and to the bloodstream, once the cells have passed beyond the endothelial barrier. Thus, lymphoid cells can be cleared from an exudate, provided lymphoid channels are intact.

F. Exudates

Most inflammatory responses are morphologically identified by the presence of proteins, salts, water, and cells outside blood vessels, giving rise to the so-called *exudate*. The cellular character of the exudate, as implied above, defines the morphologic stage of the inflammatory response as acute, subacute or chronic. The exudate may be water-rich (serous), protein-rich (e.g., fibrinous), and so forth. An exudate consisting primarily of neutrophils is termed a *purulent* exudate. One in which numerous neutrophils are associated with tissue destruction would be a *suppurative* exudate, as in the case of an *abscess*. The presence of fibrin in an inflammatory exudate has been described as a mechanism for walling off organisms that might otherwise spread to distant parts of the body. The accumulation of proteins and leukocytes in the exudate, as well as the build-up of tissue-breakdown products, leads to the problem of removal of all these materials so that the tissue can be restored to its original form.

Perhaps the most important consideration is whether the agent responsible for the induction of the inflammatory response can be neutralized, removed, or destroyed. If the responsible agent consists of bacteria, successful phagocytic destruction of the organisms will result in the disappearance of leukocytes, a reduction in permeability, and a return of the tissue to its original state. If for some reason, on the other hand, the inciting agent is not successfully dealt with, the continued accumulation of leukocytes may lead to the release of tissue-destructive enzymes from leukocytes and the subsequent liquefaction of host tissue. When this happens, an *abscess* appears. Nowhere is this complication more serious than in the central nervous system (as in the case of bacterial meningitis) or in the lung in which a lung abscess develops.

In many cases the bacterial agent is successfully coped with and the acute inflammatory process subsides, rather than increasing in intensity and/or proceeding to an abscess. Occasionally the acute inflammatory response may proceed to the subacute inflammatory reaction with granulation tissue, as in the case of pneumococcal pneumonia in which the fibrin-rich and neutrophil-rich (fibrinopurulent) exudates fail to *resolve* and becomes *organized*. The end result here would be the laying down of a collagenous scar in alveolar spaces, a catastrophic event for the patient. On the other hand, in the case of a myocardial infarct this is precisely what is desired, since necrotic muscle, having no regenerative capacity, must be replaced by a dense collagen scar if myocardial rupture is to be avoided. The sprouting network of angioblastic and fibroblastic cells in the area of necrotic heart muscle around the end of the first week is a welcome event indeed. As the scar matures, all evidence of inflammation will fade. As will be discussed below, healing by this type of progression of the inflammatory response is very important in tissues unable to regenerate. Sometimes the acute inflammatory response will proceed directly to the chronic phase with the accumulation of lymphocytes and plasma cells.

The persistence of an inflammatory exudate ("non-resolution") is a serious hazard to the functional integrity of the involved tissue. In the lung, progressive accumulation of inflammatory cells, fibrin, and granulation tissue may result in a chronic inflammatory focus. If the margin of this zone becomes sufficiently walled off with inflammatory cells and fibrin or fibrous scar tissue, a chronic festering wound develops. In the pleural cavity the consequence may be serious compression of adjacent lung tissue and/or erosion into the underlying lung parenchyma or the overlying chest wall, with discharge of debris. Rarely will the persistence of an inflammatory response over a long period of time lead to any beneficial results for the individual.

G. Control of Inflammatory Reactions

The great potential for the exacerbation of tissue injury by inflammatory responses implies the necessity for rigid regulatory controls. Unmitigated inflammatory responses invariably lead to serious disease, and this is nowhere better illustrated than in the case of rheumatoid arthritis, in which crippling deformity is a frequent outcome. A central built-in control for inflammatory responses is the regulation of inflammatory mediators. The highly active peptides such as the kinins and the anaphylatoxins are rapidly inactivated by the enzyme carboxypeptidase B in plasma. Many of the enzymes in the neutrophils are irreversibly inhibited by serum α_1 globulins (anti-trypsin and other anti-proteases). A recently described *chemotactic factor inactivator* seems to regulate the levels of leukotactic mediators. This inactivator appears to be an enzyme with the ability to hydrolyze, and thus inactivate, all the known leukotactic factors. The presence of abnormally low or high levels of this inactivator would be expected to result in abnormal inflammatory cellular responses, and there is clinical support for this statement.

Built-in control mechanisms for regulation of the complement system consist of two types. In the first, several inhibitors occur naturally in serum and will block the activated forms of various complement components (deficiency of one inhibitor and the associated clinical disease are described in a later section). A second type of regulatory factor for the complement system consists of substances that inactivate the biologically active products of the complement system. The anaphylatoxin inactivator has already been described, along with the chemotactic factor inactivator. In addition, the opsonin-promoting factor from C3 (the C3b fragment) is destroyed by a natural "C3b inactivator." If this inactivator is missing, not only will there be persistence of opsonic activity—and thus excessive red cell destruction if red cells are coated with C3b—but also the other action of C3b, which is activation of the alternate (*properdin*) pathway of the complement system, will proceed in an uncontrolled manner. Again, at least one patient with deficiency of this regulator has been described, and in him all the statements given above have been confirmed. In the coagulation system several controls suppress the rate of activation of the proteins and/or bring about inactivation or destruction of activation products. Clearly, the complement, kinin-forming, coagulation, and fibrinolytic system is very complex.

H. Consequences of Inflammation

During the development and resolution or progression of the inflammatory process, it may happen that instead of healing or repair, damage to the host occurs. It has already been shown that when an inflammatory exudate persists too long, destruction of host tissue may result. In the rejection of a homografted tissue it is the lymphocytes and monocytes of the inflammatory exudate that mediate destruction of the grafted tissue. The presence of leukocytes along glomerular capillary loops in the case of glomerulonephritis may lead to hydrolysis of the underlying basement membrane and functional aberrations in glomerular filtration (see review of Cochrane, 1969). Along the articular surface of a joint, as in rheumatoid arthritis, the presence of granulation tissue with its lysosomal-rich cells may lead to enzymatic destruction of articular cartilage. A great deal of effort in clinical medicine is expended in attempts to suppress these harmful effects of the inflammatory process.

1. Host reactions

The reaction of the stromal and parenchymal elements in a tissue that has been the site of the inflammatory response varies according to the tissue and the

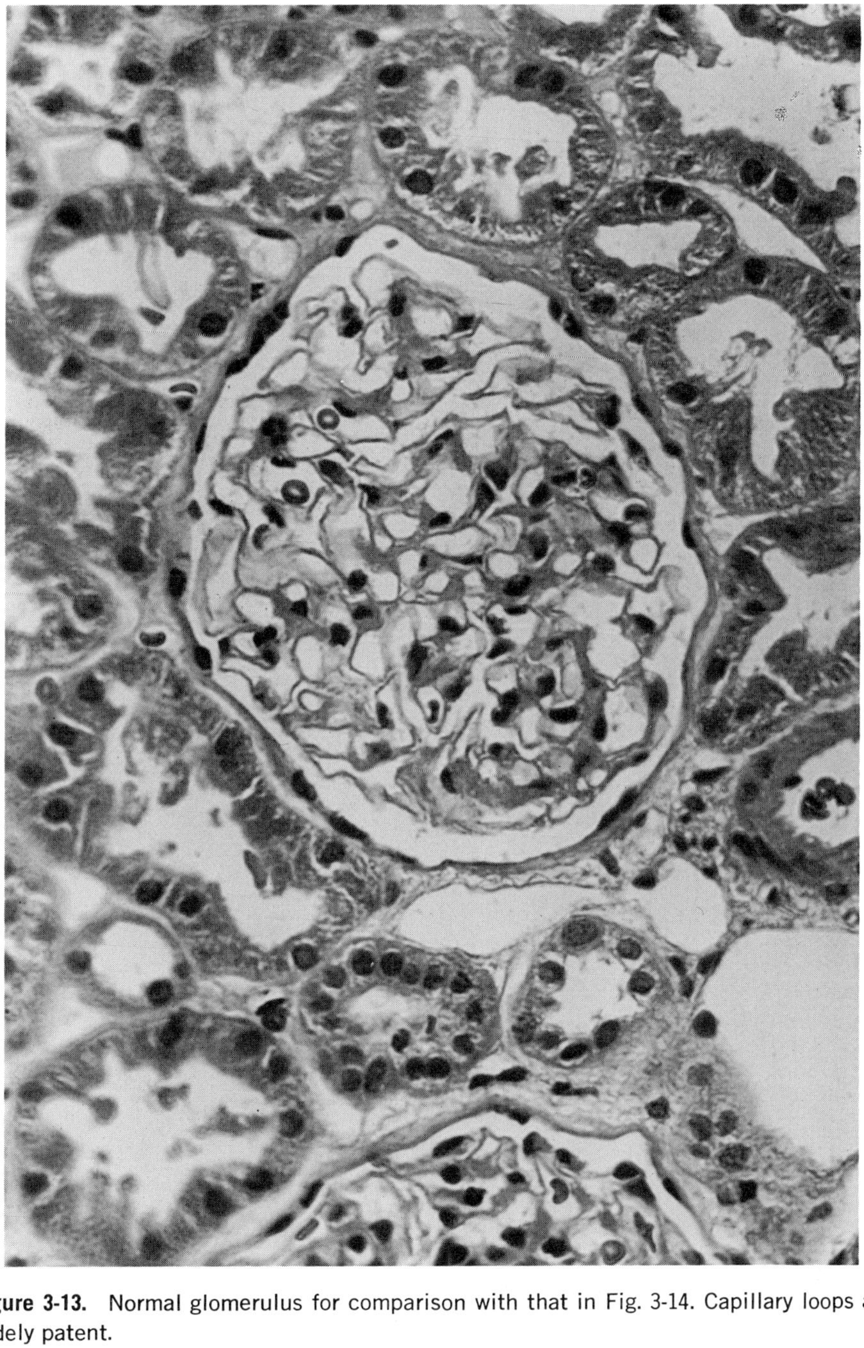

Figure 3-13. Normal glomerulus for comparison with that in Fig. 3-14. Capillary loops are widely patent.

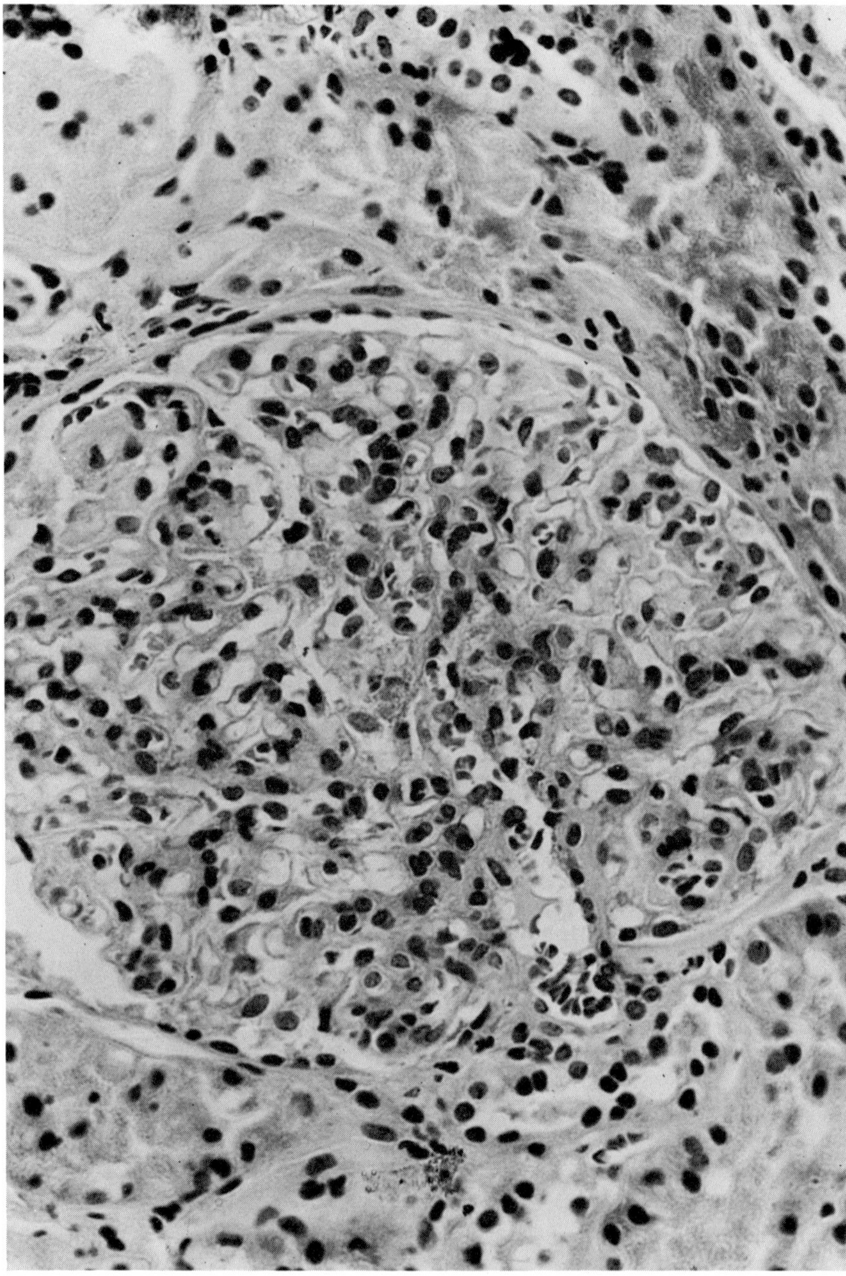

Figure 3-14. Glomerulus from a case of acute post-streptococcal glomerulonephritis. The glomerulus is enlarged due to the proliferation of endothelial and epithelial cells within capillary loops, causing partial occlusion of blood flow.

circumstances of the inflammatory episode. Both parenchymatous and stromal connective-tissue elements may be involved in a proliferative response. Following a wound in the dermis, the proliferation of fibroblastic and angioblastic elements occurs during the formation of granulation tissue. This results in the appearance of new blood vessels as well as increased numbers of fibroblastic elements capable of laying down new ground substance and collagen fibers. When inflammation in renal glomeruli takes the form of acute exudative glomerulonephritis following streptococcal infection, numerous neutrophils appear along glomerular capillary loops, and a marked proliferation of endothelial and epithelial cells frequently follows (Figs. 3-13, 3-14).

Precisely what purpose, if any, this type of response serves is unclear. It may represent an attempt by the kidney to replace damaged cells. These changes may, however, be detrimental if extensive proliferation of endothelial elements leads to occlusion of glomerular capillaries, or if rapid proliferation of epithelial cells lining glomerular loops and Bowman's capsule leads to the formation of continuous sheets of epithelial cells that obliterate the urinary spaces of surrounding individual glomeruli. The advantageous element of such proliferative activity is seen in renal tubules following destruction of tubular epithelial cells by a poison such as ethylene glycol; here the only hope for recovery of renal function is the regenerative proliferation of tubular epithelial cells.

A frequent accompaniment of the acute or chronic inflammatory response in the central nervous system is the proliferation of intrinsic supporting tissue (glial) cells. This accumulation of glial cells accompanied by a limited angioblastic response is the only way the central nervous system can respond to injury, since it lacks regenerative potential.

2. Repair—healing and regeneration

This reaction of tissue to inflammation is the basis for the phenomenon of repair, which includes healing with or without regeneration. In the repair of tissue, the area either becomes replaced with a scar, or the tissue is restored to its original state by the regenerative capacities of that tissue (see review of Schilling, 1968). The outcome of the reparative process in injured skin at the site of a laceration may be either a tissue that is indistinguishable from the original one, or an ugly scar that must be considered less than optimal repair of damaged tissue. In a laceration of the skin in which there has been the release of blood cells, protein, and fibrin from mechanically ruptured vessels, the acute inflammatory response results in a profusion of polymorphonuclear leukocytes (neutrophils)

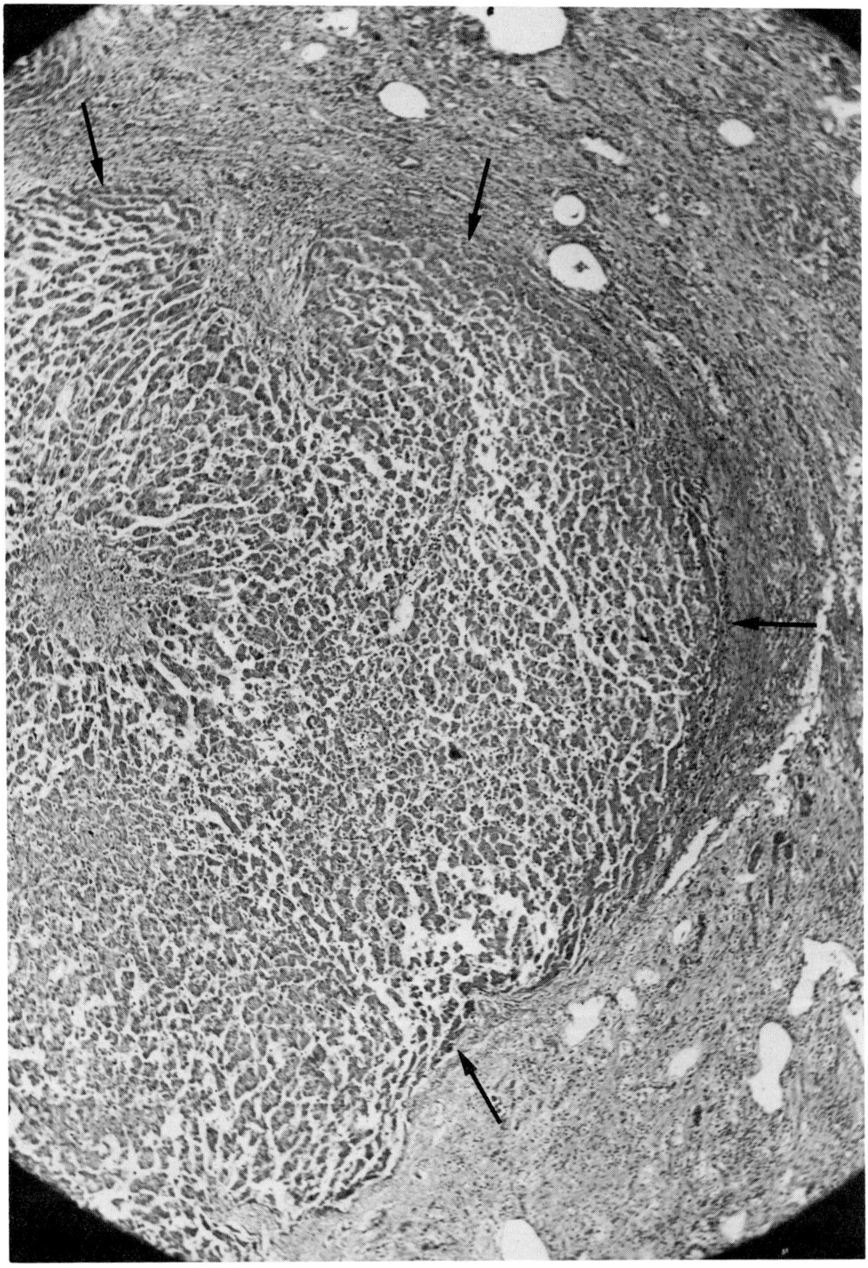

Figure 3-15. "Pseudolobule" (arrows) in the liver from a case of postnecrotic cirrhosis in a human being. The nodule contains irregular collections of liver cord cells that have undergone proliferation in an attempt to replace other destroyed liver tissue. Fibrous scar compresses periphery of lobule.

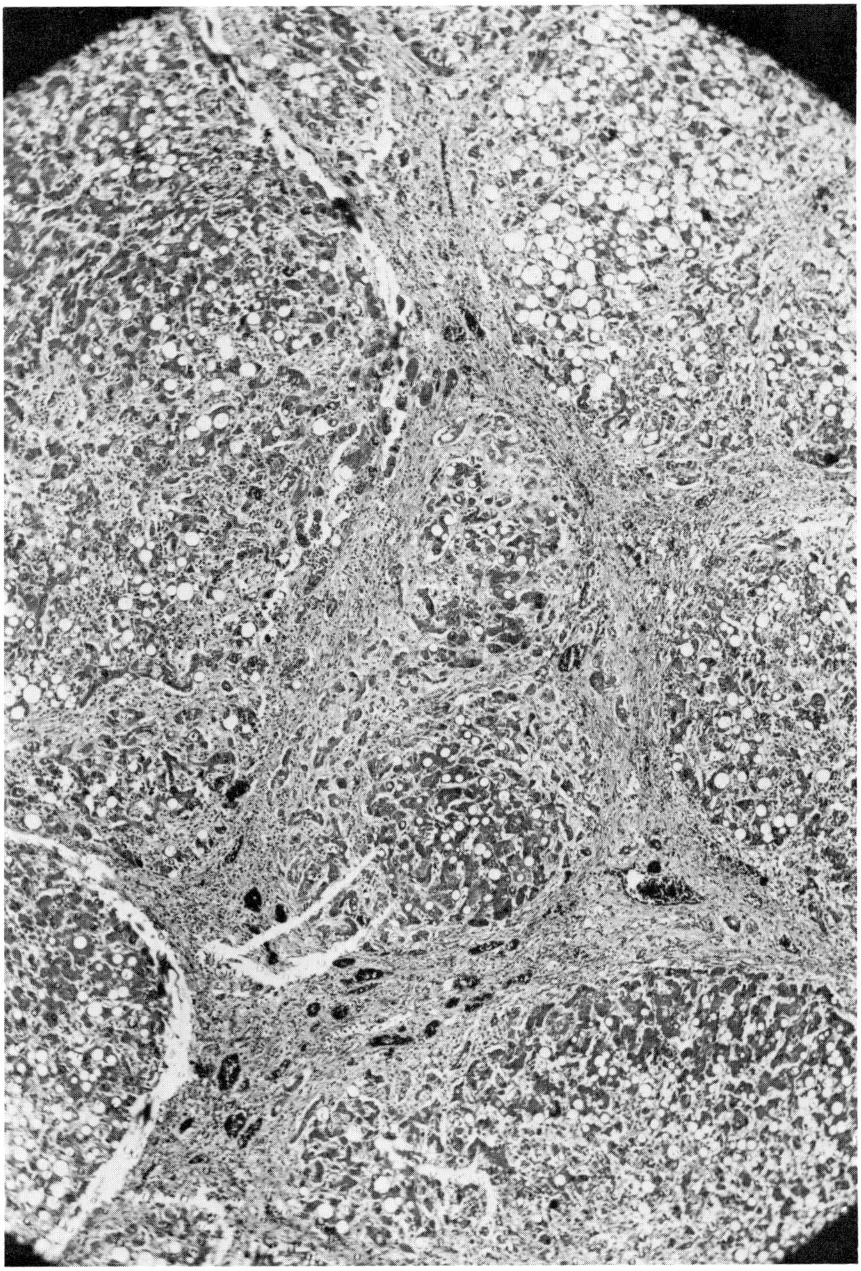

Figure 3-16. Postalcoholic cirrhosis of the liver in a human being, with residual nodules of parenchymal cells. The extensive amount of connective tissue (with interspersed bile ducts) has caused irreversible interruption of hepatic lobules. Fatty (vacuolar) changes can be seen in liver cord cells.

Table 3-6 Examples of Regenerative Capacities of Various Tissues and Organs

UNLIMITED OR MODERATE CAPACITY	LIMITED OR NO CAPACITY
epithelium of skin, gastrointestinal and genitourinary tracts	skeletal, cardiac and smooth muscle
formed elements of bone marrow (red cells, white cells, platelets)	lung parenchyma
renal tubular epithelium	renal glomeruli
liver parenchyma	neurons of central nervous system
lymphoid tissues	retinal tissue and all sense organs
endothelium	endocrine glands
bone	gonadal parenchyma
peripheral nerves	dental structures
ductal epithelium of exocrine glands	

surrounding the zone of damage. In a few days angioblastic and fibroblastic proliferation ensues, and these elements bridge the gap where disruption of tissue has occurred. Fibrin, which has formed in the exudate, will be invaded by the granulation tissue. Shortly thereafter, and probably independently, epithelial cells begin rapid proliferation and proceed to overgrow the wound area. If all goes well, within a week or so the area is completely covered by epithelial cells that have regenerated from the margins of the wounds or from retained hair follicles in the area of the injury; the tiny blood vessels that have grown into the area of the wound begin to disappear, and evidence of newly formed collagen from active fibroblasts will be seen.

In some circumstances, fibroblasts lay down an inordinate amount of connective tissue, and this may result in the formation of a scar. The continued presence of bacteria can predispose an area to this undesirable end. In the case of a liver damaged by the hepatitis virus, the region undergoing repair is often the site of competition between fibroblastic proliferation (from cells originating in portal areas) and regeneration of hepatocellular elements and bile ducts (Figs. 3-15, 3-16). The presence of fibrous scar tissue in a vital organ such as the liver is detrimental not only because it effectively precludes the expansion and regeneration of hepatic lobules, but also because it may seriously interfere with blood flow, which results in portal hypertension. There is no clear indication as to why, in certain individuals with hepatitis, the inflammatory process persists in the liver. Nevertheless, as long as it continues, there is grave danger that the process will eventuate in the laying down of dense fibrous scar tissue, giving rise to hepatic cirrhosis (fibrous scarring). It may well be the local persistence of virus that results in continued inflammation, although many have postulated the role of an auto-immune process. Whatever the cause, it is vital that the inflammatory reaction subside if the liver is to return to normal function.

Repair in the central nervous system is seen primarily in the form of scar-tissue formation because neuronal elements have little or no capacity to regenerate. As indicated above, the inflammatory process, like other injuries, may lead to a proliferation of astrocytes and the formation of large amounts of glial scar. In the peripheral nervous system, Schwann cells, which function as nutritive and supporting tissue elements around axons of peripheral nerves, participate in the laying down of new myelin sheaths after a nerve has been damaged. Table 3-6 lists the various regenerative capacities of tissues in the body. It is obvious that if an injured tissue is unable to regenerate, repair can only be accomplished by the formation of a scar.

I. Granulomatous Inflammation

Granulomatous inflammation is almost impossible to define. Originally the term *granuloma* descriptively defined the tiny, white, granular bodies that could be seen in tissues such as the peritoneum, where they appeared as a result of systemic (hematogenous) spread of the tuberculous organism and the peculiar local inflammatory reaction to the mycobacterium. The term was later redefined according to certain microscopic criteria. At the present time granulomatous inflammation usually refers to an inflammatory response characterized by the presence of lymphocytes, monocytes, and plasma cells. Monocytes or histiocytes are clustered in a characteristic elliptical formation around the causative agent or around a central necrotic area. Large histiocytic cells with abundant cytoplasm are usually referred to as *epithelioid cells,* and it seems more than likely that they are derived from circulating monocytes. It is not unusual for multiple histiocytes to unite to form giant, multinucleated cells with common cell membranes (Fig. 3-12).

Recently it has become evident that in at least one experimental model granulomatous inflammation may be dependent upon an intact immunologic responsiveness of the individual, but it is equally clear that in other situations granulomatous inflammation can occur in the face of severe immunologic suppression. When experimental schistosomiasis is induced in the mouse, it has been found that immunosuppressive agents, which preclude the development of a state of delayed hypersensitivity, will prevent the formation of granulomas in response to the infective agent or its products (Domingo, Cowan, and Warren, 1967).

Considering the multiplicity of mediators produced by contact of sensitized lymphocytes with antigen, it is not difficult to visualize the accumulation of monocytes in clusters defining a granuloma and then, by the action of enzymes released from the leukocytes as well as the elaboration of a cytotoxic factor (Perlmann *et al.*, 1968; Kolb and Granger, 1968), the subsequent death of cells in the central areas of the granuloma. This central necrosis is very characteristic of granulomas in tuberculosis and syphilis. For a long time it has been assumed that granulomatous inflammation of pulmonary tuberculosis represents an immunologic response with allergic manifestations, although at present there is little direct evidence for this conclusion. Nevertheless, the association between granulomatous inflammation and immunocompetence suggests that this assumption may be correct.

Situations also exist in which immunologic responsiveness is apparently not required for the development of granulomatous inflammatory responses. The condition of "blue velvet disease," seen in addicts who inject themselves with substances containing talc crystals, results in the formation of diffuse pulmonary granulomas. Evidence suggests, however, that no immunologic mechanism is involved in this type of cellular response. Warren and Kellermeyer (1968) have demonstrated that, in mice, granulomas may be induced by systemic injection of plastic beads in the face of severe suppression of immunocompetence; and it has been suggested that kinin formation may be necessary for the production of this type of granuloma. Histologically, it is not possible to differentiate between granulomas dependent upon or independent of immunologic mechanisms.

Most granulomatous inflammatory responses will fade as the inciting agent is removed. In the case of tuberculosis or syphilis, however, extensive destruction of cells within the central portion of the granulomas may occur. The reasons for this extensive cellular destruction are not clear (see above); but once necrotic tissue forms, there will be continuing inflammatory response unless this debris is removed. If extensive necrosis of granulomas develops in peripheral lymph nodes, rupture through the skin surface may occur with discharge of contents. Similarly, in the lung, necrotic granulomas may rupture through the bronchial wall, to lead to discharge of contents into the tracheobronchial tree or into large blood vessels. Occasionally, if the area of necrosis is not extensive, calcification and even bone formation can ensue, and the end result will be a fibrocalcific or osseous nodule.

J. Defective Inflammatory Responsiveness

Among clinical aberrations of the inflammatory response, the most obvious example occurs when cells are defective in numbers. In conditions such as severe bone marrow depression due to drugs or radiation, neutrophils, having one of the shortest life spans of any cellular element in the marrow, are the first cells to disappear from the circulation. Under such circumstances a typical acute inflammatory response is not possible, at least insofar as the cellular elements are concerned. The inability to mobilize neutrophils renders the individual susceptible to infections that may become life-threatening. In the cases of lymphopenic agammaglobulinemia (Swiss type) or thymic aplasia, the absence or severe reduction in the number of circulating lymphocytes results in a great susceptibility to infectious agents due to the loss of cell-mediated and humoral-immune defense mechanisms. It is presumed that lymphocyte precursors are absent from the bone marrow, or that they lack the thymic environment that allows them to undergo "maturation" and thus provide the individual with immunocompetent cells. In such individuals one would obviously not find lymphocytes accumulating in chronic inflammatory exudates.

An individual whose granulocytes or monocytes are functionally defective is especially vulnerable to bacterial agents. It is well known that in granulocytic leukemia, neutrophils are unable to cope with infectious agents, especially bacteria, although the basis of this defect is not known. In the so-called "stem-cell" leukemias, precursor cells are ineffective against bacterial agents and appear to crowd out the functionally (and morphologically) mature cells. It is common in autopsy specimens from leukemic patients to see colonies of bacteria in lung tissue without any significant accumulation of neutrophils in the area, in spite of the fact that lumens of vessels contain large numbers of leukocytes.

In chronic granulomatous disease of childhood, neutrophils phagocytize bacteria but fail to kill and digest them. This is especially true with *Staphylococcus* and *Serratia sp.* In this disease, both the customary burst of respiratory oxidative activity and the production of hydrogen peroxide following phagocytosis are lacking (Holmes, Page, and Good, 1967), and an oxidase for reduced nicotinamide adenine dinucleotide (NADH) is apparently lacking. Precisely how these metabolic aberrations are related to defective lysosomal function (see Chapter 2) is not known. The persistence of bacteria in various tissues of these patients leads to the progressive accumulation of mononuclear cells and lymphocytes–hence the term *chronic granulomatous disease*. This defect is most commonly a sex-linked recessive character appearing in males, whereas the carrier female has evidence of partly decreased leukocytic bactericidal activity.

The Chediak-Higashi syndrome is another condition in which neutrophilic granulocytes are defective. Morphologically the cells are recognizable by large cytoplasmic granules. For reasons that are not clear, these cells are not chemotactically normo-responsive and they do not effectively phagocytose and kill bacteria. The affected individuals frequently die after a series of bacterial infections.

Acquired defects in neutrophils resulting in inadequate chemotactic responses have been described in several disease states including diabetes mellitus, rheumatoid arthritis, severe bacterial infections, burns, alcoholism, and malignant neoplasms. The basis for these chemotactic defects has not been defined, but in each case the outcome is susceptibility to bacterial infections.

The inflammatory response may be abnormal because of functional or structural defects in blood vessels. The most common example of this defect is sunburn, which actually represents a first-degree burn. Persistent vasodilatation is caused by the actinic damage to vessels which, if severe, can result in increased capillary permeability with accumulation of water, protein, and electrolytes in extravascular areas. Ionizing radiation, especially that associated with gamma- or X-irradiation, can produce endothelial damage resulting in persistent vasodilatation and permeability changes.

Defects in plasma constituents may result in aberrations of the inflammatory response. At least two different types of impaired phagocytosis have been reported, each dependent on deficiency of a plasma opsonin. Individuals with sickle cell disease have been found lacking in a heat-labile opsonin that promotes phagocytosis of pneumococci (Winkelstein and Drachman, 1968). Miller *et al.* (1968) have reported the case of a child in whom deficiency of a plasma factor impairs the ability of leukocytes to phagocytose yeast cells and *Staphylococcus aureus.* In addition, this serum does not generate chemotactic activity when activated appropriately. These defects can be corrected by the addition of highly purified fifth component of human complement.

There has also been a study made on a child who has an *inhibitor* in his serum that renders neutrophils unresponsive to chemotactic stimuli (Ward and Schlegel, 1969). The child fails to show an accumulation of neutrophils in inflammatory sites, presumably because of the presence of this inhibitor in plasma. As a result, neutrophils are not efficiently mobilized and bacterial infections are common. This defect has now been described in several additional cases.

The loss of *homeostatic factors* in plasma may lead to uncontrolled, acute inflammatory episodes. This is especially well documented in patients who lack the natural inhibitor of the esterase of the first component (C1) of human complement (Landermann, 1962; Donaldson and Evans, 1963). The C1 esterase inhibitor may be totally lacking, or it may be present in normal quantity but in a non-functional form. In either case the individual is subjected to episodes of angioedema that may be life-threatening. It is now recognized that the C1 esterase inhibitor also acts on plasmin and kallikrein, but it is not known which mediators (products of enzymes) are most important in the associated clinical disorder. Patients with sera deficient in α1-antitrypsin develop severe pulmonary emphysema. It has been recently shown that these patients also have an associated deficiency of the chemotactic factor inactivator. Thus, with an inability to regulate the level of chemotactic mediator and, lacking the inhibitors of granulocyte proteases, it may well be that the pulmonary emphysema represents the long-term effect of inadequate control of inflammatory reactions in the lung.

Defective ability to regulate the level of C3 in humans results in disease. Three types of disorders have been described. In the first, there is a deficiency of a natural inactivator (KAF) of the C3b fragment. This presumably results in inordinate firing by C3b of the alternate complement pathway, with result in C3 consumption and loss of this phagocytic-promoting factor from C3. Another C3 defect is associated with the presence of a C3-destroying enzyme that is unrelated to any enzyme of the complement system. In the third case a genetic deficiency of C3 has been found. In each of the three conditions described, the loss of C3 abrogates the important protective phagocytic-promoting function of C3. The outcome is life-threatening bacterial infections.

"Experiments of nature" provide an array of clinical patterns, pointing out aspects of exaggerated or impaired inflammatory responses. The variety of mediators participating in the inflammatory response is formidable, but it is from such material so generously provided by nature that an understanding of the role of these mediators will eventually emerge.

References

Alpers, C. A., Abramson, N., Johnston, R. B., Jr., McCall, C. E., Jandl, J. H., and Rosen, F. S. (1968), Increased susceptibility to infection associated with a defect of complement metabolism, J. Clin. Invest., *48*:1a (abst.).

Becker, E. L., and Ward, P. A. (1967), Partial biochemical characterization of the activated esterase required in the complement-dependent chemotaxis of rabbit polymorphonuclear leukocytes, J. Exp. Med., *125*:1021.

Becker, E. L. (1969), The relation of complement to the other systems, Proc. Roy. Soc., Ser. B., *173*:188.

Boyden, S. (1962), The chemotactic effect of mixtures of antibody and antigen on polymorphonuclear leukocytes, J. Exp. Med., *115*:453.

Brocklehurst, W. E. (1960), The release of histamine and formation of a slow-reacting substance (SRS-A) during anaphylactic shock, J. Physiol. (London), *151*:416.

Cochrane, C. G. (1968), Immunologic tissue injury mediated by neutrophilic leukocytes, in Advances in Immunology, *9*:97, F. J. Dixon and H. G. Kunkel, Eds., Academic Press, New York.

David, J. (1973), Lymphocyte mediators and cellular hypersensitivity, New Eng. J. Med., *288*:143.

Domingo, E. O., Cowan, R. T., and Warren, K. S. (1967), The inhibition of granuloma formation around *Schistosoma mansoni* eggs. I. Immunosuppressive drugs, Am. J. Trop. Med., *16*:284.

Donaldson, V. H., and Evans, R. R. (1963), A biochemical abnormality in hereditary angioneurotic edema. Absence of serum inhibitor of C'l-esterase, Am. J. Med., *35*:37.

Harris, H. (1960), Mobilization of defensive cells in inflammatory tissue, Bact. Rev., *24*:3.

Hirsch, J. G. (1962), Cinemicrophotographic observations on granule lysis in polymorphonuclear leukocytes during phagocytosis, J. Exp. Med., *116*:827.

Holmes, B., Page, A. R., and Good, R. A. (1967), Studies of the metabolic activity of leukocytes from patients with a genetic abnormality of phagocytic functions, J. Clin. Invest., *46*:1422.

Hurley, J. V. (1964), Substances promoting leukocyte emigration, Ann. N. Y. Acad. Sci., *116*:918.

Karnovsky, M. L. (1962), Metabolic basis of phagocytic activity, Physiol. Rev., *42*: 143.

Keller, H. U., and Sorkin, E. (1968), Chemotaxis of leucocytes, Experientia, *24*: 641.

Kellermeyer, R. W., and Graham, R. C., Jr. (1968), Kinins–possible physiologic and pathologic roles in man, New Eng. J. Med., *279*:754, 802, 859.

Kolb, W. P., and Granger, G. A. (1968), Lymphocyte *in vitro* cytotoxicity: characterization of human lymphotoxin, Proc. Natl. Acad. Sci., *61*:1250.

Landerman, N. S. (1962), Hereditary angioneurotic edema. I. Case reports and review of the literature, J. Allergy, *33*:316.

Lepow, I. H., and Ward, P. A., Eds. (1973), Inflammation–Mechanisms and Control, Academic Press, New York.

Lewis, T. (1927), The blood vessels of the human skin and their responses, Shaw, London.

Marchesi, V. T. (1961), The site of leukocyte emigration during inflammation, Quart. J. Exp. Physiol., *46*:115.

Marchesi, V. T. (1962), The passage of colloidal carbon through inflamed endothelium, Proc. Roy. Soc., Ser. B., *156*:550.

Marchesi, V. T. (1964), Some electron microscopic observations on interactions between leukocytes, platelets, and endothelial cells in acute inflammation, Ann. N. Y. Acad. Sci., *116*:774.

Marchesi, V. T., and Florey, H. W. (1960), Electron micrographic observations on the emigration of leukocytes, Quart. J. Exp. Physiol., *45*:343.

Marchesi, V. T., and Gowans, J. L. (1964), The migration of lymphocytes through the endothelium of venules in lymph nodes: an electron microscope study, Proc. Roy. Soc., Ser. B., *159*:283.

Miles, A. A. (1961), Local and systemic factors of shock, Fed. Proc., Suppl. #9, *20*:141.

Miller, M. E., Seals, J., Kaye, R., and Levitsky, L. C. (1968), A familial, plasma-associated defect of phagocytosis, Lancet *2*:60.

Müller-Eberhard, E. J. (1968), Chemistry and reaction mechanisms of complement, *in* Advances in Immunology, *8*:1, F. J. Dixon and H. G. Kunkel, Eds., Academic Press, New York.

Orange, R. P., Valentine, M., and Austen, K. F. (1968), Antigen-induced release of slow reacting substance of anaphylasis (SRS-A^{rat}) in rats prepared with homologous antibody, J. Exp. Med., *127*:767.

Page, A. R., and Good, R. A. (1968), A clinical and experimental study of the function of neutrophils in the inflammatory response, Am. J. Path., *43*:645.

Perlmann, P., Perlmann, H., and Holm, G. (1968), Cytotoxic action of stimulated lymphocytes in allogenic and autologous erythrocytes, Science, *160*:306.

Pickles, V. R. (1969), Prostaglandins, Nature, *224*:221.

Schilling, J. A. (1968), Wound healing, Physiol. Rev., *48*:374.

Spector, W. G., and Willoughby, D. A. (1964), Vasoactive amines in acute inflammation, Ann. N. Y. Acad. Sci., *116*:839.

Volkman, A., and Gowans, J. L. (1965), The production of macrophages in the rat, Brit. J. Exp. Path., *46*:50.

Ward, P. A., Cochrane, C. G., and Müller-Eberhard, H. J. (1965), The role of serum complement in chemotaxis of leukocytes *in vitro,* J. Exp. Med., *122*:327.

Ward, P. A., Cochrane, C. G., and Müller-Eberhard, H. J. (1966), Further studies on the chemotactic factor of complement and its formation *in vivo,* Immunol., *11*:141.

Ward, P. A., and Becker, E. L. (1967), Mechanisms of the inhibition of chemotaxis by phosphonate esters, J. Exp. Med., *125*:1001.

Ward, P. A. (1968), Chemotaxis of mononuclear cells, J. Exp. Med., *128*:1201.

Ward, P. A., and Becker, E. L. (1968), The deactivation of rabbit neutrophils by chemotactic factor and the nature of the activatable esterase, J. Exp. Med., *127*:693.

Ward, P. A., and Schlegel, R. J. (1969), Defective leukotaxis in a child with recurrent infections, Lancet, *2*:344.

Ward, P. A., Remold, H. G., and David, J. R. (1969), Leukotactic factor produced by sensitized lymphocytes, Science, *163*:1079.

Ward, P. A. (1970), Neutrophil chemotactic factors and related clinical disorders, Arth. and Rheum., *13*:181.

Warren, K. S., and Kellermeyer, R. W. (1968), Foreign body granuloma as a response to chemical mediators of inflammation, J. Clin. Invest., *47*:99a.

Wilhelm, D. L., and Mason, B. (1960), Vascular permeability changes in inflammation: the role of endogenous permeability factors in mild thermal injury, Brit. J. Exp. Path., *41*:487.

Wilhelm, D. L. (1962), The mediation of increased vascular permeability in inflammation, Pharmacol. Rev., *14*:251.

Willoughby, D. A., and Spector, W. G. (1964), The lymph node permeability factor: a possible mediator of the delayed hypersensitivity reaction, Ann. N. Y. Acad. Sci., *116*:874.

Winkelstein, J. A., and Drachman, R. H. (1968), Deficiency of pneumococcal serum opsonizing activity in sickle-cell disease, New Eng. J. Med., *279*:459.

4

HOST-PARASITE INTERACTION

Charles E. McCall, M.D.

A. Introduction—Parasitism

Within the evolutionary process there has always existed a constant interplay between both the offensive and the defensive forces of all forms of life. Underlying these reactions within the biologic world are the quests of all forms of life for food and a suitable environment for self-preservation and replication. Theobald Smith (1934) in his classic discussion of parasitism has suggested that two universal habits have evolved from these biologic necessities: the predatory and the parasitic.

Parasitism does not necessarily evoke a pathobiologic reaction, for it has its foundation in the interdependence of all life. Indeed, most of man's parasites do not harm him. An inoffensive relation between host and parasite is called *commensalism.* Occasionally, mutual benefits result from host-parasite interaction (*mutualism*), as demonstrated by the production of vitamin K by the indigenous intestinal bacterial flora of man.

It is beyond the scope of this discussion to describe uneventful parasitism in any detail. Instead, the determinants that transform the host-parasite interaction in man into an abnormal or diseased state will be emphasized. These determinants do not emanate solely from properties of the parasite. They include the genotypic and phenotypic constitution of both host and parasite interacting within a specific biologic ecology. Parasitism resulting in disease is aberrant; commensalism is usually a better biologic habit for the parasite as well as the host.

Host-parasite pathobiology has itself been an evolutionary phenomenon. The contemporary state of parasitic diseases of man reflects a fascinating natural history that has been comprehensively reviewed (Burnet, 1966). In man, a relatively constant population of parasites, which usually reside in a balanced relationship with their hosts, has developed through the selection and mutation forces of evolution. Soon after birth man encounters a large number of microbes which then colonize his skin, mucous membranes, and gastrointestinal tract, establishing a pattern which, with intermittent alterations, persists throughout life. Members of this indigenous microbiota are *endogenous parasites*. Within recent years alterations of the equilibrium between these endogenous parasites and man have allowed expressions of endogenous microbial disease with increasing frequency.

The most rapidly fatal host-parasite reactions occur in unnatural hosts who are ill-prepared for the invasion, and the microbes producing such disease cannot be considered members of the normal human flora. Many of the great plagues of human history fall within this category of exogenous infection: smallpox, yellow fever, typhus, diphtheria, typhoid fever, malaria, bubonic plague, and cholera. This truly infectious kind of microbial disease caused by *exogenous parasites* is still immensely important throughout the world, although medical and socioeconomic advances have decreased the incidence in more developed countries.

The evolutionary development of host-parasite relations and the advances of civilization have not resulted in the so-called perfect parasitic state in which parasitism exists without disease, for many endogenous as well as exogenous parasitic diseases still plague man. Thus, we are led to the questions that are fundamental to this chapter: What are the specific and nonspecific mechanisms of host response to aberrant parasitism which produce disease? What are the assailants and how do they attack? Why are peaceful parasites, which normally can be held so easily in check, sometimes able to invade host tissue without hindrance?

B. Host Determinants of the Pathobiology of Parasitism

It is axiomatic that host-parasite pathobiology will depend upon both the microorganism and the host. At the present stage in the evolution of the infectious diseases, except for cases of extremely aberrant parasitism, the state of the host is of greater importance in determining the reaction than the parasite itself. The local and systemic host determinants of disease, therefore, will be discussed first.

1. Local interactions

a. Inflammatory injury

Although inflammation is described extensively in Chapter 3, certain aspects merit repetition because of their fundamental importance in infectious disease.

Indeed, the inflammatory process is undoubtedly the most basic of the pathobiologic host-parasite reactions. It involves the primary mechanisms by which the anti-parasitic properties of the host, particularly the phagocytic cells, are mobilized at the site of parasite invasion in an attempt to erect a defense barrier, sequester, and then destroy the parasite. Although an effective defense mechanism, inflammation is a host-parasite reaction that may harm the host as well as the parasite, thus producing disease.

The types of inflammation that follow parasitic invasion are nonspecific responses to parasites, which are adapted to either an extracellular or an intracellular existence within host tissues. *Extracellular parasites* evoke primarily an acute inflammatory response in which the neutrophilic phagocyte is the predominating cell. Through the sequence of altered microcirculation, transudation of serum factors, and active transmigration of neutrophils toward the invader, the parasite encounters this first line of defense (Spector and Willoughby, 1963). The neutrophil attempts to phagocytose and then to destroy intracellularly the invading microorganism. These ingestion and killing phases are controlled by separate metabolic and biochemical events. Intracellular bactericidal activity probably involves also at least two mechanisms: the production of hydrogen peroxide via the hexose monophosphate shunt (Klebanoff, 1967) and the release of bactericidal substances from lysosomes into the phagocytic vacuole (Zeya and Spitznagel, 1963).

Other mechanisms participate in the acute inflammatory reaction to parasites. These include interactions of: (1) specific antibody with parasite antigen

Table 4-1a Microorganisms Adapted to Extracellular Parasitism of Man

GRAM-POSITIVE BACTERIA	GRAM-NEGATIVE BACTERIA
Streptococcus	Meningococcus*
Staphylococcus	Gonococcus*
Pneumococcus	Hemophilus
Clostridia	Enteric bacilli
Diphtheria	Bordetella
Anthrax	Pasteurella
	Bacteroides
	Shigella
	Cholera vibrio

* May also be facultative intracellular parasites.

that prepares the invader for ingestion by neutrophils (opsonization); (2) components of complement, together with specific antibody, which may lyse Gram-negative bacteria; (3) substances such as lysozyme and beta lysin, which may destroy some microorganisms extracellularly (Myrvik and Leake, 1960).

Most extracellular parasites to which the host responds with acute inflammation are bacteria. Those that man commonly encounters are listed in Table 4-1a.

It is not surprising that acute inflammation results in cell injury and cell death that is harmful to the host as well as to the parasite. Constituents of the cytoplasm of cells participating in the inflammatory process are released into the

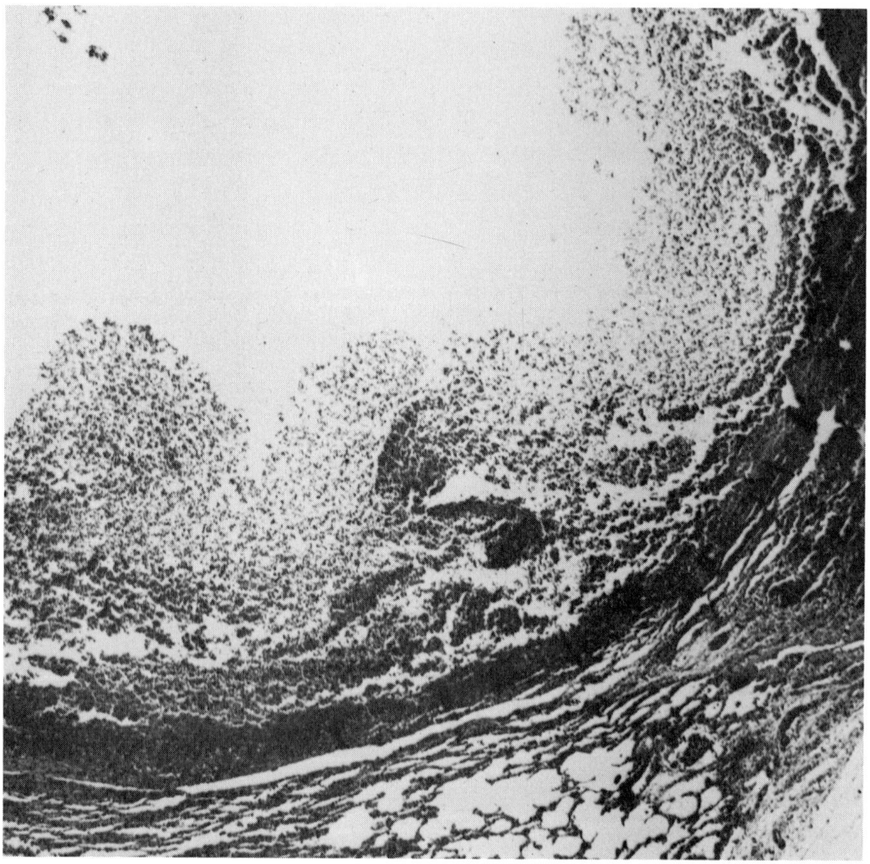

Figure 4-1. Microscopic view of an abscess in the skin due to infection with the extracellular parasite **Staph. aureus.** The subcutaneous tissue seen at bottom right is replaced elsewhere by pus, a mixture of dead and dying neutrophils and products of tissue digestion. Some of this pus has fallen out of the section, leaving an empty space.

environment. Included are vasoactive polypeptides such as bradykinin, and vasoactive amines such as histamine and 5-hydroxytryptamine (Wilhelm *et al.,* 1965). In addition, a sequence of steps following the activation of the complement system results in elaboration of anaphylatoxin which increases capillary permeability and causes constriction of smooth muscle (Nelson, 1965). Enzymes capable of causing tissue necrosis and ordinarily held in an inactive state within the granules (lysosomes) of neutrophils, may be released into the immediate environment (Weissmann, 1965). These enzymes display powerful proteolytic, lipolytic, and collagenolytic properties that may operate in the immediate vicinity of inflammation.

The host-parasite interaction following invasion by pyogenic bacteria such as *Staphylococcus aureus* is typical of acute inflammatory injury caused by extracellular parasites. An example of this type of infection, which is characterized by abscess formation (liquefaction necrosis containing the cellular and tissue debris of inflammation), is given in Figure 4-1.

Another type of local tissue inflammation is characterized by the host's attempt to sequester and completely destroy a parasite that is partially or totally adapted to an intracellular existence. These *intracellular parasites,* which include certain bacteria (*Mycobacterium tuberculosis,* Brucellae, *Listeria monocytogenes,* and Salmonellae), most fungi, protozoa, and all viruses (Table 4-1b), will be discussed in greater detail later. The reaction to these parasites is somewhat delayed in comparison to the response of the acute inflammatory process, which

Table 4-1b Microorganisms Adapted to Intracellular Parasitism of Man

FACULTATIVE INTRACELLULAR PARASITES		
BACTERIA	FUNGI	PROTOZOA
Mycobacteria	Histoplasma	Pneumocystis
Brucella	Blastomyces	Toxoplasma
Salmonella	Coccidiomyces	Leishmania
Listeria	Cryptococcus	Trypanosoma
Streptobacillus	Candida	
	Nocardia	
OBLIGATE INTRACELLULAR PARASITES		
VIRUSES	RICKETTSIAE	PROTOZOA
All	All	Plasmodia (malaria)

may at times precede it; and it is characterized by the predominance of lymphocytes, monocytes, and fibrocytes, rather than neutrophils.

The sequence of events that brings the activated lymphocytes and mononuclear phagocytes to the intracellular parasite is similar to the dynamics of acute inflammation. It includes changes in microcirculation, chemotaxis, transmigration, phagocytosis, and intracellular killing. The pathologic lesion which develops, particularly if the phagocyte is unable to destroy all the invaders quickly, is frequently characterized by the formation of granulomata (Fig. 4-2). As in acute inflammation, the defense process becomes an expression of disease.

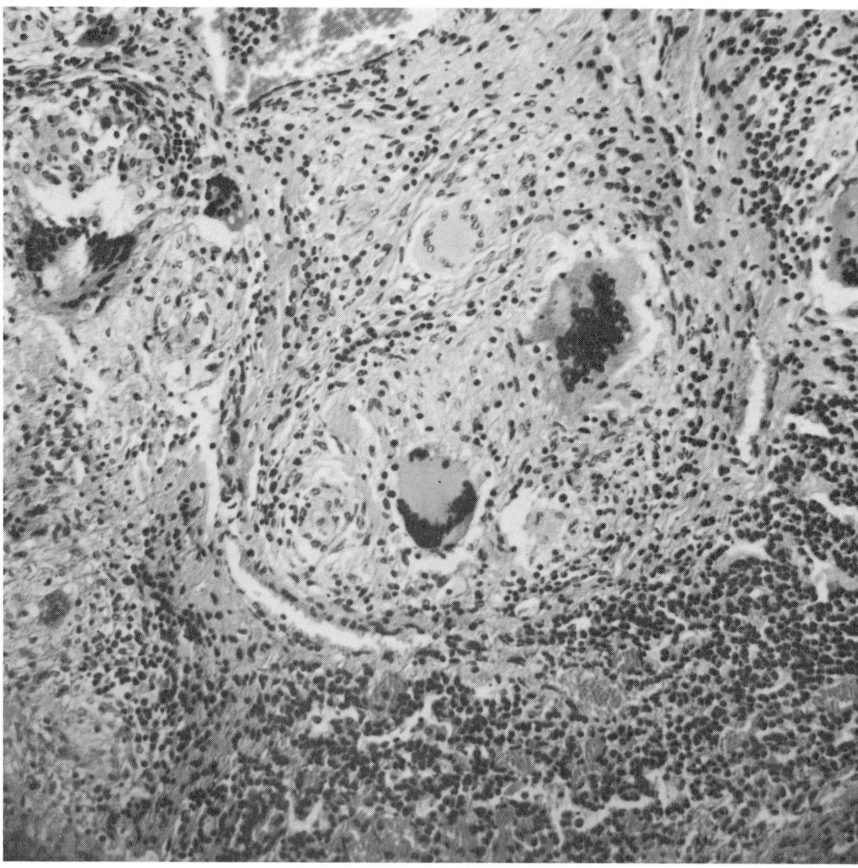

Figure 4-2. Granulomatous inflammation in the lung, caused by reaction to the facultative intracellular parasite, **M. tuberculosis.** But most of the tissue is replaced by epithelioid cells, giant cells, and lymphocytes. For a higher power view, see also Figure 3-12.

In some granulomatous inflammation, particularly that due to tuberculosis, necrosis develops within the center of the granuloma. Secondary enzymatic injury from the lysosome constituents of monocytes and lymphocytes may be responsible.

The cellular picture of the delayed inflammatory reaction may at times be equated with delayed hypersensitivity. Thus one may also categorize delayed inflammation as a form of immunologic injury.

b. Immunologic injury

The mechanisms of immunologic (allergic) injury are described in detail in Chapter 5. The expression of allergic injury, at least in part, involves elements of the types of inflammation just discussed, but these hypersensitivity reactions should be considered separately, for in parasitism they are secondary rather than primary responses. Presensitization, usually with the formation of antibody, is a prerequisite.

Since parasites, either alive or dead, are fertile sources of antigen, one might expect the antigen-antibody interaction, which is based upon the specific antigenic nature of the parasite, to be frequent. At times, this interaction activates a train of cellular and biochemical events in which tissues are injured. Our knowledge in this area is incomplete, but it is probable that all major categories of parasites, which include bacteria, fungi, viruses, protozoa, and metazoa, are at times agents of allergic injury.

Following invasion of *Mycobacterium tuberculosis,* the development of delayed hypersensitivity, which in itself is an immune response, also becomes a pathologic process. Similar injury may be associated with deep fungal infections such as histoplasmosis, blastomycosis, cryptococcosis, and coccidiomycosis. The tissue damage in postviral encephalitides and polyneuropathies may involve also the delayed hypersensitivity process (Epstein, 1967).

Allergy may play a role in the symptomatology of measles. Whether the rash, which develops at about the time antibodies are detectable in the serum, is due to a direct viral effect on epithelium and vascular endothelium or to an immune reaction is not clear. Support for the latter theory is found in the fact that when children acquire fatal giant-cell pneumonia, they do not form neutralizing antibodies and do not develop a rash. Infection with certain rickettsiae is also characterized by a rash. In the case of epidemic typhus, after an incubation period, fever develops and persists until the infection resolves. Between the fourth and the seventh day of the disease process, a characteristic rash appears. Since rickettsiae are demonstrable in this lesion, one might assume that it results from a direct toxicity of the localized rickettsiae. It is of interest, however, that the rash occurs about five to seven days after the onset of the fever. Together with the accumulation of cells of the lymphoid series, this observation suggests that an immune reaction may also participate in the pathogenesis of this rash.

The sequelae of Group A streptococcal infections resulting in the syndromes of acute rheumatic fever, acute glomerulonephritis, and vascular (Schönlein-Henoch) purpura have long been a part of the annals of medicine (Cluff and Johnson, 1965). Although the mechanisms underlying these syndromes have not been established with certainty, antigen-antibody reactions are probably operative. The M-protein antigens (see below) of the streptococci have been strongly suspected as possible agents. One possible explanation for tissue damage in these syndromes is that specific antibodies cross-react with antigens of streptococci and similar antigens of target tissue (Kaplan, 1964). The pathobiologic reactions also suggest similarities between these syndromes and experimental serum sickness, in which soluble antigen-antibody complexes are deposited in target tissue, causing damage by an Arthus-like reaction (Dixon *et al.*, 1961).

c. Hyperplasia

Local parasitic invasion frequently results in hyperplasia of neighboring lymphoid tissue, a manifestation of disease. This reaction may extend throughout the entire reticuloendothelial system and cause enlargement of the liver and spleen. The stimulus to such hyperplastic reaction within lymphoid and reticuloendothelial tissue has not been adequately delineated, but it probably involves the recognition and processing of parasite antigens, which in turn directly or indirectly stimulate the cells that participate in antibody formation and other immune processes. Virtually all parasites are capable of eliciting such a hyperplastic response. The extracellular parasites more frequently cause local reactions, whereas the intracellular parasites cause hyperplasia, both locally and systemically.

d. Neoplasia

The oncogenic potential of viral host-parasite interaction is described in Chapter 6. The alterations by viruses of the basic replicating mechanisms of human cells immediately suggest that viruses might have oncogenic potential. Indeed, viruses have been clearly implicated as the cause of animal neoplasia; examples are the polyoma virus of mice and the SV_{40} virus of monkeys. Moreover, human viruses such as adenoviruses have caused neoplasia in animals.

As yet the evidence that viruses cause human neoplasia is at best circumstantial. The possibility that a herpes-like virus causes Burkitt's lymphoma, a neoplasm endemic in Africa, is explored in Chapter 6.

Interactions between host and potential oncogenic viruses can result in virus multiplication with or without transformation of the cell. In animals infected with leukoviruses, for example, infectious virus is produced in most infected cells. Some cells, however, are transformed into neoplastic cells. This results from the presence of virus genetic information that does not lead to virus replication, but instead causes alterations in the cell plasma membrane, cell morphology, and orientation: tumor-specific antigens appear and the cell grows at an uncontrolled rate. During this neoplastic transformation there may be alterations in the immune status of the host, or an alteration in the host's immunologic surveillance may permit expression of the oncogenic potential (see Chapter 6).

The problems of paramount importance in the theory of the viral etiology of neoplasia are the elucidation of the mechanisms of transformation of supposedly normal cells into neoplastic cells and the determination of the fate of the viral genome in neoplastically transformed cells. A general concept of transformation by polyoma and SV_{40} DNA tumor-producing viruses is that their viral DNA enters the infected cell and activates cellular activities to produce one or more proteins required for the transformation (Eckart, 1969). Viral genetic material becomes a part of the heredity of the transformed host cells, and as transformed cells develop, neoplastic potential emerges. The RNA tumor viruses apparently replicate by means of an RNA-dependent DNA polymerase (reverse transcriptase) that produces virus-specific DNA, which presumably is integrated into the host genome.

2. Systemic reactions

It hardly needs to be mentioned that systemic reactions occur in infectious disease as well as in local injury at the site of the parasite invasion. These are the cardinal symptoms and signs of advanced host-parasite interaction: malaise, headache, alterations in pulse rate, shock, fever, negative nitrogen balance, electrolyte imbalance, elevated serum glucose, and leukocyte responses. As in the case of local reactions, these phenomena are frequently called non-specific, although such a classification may reflect our ignorance of the specific mechanisms responsible. Indeed, there is much to be learned concerning the mechanisms by which a local invasion of parasites precipitates a chain of events leading to systemic symptoms and sometimes to death.

a. Metabolic and hormonal reactions

Host-parasite interaction elicits many metabolic and biochemical events that may be responsible for certain generalized symptoms of infection, for they are qualitatively similar, relatively stereotyped, and apparently not specifically related to the etiology of the infection. For the most part these reactions are systemic, although it is obvious that infections involving particular organ systems, such as hepatitis, myocarditis, and pneumonitis, would cause local metabolic changes and impairment of organ function secondary to tissue invasion.

Protein catabolism with a negative nitrogen balance is a prominent systemic reaction in infection and is probably a result of fever and decreased dietary intake (Beisel *et al.,* 1967). This persistent catabolism during chronic infections such as tuberculosis probably causes the wasting state which characterizes these diseases. In contrast, selective anabolism occurs also during host-parasite interaction, as increased synthesis of interferon, alpha globulins, specific enzymes, and antibody proteins indicates. During certain experimental bacterial and viral infections, there is increased synthesis of ribonucleic acid, perhaps reflecting a need to produce proteins utilized in host defense mechanisms.

Through increased aldosterone output, there is renal retention of salt, with secondary depression of serum sodium and chloride during infection. Increased elaboration of the adrenocortical hormones and/or growth hormone during infection may be responsible for the glucose intolerance that sometimes occurs during severe host-parasite interaction. This may be followed by depletions in tissue carbohydrates and a terminal hypoglycemia.

It is likely that specific systemic metabolic events may be associated with specific parasitic infections. One such mechanism has recently been elucidated. During Gram-negative but not Gram-positive bacterial infections, there is an elevation of plasma-free fatty acids, triglyceride, and phospholipid (Gallin *et al.,* 1969). An increase in pre-beta lipoprotein appears to be responsible for this elevation. As a consequence there may be increases in gluconeogenesis, conversion of glucose to lactate, suppression of glycolysis, and activation of clotting processes.

b. Cardiovascular reactions

During severe host-parasite pathobiologic processes, altered cardiovascular reactivity is frequently seen (Weil *et al.,* 1964). The peripheral vascular resistance decreases, the pulse becomes rapid, and the cardiac output increases. Although the blood pressure falls, this generalized reaction, sometimes referred to as *warm shock* because of the peripheral vasodilatation, is usually reversible. At times, however, an irreversible shock-like state (*cool shock*) appears, which in contrast is characterized by a decrease in cardiac output and an increase in peripheral vascular resistance. Occurring distant from the site of host-parasite interaction, these changes still defy simple explanation. It has been postulated that the vasoactive substances released at the site of host-parasite reactions are responsible. It has also been postulated that specific parasite toxins, acting directly on the heart and blood vessels, or mediated through the central nervous system, precipitate these drastic systemic reactions. Recent evidence links disseminated intravascular coagulation with shock caused by infection (Corrigan *et al.,* 1968). Since most fatalities in host-parasite disease are the result of cardiovascular collapse, the need for a specific explanation is apparent.

c. Fever

Recognition of the elevation of body temperature in most forms of parasitic disease dates back to ancient history. Indeed, this is perhaps the most common and best known manifestation of infectious disease. Yet it is only recently that the pathogenesis of fever has been somewhat clarified. Most evidence suggests that parasites induce fever primarily by stimulating certain cells (usually neutrophils and monocytes) to elaborate a substance that acts on the thermoregulatory

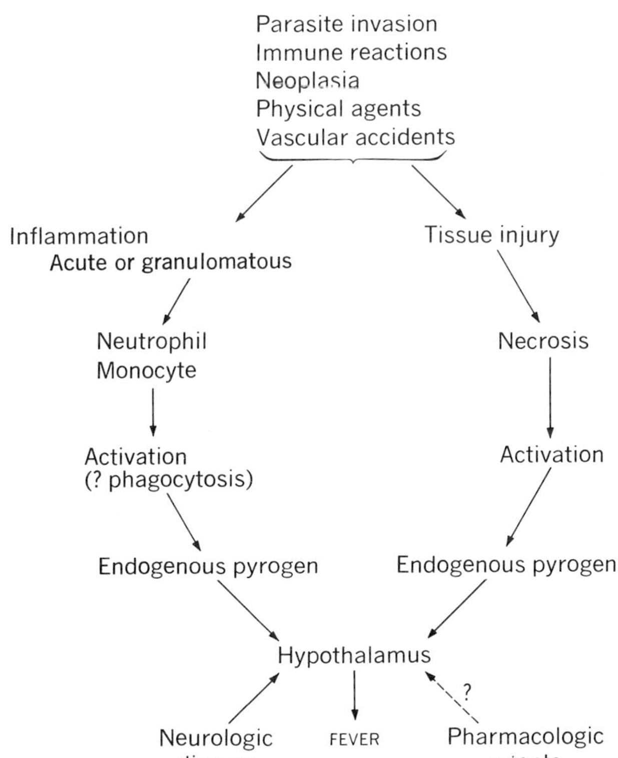

Figure 4-3. Pathways in the pathogenesis of fever.

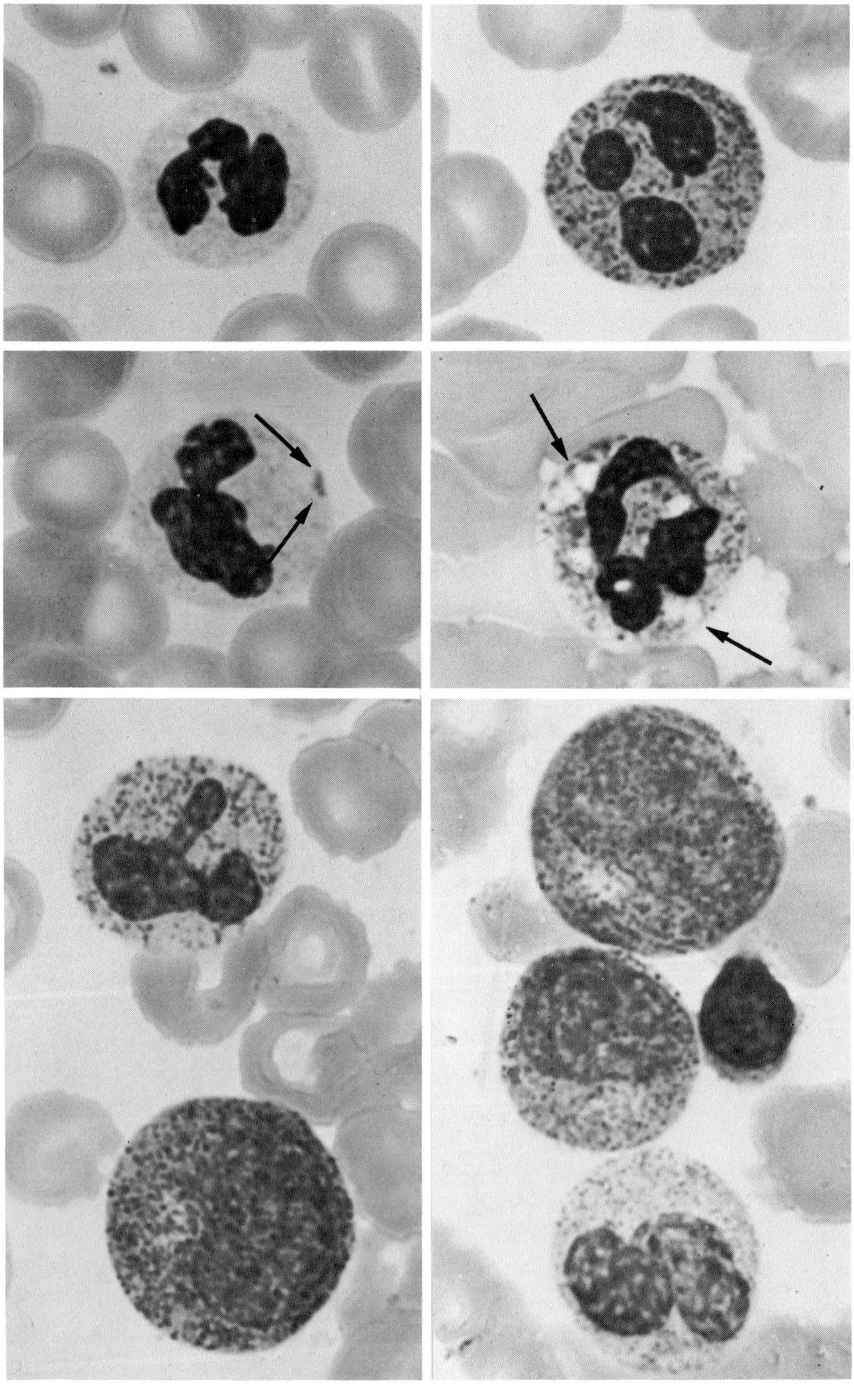

a b c d e f

centers of the brain (Atkins and Snell, 1965). This *endogenous pyrogen* has not been purified but is probably a lipoprotein. The process of phagocytosis is in many situations associated with and perhaps responsible for the release of endogenous pyrogen, after which there is a latent period before the host increases body temperature by vasoconstriction and increased muscular activity. This chill phase is later followed by vasodilatation and diaphoresis in an attempt by the host to return body temperature to its closely held norm.

The release of endogenous pyrogen is not specific to host-parasite interaction, for allergic fevers are probably generated in a similar fashion. (Furthermore, neither a beneficial nor a deleterious effect of fever has been established.) A schematic diagram of known and hypothetical mechanisms of the pathogenesis of fever is given in Figure 4-3.

d. Hematologic reactions

Another classic, generalized response to host-parasite interaction is the alteration in the quantity and quality of blood neutrophils which occurs during serious bacterial infection. Although nonspecific to many types of bacterial host-parasite infection, these changes in blood neutrophils occur infrequently in viral, protozoan, and fungal infections. Perhaps the determinant of this response is extracellular parasitism in which the primary inflammatory cell is the neutrophil. It has been suggested that certain leukotactic factors are elaborated at the local inflammatory site and that these substances then act as a stimulus to the production and release of neutrophils from the bone marrow (Menkin, 1956). Teleologically, the reason for an increase in total neutrophils is clear—a need for more phagocytes.

The increase in quantity of neutrophils is accompanied also by an increase in the proportion of immature cells and by specific changes within cell cytoplasm. When observed with a Romanowsky stain, these cytoplasmic changes appear as heavily stained granules called *toxic* granules, vacuoles, and inclusions of rough endoplasmic reticulum called *Dohle bodies* (McCall *et al.,* 1969) (Fig. 4-4). The morphology of these toxic neutrophils reflects alterations in the constituents and activity of lysosomes and in cytoplasmic autophagy. The neutrophils so affected are dysfunctional, having decreased migratory, chemotactic, phagocytic, and bac-

Figure 4-4. Stained blood films from human blood and bone marrow:

a. Normal blood neutrophil.

b. Blood neutrophil with toxic granulation.

c. Dohle body (arrows).

d. Vacuoles (arrows) in a toxic neutrophil.

e. Toxic granulation in a mature blood leukocyte and metamyelocyte.

f. Toxic neutrophil and precursors in bone marrow. (Courtesy of McCall, Katayama, Cotran, and Finland, 1969)

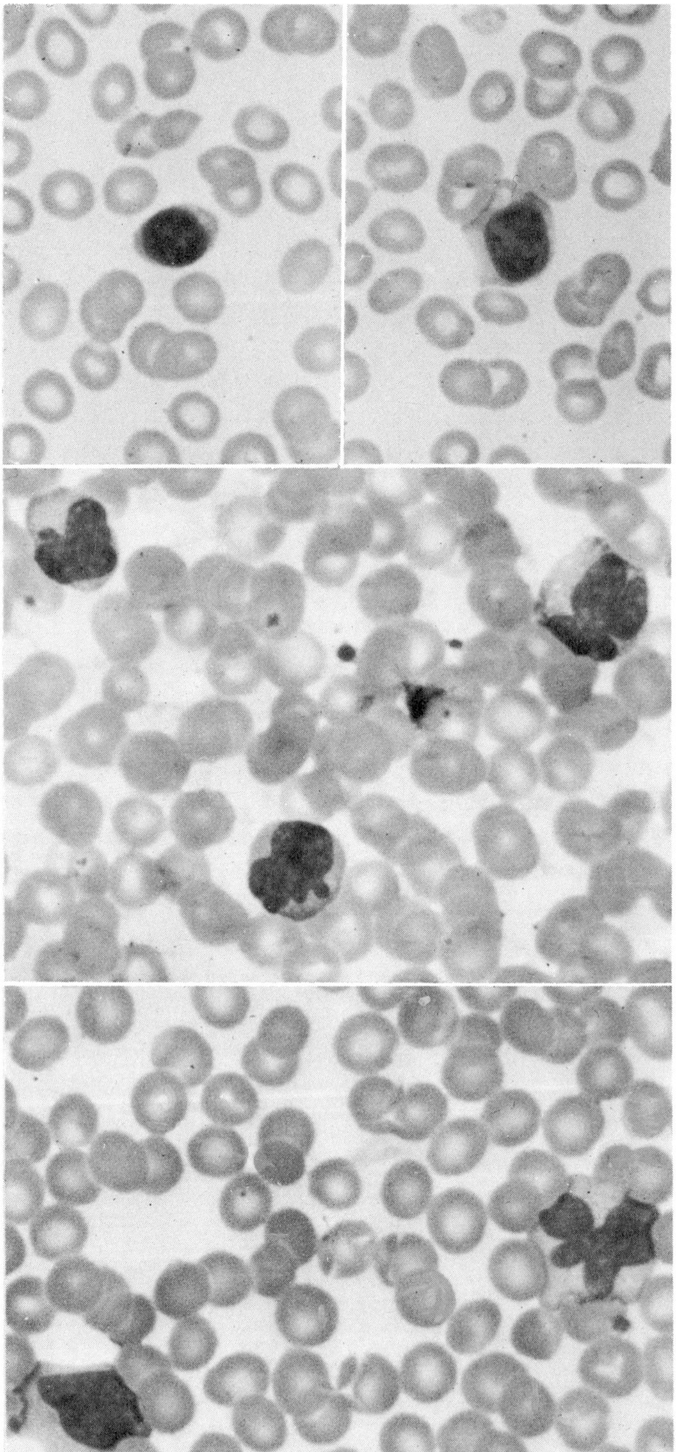

a b c d

tericidal activities (McCall and Caves, 1970). Collectively, the pathobiology of toxic neutrophilia may reflect cellular immaturity, a reaction to cellular injury, or a stimulus of infection. The phenomenon probably is not specific to bacterial infection, for such changes have been described in other severe inflammatory states.

Hematological changes occur also in intracellular parasitism. As in the case of the neutrophil response, the cells involved are those participating in the specific defense reaction. For example, in tuberculosis there may be an increase in the number of circulating monocytes, the cytoplasm of these cells may become vacuolated, and there is an increase in the quantity of certain of their lysosomal enzymes. In infectious mononucleosis, presumably a viral disease, the cytopathologic reactions of the circulating lymphocytes are highly characteristic. These *atypical lymphocytes* are morphologically and metabolically distinct from lymphocytes of uninfected hosts, reflecting an increase in the synthesis of lysosomal enzymes, rough endoplasmic reticulum, and RNA (Wood and Frenkel, 1967) (Fig. 4-5).

Other blood constituents may be altered during host-parasite interaction. Anemia due to decreased red cell production and/or increased red cell destruction is common. There may be destruction or decreased production of blood platelets. At times there is a disorder in the clotting mechanism in which many of the essential clotting factors are consumed (McKay, 1965). The ensuing disseminated intravascular coagulation, which results in both thrombosis and bleeding, has been implicated as a cause of shock and death in a number of severe infections both by extracellular and intracellular parasites. The initiating factors in this injury are unclear, but immunologic interaction of host and parasite may precede the event. The generalized Schwartzman reaction in animals, which is a response to the endotoxin of certain bacteria, has been equated with the same process in humans.

C. Parasite Determinants of the Pathobiology of Parasitism

1. Concepts and definitions

The emphasis in the preceding discussion upon the host's response in aberrant parasitism was not meant to imply that the parasite is a neutral element. In-

Figure 4-5. Stained blood films from human blood.
a. Normal small lymphocyte.
b. Normal large lymphocyte.
c, d. Atypical lymphocytes from patients with infectious mononucleosis.

deed, the popularity of Robert Koch's germ theory of disease, which emphasizes the parasite, has continued to foster extensive research into the specific mechanisms whereby parasites cause disease. Three concepts which permit biologists to understand better the offensive capacity of the parasite have evolved. To satisfy the need for food, self-preservation, and replication, the parasite must: (1) have a natural habitat (reservoir); (2) be able to move to a new reservoir or susceptible host by means of spread; and (3) be able to penetrate host tissue and thereafter either subsist or be excreted. Since this discussion is primarily concerned with direct host-parasite interaction, the third category will be stressed.

The pathogenic potential of a parasite, however, cannot be separated from the first two concepts of reservoir and spread to a susceptible host which are epidemiologic features of parasitism. If man is an unnatural host, for example, contracting the disease depends upon his proximity to a natural reservoir and to a vehicle that can transmit the parasite to the susceptible tissues in his body. In Rocky Mountain Spotted Fever, which is caused by a rickettsia, the prevalence of disease in man depends upon the prevalence of parasites in the natural reservoir (e.g., wild animals), the availability and prevalence of carriage within the vector (e.g., tick), and the exposure of the susceptible host to these epidemiologic determinants.

In concert, the forces underlying transmission from a reservoir through a vehicle of spread to a new host constitute *communicability*. Communicability does not mean that after transfer to a new host the parasite is necessarily capable of eliciting a pathologic interaction. The capacity to cause disease is a separate property called *pathogenicity*. The variability in pathogenicity among strains within a group of parasites reflects individual *virulence*.

The most pathogenic parasites usually cause disease in an unnatural host. In a natural host the pathobiologic reaction depends upon a change in the dynamics of commensalism, which renders the parasite a potential pathogen. The ensuing host-parasite interaction is called *opportunistic infection*. These infections by parasites within natural hosts are of paramount importance, and they will be discussed in greater detail later.

2. Extracellular parasitism

a. Invasive properties

The interactions of pathogenic parasites with the host may be conveniently divided into two categories: those that occur extracellularly and those that occur intracellularly. The extracellular parasites include most pathogenic bacteria (Table 4-1a).

Pathogenic bacteria arrive at the site of host-parasite interaction either by primary penetration, by secondary inoculation from vectors (such as insects) or accidental breaks in environmental barriers (such as skin, mucous membranes). Unfortunately, the characteristics of primary tissue penetration by pathogenic bacteria are for the most part unknown. It has been clearly shown, for example, that salmonellae can invade epithelium of the small intestine of man and make their way into the lamina propria, where they then elicit the inflammatory response. How they are able to do this is an enigma, but it must reflect an offensive property of the parasite.

Once in an appropriate environment for multiplication, bacteria produce disease by two mechanisms (Davis *et al.,* 1968): invasion of tissue and elaboration of toxins.

The capability of invading tissue usually reflects the pathogen's defensive mechanisms against the host's own defenses. A common defense in bacteria is the formation of a thick capsule of gummy material which effectively repels the phagocyte. This is advantageous for extracellular parasites, most of which are unable to maintain life once they have been ingested.

Capsules are heterogeneous in composition. For example, the capsule of the pneumococcus is a complex of a high-molecular-weight polymer of glucose and glucuronic acid, and that of the anthrax bacillus contains a polypeptide of glutamic acid. That these capsules are indeed virulence factors is clearly exemplified in the case of pneumococcal infections. The smooth, fully encapsulated strains cause disease, whereas the unencapsulated, rough strains do not (MacLeod and Krauss, 1950). Moreover, specific host antibody against the capsule reduces or abolishes the virulence of the bacteria. In human disease the heavily encapsulated Type 3 pneumococcus is more virulent than the less encapsulated types of pneumococcus. Likewise, the capsule size of *Klebsiella pneumoniae* varies, and strains with thicker capsules are more virulent than those with thin capsules.

Little is known of the molecular mechanisms by which capsules inhibit phagocytosis. One hypothesis has been that the hydrophobic lipid components of neutrophil membranes are prevented from making intimate contact with the hydrophilic capsular gel. Another is that there are repelling electrical forces between capsule and neutrophil.

Not all antiphagocytic substances in microorganisms are capsules. For example, the streptococcus has a virulent antiphagocytic protein that resides in the cell wall. This is called M-protein and is both antiphagocytic and antigenic.

Some bacteria elaborate extracellular enzymes that would appear to directly facilitate invasion and spread in host tissue. Many Gram-positive bacteria produce hyaluronidase that promote diffusion by depolymerization of hyaluronic

Table 4-2 Invasive Factors That Influence Pathogenicity of Some Bacterial Parasites of Man

INVASIVE FACTOR	SOURCE	ACTIVITY
Capsules	*Diplococcus pneumoniae* *Hemophilus influenzae* *Klebsiella pneumoniae* *Bacillus anthracis* *Staphylococcus aureus* *Pasturella pestis*	Antiphagocytic
M-protein at cell surface	Streptococci-Group A	Antiphagocytic
Extracellular enzymes*		
hyaluronidases	Streptococci-Group A	Lysis of tissue ground substance
coagulases	*Staphylococcus aureus*	Clots fibrin
kinases	Staphylococci, Streptococci	Lysis of fibrin
collagenase	*Clostridium perfringens*	Lysis of collagen

* The role of extracellular enzymes in the pathogenesis of human infections is uncertain.

acid in the tissue ground substance. Staphylococci elaborate coagulases that clot plasma by converting fibrinogen to fibrin. Both streptococci and staphylococci elaborate kinases that catalyze plasminogen to plasmin, which then lyses fibrin. In contrast with the enzymes mentioned above, about whose *in vivo* potential we still speculate, there is some clinical evidence that collagenases facilitate the invasion of the *Clostridia* bacilli that cause gas gangrene. Invasive factors that influence the pathogenicity of some bacterial parasites of man are listed in Table 4-2.

b. Exotoxins

A small but significant group of bacterial pathogens cause pathologic host-parasite interaction by elaborating exotoxins (van Heyningen, 1955). Although one might define bacterial enzymes that act locally as *toxins,* the term is usually confined to substances acting at a distance from the site of invasion. The toxin production may depend upon penetration, invasion, and replication, but it is independent of bacterial autolysis. Bacteria producing exotoxins that cause human disease are listed in Table 4-3. The diseases include diphtheria, tetanus, gas gangrene, botulism, food poisoning, whooping cough, cholera, and scarlet fever.

Table 4-3 Exotoxins That Determine Pathogenicity of Some Bacterial Parasites of Man

DISEASE	SOURCE OF EXOTOXIN	ACTIVITY
Diphtheria	*Corynebacterium diphtheriae*	Inhibits protein synthesis; inhibits oxidative processes
Botulism	*Clostridium botulinum*	Anticholinergic
Tetanus	*Clostridium tetani*	Anticholinergic; ? blocks inhibitory synapses
Gas gangrene	*Clostridium perfringens*	Cytolytic
Staphylococcal food poisoning	*Staphylococcus aureus*	? Stimulates brain or peripheral nerves to produce vomiting
Scarlet fever	Streptococci, Group A	Cytotoxic to blood vessels
Whooping cough	*Bordetella pertussis*	Necrotizing to bronchial epithelium; produces lymphocytosis
Cholera	*Vibrio cholera*	Alters water and electrolyte balance in intestine by activating adenylcyclase

Exotoxins, which are heat-labile proteins, include the most powerful poison known. One ounce of diphtheria toxin, for example, could kill every inhabitant of New York City. Diphtheria toxin inhibits protein synthesis and thus damages many types of cells. A strange phenomenon in the production of diphtheria toxin is that a bacteriophage, which is in itself a viral parasite of the bacteria, determines the synthesis of toxin.

The virulent alpha toxin of *Clostridium perfringens* is a lecithinase, which splits lecithin into diglyceride and phosphorylcholine. Since lecithin is probably important in maintaining the structure of cell membranes, its removal results in collapse of the membrane and lysis of the cell.

The exotoxins responsible for botulism and tetanus are neurotropic. Botulism toxin affects production and/or release of acetylcholine at the preganglionic and postganglionic synapses in the autonomic nervous system, in addition to affecting cholinergic mechanisms in peripheral nerves. In contrast, tetanus toxin appears to act within the central nervous system, probably causing spasm by blocking inhibitory motor neurons.

Staphylococci may produce an enterotoxin that acts on the central nervous system or peripheral nerves to produce severe vomiting. Some streptococci produce an erythrogenic toxin that causes injury of small blood vessels to produce the scarlet-fever syndrome. The exotoxin produced by *Bordetella pertussis,* the cause of whooping cough, is necrotizing to the bronchial epithelium and is responsible for the unusual lymphocytosis associated with the disease. The cholera toxin alters fluid and electrolyte balance in the gastrointestinal tract through activation of adenylcyclase at the cell surface, thus increasing the level of cyclic adenosine monophosphate.

c. Endotoxins

In contrast to exotoxins, which are produced primarily by Gram-positive bacteria, most Gram-negative bacteria contain a complex macromolecular phospholipid and polysaccharide moiety within their cell wall which is toxic. In contrast with exotoxins, these endotoxins are released only after bacterial lysis, and the reactions with the host are less potent and less specific than those of the exotoxins. Indeed, the role of endotoxins in human host-parasite pathobiology has not been established with certainty. Nevertheless, their implication in human disease has long been suspected and the literature is replete with studies of endotoxins (Westphal *et al.,* 1961).

The biologic effects of bacterial endotoxins are numerous, but we shall mention only the two that are most likely to be associated with pathobiology in man. First is the production of fever due to either primary alteration of hypothalamic activity or elaboration of endogenous pyrogen, perhaps through the phagocytosis of the macromolecules of endotoxin or from its effect at the cell surface. Second, in experiments, endotoxins produce a shock syndrome; the cause of this syndrome is not yet clear. Investigators debate whether the cardiovascular collapse results from direct effects of the toxic lipid moiety on the peripheral vascular system, or whether it is secondary to a generalized Schwartzman reaction in which vasoactive substances are released from cells and the clotting mechanism is activated. The shock and massive bilateral adrenal necrosis which sometimes occur in meningococcal sepsis have been attributed to the Schwartzman-like effects of endotoxin. Whatever the mechanisms, shock and cardiovascular collapse are an ominous and frequent occurrence in severe Gram-negative sepsis.

3. Intracellular parasitism

In contrast to extracellular parasites that cannot live within cells, certain parasites are adapted to intracellular existence. Within this group are *facultative* intracellular parasites, which can live and replicate either inside or outside cells, and *obligate* intracellular parasites, which can live only inside cells because they require certain cellular events for subsistence and replication (Table 4-1b). Examples of facultative intracellular parasites include the bacilli causing human tuberculosis, salmonellosis, and brucellosis, and many of the pathogenic fungi. The obligate intracellular parasites include all rickettsiae, all viruses, and some protozoa. How these microorganisms are able to maintain intracellular existence is a fundamental question regarding intracellular parasitism.

a. Facultative intracellular parasites

The facultative intracellular parasites are perhaps more puzzling than the obligate. Virulent tubercle bacilli are able to live within cells while avirulent tubercle bacilli cannot. The virulent bacilli may either neutralize the destructive forces within the cell or repress the mechanisms that activate them. Both Brucella and *Mycobacterium tuberculosis* have been subclassified on the basis of catalase production. The virulent strains that multiply freely within host cells produce considerably more catalase than those that are avirulent and cannot multiply intracellularly. The role of catalase is uncertain, but since the peroxides of host cells are probably important in the intracellular bactericidal reaction, the bacterial catalase may control the amount of hydrogen peroxide produced. Whatever the mechanisms, the ability to resist rapid intracellular destruction is a property of all facultative intracellular parasites, which perhaps by this resistance then cause the tissue inflammation characterized by formation of granulomata. Support for this theory can be seen in chronic granulomatous disease of children. In this unusual disease, the neutrophils and the monocytes can ingest but can not intracellularly destroy certain bacteria (Quie *et al.,* 1967). The host-parasite tissue reaction in this disease is characterized by the formation of granulomata. Instead of acute inflammation with abscess formation, granulomatous inflammation follows infections with extracellular parasites such as staphylococci, which because of a defect in host defense have become adapted to intracellular existence.

b. Obligate intracellular parasites

The obligate intracellular parasites include certain protozoa, all rickettsiae, and all viruses. The obligate intracellular parasites require either a host substrate or a host metabolic activity or both, for subsistence and replication (Moulder, 1962). An example of the use of host-cell substrate by an obligate intracellular parasite can be seen in malaria, caused by the protozoan *Plasmodium vivax.* When within a red cell, malarial sporozoites are capable of completing all the intermediate pathways in carbohydrate, nucleic acid, and lipid metabolism of free living microorganisms. Outside the host cell, the sporozoite is apparently unable to synthesize co-enzymes that are necessary to many metabolic reactions in the organisms. The intracellular environment of the host cells provides these important enzymes for the parasite. Another interesting observation is that the malarial parasites have developed a unique manner of obtaining amino acids for protein synthesis. The plasmodium phagocytoses a portion of the red cell's cytoplasm, secretes hydrolytic enzymes into the vacuole, and absorbs from the vacuole the amino acids provided through the digestion of hemoglobin. The iron pigment remains in the vacuole until the red cell ruptures.

Rickettsiae cannot metabolize glucose or glucose-6-phosphate, apparently because they lack a complete set of glycolytic enzymes. Therefore, instead of using glucose as a primary substrate, rickettsiae utilize glutamate, most likely by oxidative deamination to oxaloacetate. The oxaloacetate then enters the Krebs cycle. Apparently the electrons derived from glutamate oxidation can be carried to oxygen thus providing the energy source for rickettsiae through oxidative phosphorylation. Another weakness of rickettsiae is the instability of their membranes and their transport mechanism. When rickettsiae are removed from host cells, their membranes lose essential substances such as adenosine diphosphate and triphosphate. Thus, rickettsiae seem to depend on the host cell for structural as well as metabolic integrity.

Viruses are the most intriguing of the obligate intracellular parasites. One may still wonder what they represent within the order of biology. Composed of a block of genetic material without metabolic machinery and surrounded by a protective protein envelope (capsid) which serves as a vehicle of transmission, does a virion qualify as a living organism? Indeed, the composition of the envelope may at times contain specific components of the host cell and therefore might be considered a part of the host. Regardless of the position we espouse, we must accept that viruses are probably the most common parasites of man. More than forty different disease syndromes result from the interactions of viruses with their hosts. These reactions are so varied and so many of them depend upon poorly defined mechanisms, that our discussion must be confined to generalizations and examples.

Viruses contain either RNA or DNA which carries into the host cell new genetic information. When functioning, this viral genetic material leads to synthesis of new virus within the nucleus or cytoplasm of the host cell. This cycle of virus synthesis can be divided into a series of steps (Buddingh, 1965). The virus particles first establish contact with the host cells. Viruses such as influenza and some of the picornaviruses may attach to specific receptors on the host cell surface. One view broadly accepted is that the majority of viruses are taken into the cells by a process of phagocytosis or viropexis. Some viruses, however, may pass directly through the cell membrane without being engulfed into a phagocytic vacuole. After attachment and entry into the cell, the nucleic acid (RNA or DNA) reaches a replicating site (see Figure 2-29). The nucleic acid then "instructs" replication of itself into protein units that constitute its envelope. These basic units are then assembled into virus particles (maturation), and the mature viruses may then be freed from the host cell (release) to repeat the cycle. If the viruses are released it is a *productive infection,* but if they do not complete the cycle of reproduction and release it is an *abortive infection.*

Not all of these steps necessarily follow a chronological sequence. For example, some viruses may not reproduce for a period of time during which the viral molecules and cellular molecules are in intimate but inapparent interplay, known as latency.

The host-parasite interactions with viruses can be subdivided into the following major types: *inapparent* (subclinical), *apparent* (acute and chronic), and *latent* infection. An *inapparent* infection is defined as one not associated with any clinical signs of disease, although there is replication of the infectious virion. In contrast, in *apparent* infections there are obvious clinical signs of disease in the host. The apparent infections may be acute and last for a relatively short period of time, or they may be chronic and persist for months or years. A *latent* infection is a type of inapparent infection in which the production of infectious viruses cannot be detected during a time in which the host and virus cells are at equilibrium with each other. This equilibrium, however, may be disturbed, after which infectious virus units are produced and clinical disease results.

Examples of *inapparent* viral infection are seen when at times the respiratory syncytial or the lymphocytic choriomeningitis virus multiplies without producing specific immunity or clinical disease in the host. Cytomegaloviruses, reoviruses, herpes simplex, and varicella have been isolated at times from normal kidneys.

Influenza infection is an example of acute *apparent* viral infection due to direct cytotoxicity. The virus enters the body in the form of a wet or dry aggregate (droplet) and localizes in the respiratory tract. By attaching to the n-acetyl neuramic acid receptor on the cell surface of the epithelial cells of the upper and lower respiratory tracts, the nucleocapsid enters the cell and establishes infection. The consequence of virus multiplication is host-cell necrosis with desquamation of the epithelium of the respiratory tract. Multiplication of the virus and its subsequent spread to cells in the respiratory tract may be restricted by secretory IgA antibody, the production of interferon, or a natural antiviral component of mucus containing a glycoprotein that can neutralize influenza infectivity. Another example of *apparent* viral infection and a chronic injury to the host is that due to the papilloma or wart virus.

The so-called "slow" viruses replicate chronically in the host and apparently avoid inducing an immune response whatsoever until the time they cause disease (Gajdusek, 1967). Such reactions are often localized to a single organ such as the brain. These diseases include scrapie in sheep, transmissible mink encephalopathy, and kuru, subacute sclerosing panencephalopathy, and Jakob-Creutzfeldt diseases in humans. Such viruses perhaps can be regarded as nonantigenic substances that are associated with host-cell membranes and somehow induce the host cell to replicate them. Once symptomatology begins, the "slow" virus diseases frequently progress inexorably to death. The unusual host-parasite interaction has suggested that slow viruses may cause diseases that hitherto have been considered fundamentally genetic, immunologic, neoplastic, or metabolic disorders.

Latency is a condition in which viruses persist in the body despite an immune response with continued production of circulating antibody. During the latent period the production of infectious virus cannot be detected, and the virus and host cells appear to be in equilibrium. Examples are varicella-zoster and Herpes simplex. Varicella-zoster virus is probably maintained in the cells of dorsal root ganglia following primary infection, and subsequently it is activated and liberated from these sites to produce the skin lesions called shingles. The viruses may be activated by suppression of cellular immune reactions by therapeutic agents such as adrenocorticosteroids and cytotoxic drugs, or by certain neoplasms such as Hodgkin's disease. Another classic example of latency in man is *Herpes simplex* infection of the lip. The lesion we call the fever blister disappears, only to recur at irregular intervals under certain conditions (fever, stress, ambient heat) that activate the virus to complete its reproductive cycle.

As previously discussed, the immune mechanism of the host may be responsible for the pathogenesis of virus-induced disease (Webb and Hall, 1972). One such example is the severe form of obstructive bronchiolitis associated with respiratory syncytial virus infection of infants. The presence of maternal serum antibody (IgG) results in a severe form of the disease which is not present during infection beyond two years of age or when the antibody disappears. In pox virus infections the pox itself is caused by virus multiplication in the skin. Later, however, erythema surrounds the lesion, and this is probably related to an immunopathologic process. The occasional severe complications of pancreatitis, orchitis, and meningoencephalitis of mumps may be associated with immunopathologic reactions.

Virus-induced immunologic alterations may play a role also in the pathogenesis of certain chronic virus infections like serum hepatitis and chronic viral glomerulonephritis. It is possible also that certain hypersensitivity diseases such as systemic lupus erythematosus are caused by viral infection either by direct multiplication or by the virus infection's acting as an immunologic adjuvant. There is strong evidence that delayed hypersensitivity to viral antigens is important in the pathogenesis of certain viral diseases. For example, a small proportion of patients with measles develop encephalitis, during which time the brain is infiltrated by lymphocytes. Demyelination of nerve fibers results, and this is thought to represent a delayed hypersensitivity response.

An allergic response may be contributory in "slow" virus disease, where there is both a destructive and a proliferative phase. There are two ways in which this autohypersensitivity reaction may be induced. First, the host cell membrane may be incorporated into the new virus; and second, the process of viral infection may induce the formation of neoantigens at the surface of the host cell. The normal membrane determinants may then become immunogenic and later the target of immunologic attack. Complement may participate in the destructive reaction.

The implications of neoplasia resulting from virus infection are discussed on pages 148–49 and in Chapter 6.

In summary, it is likely that the complex events associated with virus-induced disease are the result of host-parasite interactions involving a combination of biochemical, physiologic, cytologic, and immunologic and neoplastic changes. The multiplication of a virus in the host cell is a prerequisite for the development of disease, but virus multiplication does not always lead to disease. Moreover, not all of the steps of viral multiplication proceed in an orderly fashion. The actual process of viral replication can cause damage to cells by viral components made in excess; it may produce substances causing cell death without viral multiplication; and at times an allergic response to the infection by viruses may be more damaging to the host than the cytopathic effects of the virus itself. Finally, the virus may cause fundamental changes in the cell leading to neoplastic transformation.

4. Organotropism

Many parasites not only select a specific host but may select the tissue they invade. For example, both meningococci and pneumococci frequently reside in the human nasopharynx; yet of the two, only pneumococci consistently invade the lower respiratory tract to cause pneumonia. Whereas the meningococci usually infect the upper respiratory tract of man before they invade the meninges, the closely related species that causes gonorrhea invades the genitourinary tract. This phenomenon of tissue preference is called *organotropism* and is seen with all types of parasites. Examples of this phenomenon in common bacterial, viral, and rickettsial pathogens are listed in Table 4-4.

When *Bordetella pertussis,* the agent of whooping cough, is introduced in

Table 4-4 Parasites Displaying Specific Organotropism in Host-Parasite Interactions

PARASITE	ORGANOTROPISM
Bacteria	
Meningococcus	meninges
Pneumococcus	lower respiratory tract
Gonococcus	genitourinary tract
Mycobacteria	lower respiratory tract
Cholera bacillus	gastrointestinal tract
Salmonella and Shigella	gastrointestinal tract
Mycoplasma	
Mycoplasma pneumoniae	lower respiratory tract
Rickettsiae	blood vessels
Metazoa	
Trichinella	muscle
Filaria	blood vessels and lymphatics
Protozoa	
Malarial protozoa	red blood cells
Trypanosomes	blood vessels and brain
Viruses	
Enteroviruses (polio, coxsackie, ECHO)	GI tract, central nervous system
Reoviruses, rhinoviruses, adenoviruses, myxovirus (influenza)	respiratory tract
Myxovirus (measles)	skin
Arboviruses	central nervous system, liver (yellow fever)
Herpes viruses	skin, nervous system
Poxviruses	skin
Rabies virus	central nervous system
Hepatitis viruses	liver
Mumps	salivary glands

chick embryos, the microorganisms, in addition to producing a local lesion on the membrane, frequently invade the embryo and eventually localize on the ciliated epithelium of the bronchial mucosa. If they are injected into the amniotic cavity, the same localization results. When, on the other hand, inoculation occurs before ciliated cells have appeared, infection of the bronchial epithelium fails to occur. These findings are in keeping with the pathobiology of whooping cough in humans. Similarly, *Neisseria meningitidis,* which causes bacterial meningitis in man, localizes in the meningeal tissues of embryos.

The obligate intracellular parasites also have tissue preferences. Of the examples listed in Table 4-4, the neurotropic viruses have received the greatest attention. Dissemination to the nervous system may occur by transmission along the axial structure of peripheral nerves as well as through the blood (viremia). The centripetal transmission of herpes simplex virus in mice can be followed by making serial sections of nerves. The virus may diffuse within the axon or multiply in endoneural cells. In the case of herpes simplex, there is organotropism of both skin and nervous system. Similarly, some Echo viruses and Coxsackie viruses prefer both respiratory and nervous tissue. Although infections in two tissue sites may reflect dissemination by viremia, this is perhaps not always the case. The nature of tissue preference remains an enigma.

D. Opportunistic Host-Parasite Interactions (Table 4-5)

While great progress in medical therapy has resulted from research on host-parasite pathobiology, and while we no longer face with frequency most of the grave infectious diseases of history, a new challenge has evolved. The forces underlying the equilibrium of uneventful parasitism have been so altered that interactions have developed which favor an aberrant course. These are called *opportunistic* infections, and in the prosperous countries most are caused by invasion of endogenous parasites.

Two primary changes underlie opportunistic, aberrant host-parasite interactions and lead to infection by endogenous parasites: altered microbial ecology and compromised host defense.

As previously discussed, man's microbial ecology is composed of indigenous microbiota that develop soon after birth (Rosebury, 1962). These parasites are accepted as natural inhabitants, residing at the interphase between tissue and external environment. Included are many bacteria and fungi, and at times protozoa, metazoa, and viruses. If the number of one of these parasites becomes great enough, the state of commensalism is transformed into pathogenicity. When such

Table 4-5 Indigenous Microbiota That Produce Disease by Opportunistic Host-Parasite Interactions

SKIN	UPPER RESPIRATORY TRACT	LOWER INTESTINE	GENITOURINARY TRACT (VAGINA AND ANTERIOR URETHRA)
Coagulase-negative staphylococci	Coagulase-negative staphylococci	Coagulase-negative staphylococci	Coagulase-negative staphylococci
Coagulase-positive staphylococci	Coagulase-positive staphylococci	Coagulase-positive staphylococci	Coagulase-positive staphylococci
Candida species	Group A streptococci*	Anaerobic streptococci	Anaerobic streptococci
	Microaerophilic streptococci	Enterococci	Candida species
	Meningococci*	*Clostridium perfringens*	
	Corynebacteria	*Escherichia coli*	
	Hemophilus influenzae	Klebsiella-Enterobacter-Serratia Group	
	Bacteroides	Proteus species	
	Actinomyces	*Pseudomonas aeruginosa*	
	Candida species	Bacteroides	
		Candida species	

* Intermittent carrier states

an opportunity arrives, one cannot rightly say that the acquired pathogenicity resides only in specific offensive properties of the parasite. A better explanation is that an unnatural interaction occurs between a natural parasite and a natural host.

Opportunistic host-parasite interactions became increasingly evident following the introduction of antibiotics. Optimists had prematurely looked upon this group of drugs as a panacea that would rid man of all pathogens, if not all parasites. The medical profession did not readily appreciate that along with suppression of the pathogen the antibiotics induced suppression of many members of the normal indigenous flora. The more resistant organisms thereafter could multiply to the extent that their sheer quantity and the lack of interference by other microorganisms apparently made them pathogenic. The result has been a rising incidence of many Gram-negative infections (coliform, Klebsiella, Proteus, Pseudomonas) and some Gram-positive infections (staphylococcal, enteric streptococcal) (Finland *et al.,* 1959), usually occurring in the hospitalized patient. At present the new microbial ecology, consisting of both the altered flora of hospital environs and the altered flora within patients, serves as a constant source of endogenous opportunistic infection.

Compromises in host defense have been as forceful as alterations in indigenous flora in causing endogenous infections. A number of factors associated with depression of host-defense mechanisms can be listed: increased age of the host; frequent use of medical instruments that act as foreign bodies in host tissues (such as urinary catheters, intravenous catheters, heart valves); prevalence of chronic disease states such as diabetes, alcoholism, chronic bronchitis, congestive heart failure, cirrhosis of the liver, and neoplasia; and use of immunosuppressive drugs such as adrenocorticosteroids, antimetabolites, and alkylating agents. The mechanisms responsible for the suppression of normal host defense in these states still confuse the investigator. It is clear, however, that drugs such as adrenocorticosteroids, antimetabolites, and alkylating agents do suppress immunity, perhaps by compromising a number of immunologic reactions, including acute and delayed inflammation, antibody synthesis, and phagocyte production and function (Schwartz, 1969).

Other examples of opportunistic interactions somewhat different from those listed above can be cited. An infection involving the influenza virus in the lung also predisposes the host tissue to infection by bacteria. In this instance of supra-infection it appears that the influenza virus specifically blocks the metabolism of glucose at the phosphohexose-isomerase level (Fisher and Ginsburg, 1956). Since phagocytosis depends upon glycolysis, the inhibition of the metabolic event depresses this mechanism of host defense.

Another opportunistic infection occurs when certain bacteria acquire a symbiotic pathogenicity. For example, staphylococci and streptococci may together cause a necrotizing skin infection that cannot be produced by either organism alone. Similarly, certain members of the mouth flora (streptococci, bacteroides, fusiforms) may in concert cause a necrotizing, anaerobic infection within the lung or pleural cavity, an effect that cannot be produced by any one of the organisms.

Although in contemporary usage the term *opportunistic infection* usually refers to endogenous infections, it would be unfair to history and disrespectful of the future not to mention the role of opportunism in exogenous infections. The most vigorous and lethal host-parasite reactions occur between an exogenous pathogen and a population of hosts that has neither the acquired nor the genetic gift of self-defense against the parasite. History is replete with examples. After the Spanish conquest the Indians were ravaged by smallpox. Microbial diseases became rampant among South Sea islanders soon after Captain Cook arrived. Albert Schweitzer recorded that when African trypanosomiasis, also known as sleeping sickness, moved from Loango where it was endemic, to Uganda where it was unknown, one village lost most of its inhabitants.

References

Atkins, E., and Snell, E. S. (1965), Fever, *in* The Inflammatory Process, p. 495, B. Zweifach, L. Grant, and R. T. McClusky, Eds., Academic Press, New York.

Beisel, W. R., Sawyer, W. D., Ryll, E. D., and Crozier, D. (1967), Metabolic effects of intracellular infections in man, Ann. Int. Med., *67*:744.

Buddingh, G. J. (1965), Pathogenesis and pathology of viral infections, *in* Viral and Rickettsial Infections of Man, p. 339, F. L. Horsfall and I. Tamm, Eds., J. B. Lippincott Co., Philadelphia.

Burnet, F. (1966), Natural History of Infectious Disease, 3d ed., Cambridge University Press, New York.

Cluff, L. E., and Johnson, J. E. (1965), Post-streptococcal disease, *in* Immunologic Diseases, p. 418, M. Samter, Ed., Little, Brown and Co., Boston.

Corrigan, J. J., Jr., Ray, W. L., and May, N. (1968), Changes in the blood coagulation system associated with septicemia, New Eng. J. Med., *279*:851.

Davis, B. D., Dulbecco, R., Eisen, H. N., Ginsburg, H. S., and Wood, W. B., Eds. (1968), Pathogenic properties of bacteria, *in* Principles of Microbiology and Immunology, p. 574, Harper & Row, New York.

Dixon, F. J., Feldman, J. D., and Vazquez, J. J. (1961), Experimental glomerulonephritis. The pathogenesis of a laboratory model resembling the spectrum of human glomerulonephritis, J. Exp. Med., *113*:899.

Eckart, W. (1969), Cell transformation by polyoma and S.V.^{40}, Nature, *224*:1065.

Epstein, W. L. (1967), Granulomatous hypersensitivity, Prog. in Allergy, *11*:36.

Finland, M., Jones, W. F., Jr., and Barnes, M. W. (1959), Occurrence of serious bacterial infections since introduction of antibacterial agents, J. Am. Med. Assoc., *170*:2188.

Fisher, T. N., and Ginsburg, H. S. (1956), The reaction of viruses in guinea pig polymorphonuclear leukocytes, Virology, *2*:618, 637, 656.

Gajdusek, D. C. (1967), Slow-virus infections of the nervous system, New Eng. J. Med., *276*:392.

Gallin, J., Kaye, D., and O'Leary, W. M. (1969), Serum lipids in infection, New Eng. J. Med., *281*:1081.

Kaplan, M. H. (1964), Immunologic cross-reaction between Group A streptococcal cells and mammalian tissues–possible relationship to the induction of autoimmunity in rheumatic fever, *in* The Streptococcus, Rheumatic Fever, and Glomerulonephritis, p. 169, J. W. Uhr, Ed., Williams & Wilkins Co., Baltimore.

Klebanoff, S. J. (1967), Iodination of bacteria: a bactericidal mechanism, J. Exp. Med., *126*:1063.

MacLeod, C. M., and Krauss, M. R. (1950), Relation of virulence of pneumococcal strains for mice to the quantity of capsular polysaccharide formed *in vitro,* J. Exp. Med., *92*:1.

McCall, C. E., and Caves, J. (1970), Dysfunction of human neutrophils during severe bacterial infection, Clinical Research, *18*:49.

McCall, C. E., Katayama, I., Cotran, R. S., and Finland, M. (1969), Lysosomal and ultrastructural changes in human toxic neutrophils during bacterial infection, J. Exp. Med., *129*:267.

McKay, D. G. (1965), Disseminated Intravascular Coagulation: An Intermediary Mechanism of Disease, Paul B. Hoeber, Inc., New York.

Menkin, V. (1956), Biochemical Mechanisms, *in* Inflammation, Charles C Thomas Co., Springfield, Ill.

Moulder, J. W. (1962), The Biochemistry of Intracellular Parasitism, University of Chicago Press, Chicago.

Myrvik, Q. N., and Leake, E. S. (1960), Studies on antibacterial factors in mammalian tissues and fluids. IV. Demonstration of two nondialyzable components in the serum bactericidal system for *Bacillus subtilis,* J. Immunol., *84*:247.

Nelson, R. A. (1965), The role of complement in immune phenomena, *in* The Inflammatory Process, p. 819, B. W. Zweifach, L. Grant, and R. T. McClusky, Eds., Academic Press, New York.

Quie, P. G., White, J. G., Holmes, B., and Good, R. A. (1967), *In vitro* bactericidal capacity of human polymorphonuclear leukocytes: diminished activity in chronic granulomatous disease of childhood, J. Clin. Invest., *46*:668.

Rosebury, T. (1962), Microorganisms Indigenous to Man, McGraw-Hill, New York.

Schwartz, R. S. (1969), Immunosuppression: challenge of selectivity, Hospital Practice (February), p. 42.

Smith, T. (1934), Parasitism and Disease, Princeton University Press, Princeton, N.J. Reprinted 1963, Hafner Publishing Co., New York.

Spector, W. G., and Willoughby, D. A. (1963), The inflammatory response, Bact. Rev., *27*:117.

van Heyningen, W. E. (1955), The role of toxins in pathology, *in* Society of General Microbiology, Symposium No. 5, Cambridge University Press, p. 17.

Webb, H. E., and Hall, J. G. (1972), An assessment of the role of allergic response in the pathogenesis of viral diseases, *in* Microbial Pathogenicity in Man and Animals, p. 383, H. Smith and T. H. Pearce, Eds., Cambridge University Press, Cambridge.

Weil, M. H., Shubin, H., and Biddle, M. (1964), Shock caused by Gram-negative organisms. Analysis of 169 cases, Ann. of Int. Med., *60*:384.

Weissmann, G. (1965), Lysosomes, New Eng. J. Med., *273*:1084.

Westphal, O., Luderitz, O., and Staub, A. M. (1961), Bacterial endotoxins, J. Med. Pharm. Chem., *4*:497.

Wilhelm, D. L., Spector, W. G., and Willoughby, D. A. (1965), Chemical mediators, *in* The Inflammatory Process, p. 389, B. W. Zweifach, L. Grant, and R. T. McClusky, Eds., Academic Press, New York.

Wood, T. A., and Frenkel, C. P. (1967), The atypical lymphocyte, Am. J. Med., *42*:923.

Zeya, H. I., and Spitznagel, J. K. (1963), Antibacterial and enzymic basic proteins from leukocyte lysosomes: separation and identification, Science, *142*:1085.

5

IMMUNOLOGIC INJURY

Mariano F. La Via, M.D.

A. Introduction

Administration of antigen to an animal usually leads to the formation of antibody, which is characterized by the capacity to combine specifically with the antigen eliciting its production. This immune response, as we understand it today, is restricted to the vertebrate species and is typical of the integrated cellular responses of higher organisms to external stimuli.

The most obvious function of the immune response is in resistance to infectious disease. Antibodies produced against bacterial capsules facilitate phagocytosis and destruction of many organisms, combine with and neutralize bacterial toxins, and combine with viral protein to prevent entry of viruses into cells (Abramoff and La Via, 1970).

The immune response plays an opposite role in the pathogenesis of disease. *Immunologic injury* encompasses a number of reactions injurious to the host. In some of these the antigen is external, and in others the host becomes sensitized to its own tissues or to cross-reacting antigens, and *auto-immune* diseases with widespread pathologic manifestations may result (Medawar, 1957; Shaffer *et al.*, 1959; Gell and Benacerraf, 1961; Mackay and Burnet, 1965).

This chapter will deal primarily with this second aspect of immune responses. First, however, it will be useful to review briefly the process of immunological responsiveness and some of the damaging consequences of its faulty development.

B. The Immune Response

1. Phylogeny and ontogeny of the immune response

The development of immunological competence parallels the differentiation of the lymphoreticular system, and antibody production is a function of this system. Defense mechanisms in invertebrates depend mainly upon phagocytosis, and only in the lower marine vertebrates is a rudimentary adaptive immunity found. The well-defined, adaptive immune response with development of serum immunoglobulins starts in the elasmobranchs (Smith *et al.,* 1966).

Paralleling the phylogenesis of immune responses, no antibody is produced during fetal life until thymic and lymph node lymphocytes are present (Smith *et al.,* 1967). In fact the development of immune responses is a function of differentiation of thymus-dependent (T) and bone marrow (or bursa)-dependent (B) lymphocytes. This differentiation occurs during fetal development and provides the cellular basis for the progression of immune competence. The thymus develops first in all species examined except the cat (Ackerman, 1967). Lymph nodes, spleen, bone marrow, and other lymphocytes appear subsequently, probably under the influence of the thymus. At birth, human infants have a gamma globulin level that is usually at least equal to that of the mother. This immunoglobulin, in fact, is almost entirely maternal antibody that has been transferred to the fetus *in utero* (Koch *et al.,* 1959). For a period of from three to ten weeks after birth, the gamma globulin level declines and then levels off, subsequently rising until adult levels are reached at between one and four years of age. The decline after birth can be ascribed to failure of synthesis by the infant, natural decay of maternally derived protein, and growth of the infant with increase in the blood volume. The ability to respond to antigenic stimulation thus develops during fetal life and is completed after birth.

There is considerable variation among different species in the degree of maturation of the immune response at birth. In fetal lambs, for example, an antibody response can be induced against some antigens as early as the sixty-sixth day of gestation (normal gestation period is 150 days) (Silverstein *et al.,* 1963). On the other hand, chickens show a lack of response to antigenic stimulation until approximately four to five weeks after birth (Wolfe *et al.,* 1957). In man, although natural antibody synthesis does not normally occur until after birth, there is evidence that under appropriate artificial stimuli immunocompetence can be demonstrated as early as the fourth month of gestation (Koch *et al.,* 1959).

The studies on fetal lambs have suggested that the ability to respond to different antigens develops at different times during gestation. For instance, the capacity to reject homografts appears earlier than other immunologic phenomena, and the ability to exhibit a delayed hypersensitivity reaction develops later (Cannon *et al.*, 1958; Fowler *et al.*, 1960; Schinckel and Ferguson, 1953).

2. Characteristics of the immune response

Specificity, memory, and *self-recognition* are three fundamental characteristics of immune responses.

Immunologic specificity is of a very high order. It is dependent on the recognition mechanism by which an antibody reacts with the antigenic configuration most complementary to its combining site. An antibody induced by an antigen *A*, however, will cross-react with a second antigen *B* if antigen *B* contains antigenic determinants very similar to those of antigen *A*.

Immunologic memory accounts for two very important features of the immune response: (1) the more vigorous "anamnestic" reaction elicited by antigen when it is administered to an animal for the second time, even after apparent cessation of antibody synthesis in response to the first stimulation; and (2) the phenomenon of tolerance in which the initial treatment with antigen leads to a state of non-reactivity to subsequent stimulation with the same antigen. This can be considered "negative" memory (Abramoff and La Via, 1970).

Self-recognition is essential to the integrity of the animal. Antibodies are not normally made to one's own proteins although these may be highly antigenic in other individuals. This implies that a mechanism exists by which one is capable of discriminating at a very high level of recognition between one's own and very similar but foreign macromolecules (Medawar, 1957).

3. Antigens and antigenicity

Antigens are substances capable of inducing antibody production and of reacting specifically with the antibody. They may be proteins, polypeptides, polysaccharides, or nucleic acids. Although most antigens are complex macromolecules, a compound need not be extremely complex to be antigenic. Polypeptides composed of only two or three amino acids, and dextran composed only of glucose units, are antigenic (Maurer *et al.*, 1963; Mage and Kabat, 1963).

Antigens are characterized by determinant groups, i.e., those parts of the molecule which react with antibody and thus impart specificity to the antigen.

Low-molecular-weight compounds may be antigenic if they are conjugated to a carrier (usually a protein). These compounds are called *haptens.* The hapten is the determinant group when it is coupled to a carrier and acts as the inducer of antibody specificity. Thus, it will be capable of subsequently reacting with the antibody even when not coupled to the carrier (Landsteiner, 1936).

4. Antibodies

The term *antibodies* is applied to a family of serum proteins which have been well characterized structurally and functionally and which are important in a number of immunologic phenomena. These antibodies have been shown to migrate electrophoretically in the γ and slow β globulin regions and are also termed *immunoglobulins.* Five types of immunoglobulins are most commonly found: IgM or macroglobulin, IgG, IgA, IgD, and IgE. They are responsible for the neutralization of toxins, for bacterial agglutination, for cell lysis, and for some allergic reactions. Their production is therefore primarily a defense mechanism (Edelman and Gall, 1969).

In delayed hypersensitivity, in homograft rejection, and in some autoimmune diseases, specific humoral antibody is either not present or can account only for some of the observed reactions. A striking phenomenon seen in these situations is the accumulation of lymphoid cells in large numbers at the reaction sites. When the accumulation of lymphocytes is prevented, these reactions are inhibited. Attempts to isolate an antibody which could be the mediator of injury in lymphoid cells of hypersensitive reactions have thus far yielded inconclusive results. While the phenomena are undoubtedly immunological, the presence of lymphocytes is necessary for injury to occur and for passive transfer of immunity. In referring to lymphocyte-dependent immunological phenomena, however, the term *cell-bound (cellular) antibodies* is sometimes used for convenience (Bloom, 1971).

5. Antibody synthesis

The production of antibody in response to antigenic stimulation is a complex response that can be divided into three major phases: (1) afferent, with "processing" of antigen and induction of the immune response; (2) central, with multiplication and differentiation of antibody-producing cells and synthesis of antibody; and (3) efferent, with interaction of antibody or effector cells with antigen.

Considerable progress has been made in understanding the cellular and molecular events that occur during antibody production. Introduction of antigen induces proliferation and differentiation of precursors of lymphocytes of the B or the T type to yield, on the one hand, immunoglobulin-producing plasma cells and, on the other, "sensitized" lymphocytes. During the afferent limb of B-type responses and during the efferent limb of T-type responses cell interactions also occur which are of paramount importance for the completion of immune responses (Katz and Benacerraf, 1972; Unanue, 1972).

During cellular proliferation and differentiation, immunoglobulins are synthesized in plasma cells and lymphokines in "sensitized" lymphocytes. Immunoglobulins are secreted and accumulate in the serum, reaching a detectable level a few days after immunization. They are responsible for the events seen during the efferent phase of the immune response. The role of lymphokines in T-cell-type responses is still not completely clear, although it appears that they may be responsible for the effects seen during the efferent phase of cell-mediated immunity (Bloom, 1971).

If an animal which has received a single immunizing dose of antigen is left to rest for a few weeks or months and is then injected with the same antigen, the response to this second injection is somewhat different from that seen after the first antigen administration. The lag period will be shorter, the rise of antibody titer more rapid and to higher levels, the titer will persist for a longer time, and antibody avidity will increase. This is called an anamnestic response to indicate that the cell "remembers" some event that has taken place in the past and is now capable of repeating the operation with greater speed. It seems logical that if information necessary for antibody synthesis is somehow encoded in a cell, after the first exposure this cell will be better able to respond the second time (Abramoff and La Via, 1970).

6. Antigen-antibody interactions

The hallmark of these interactions is their great specificity. An antibody reacts best with the antigen used to induce the production of the antibody; however, some antibody will cross-react with other antigens that have similar determinant groups. In general, cross-reactions are not as strong as homologous reactions. The specificity of antigen-antibody reactions is exquisite enough to allow use of antibodies as reagents to detect very small chemical differences between antigens (Landsteiner, 1936).

The reaction between antigen and antibody is reversible and can be visualized as a series of bimolecular reactions.

$$\mathrm{Ag} + \mathrm{Ab} \rightleftharpoons \mathrm{AgAb}$$
$$\mathrm{Ag} + \mathrm{AgAb} \rightleftharpoons \mathrm{Ag_2Ab}$$

The equilibrium of the reaction is usually in favor of complex formation. Physical-chemical studies have shown that covalent bonds are not formed when antigen and antibody combine. Instead, the reaction probably involves hydrogen bonds, hydrostatic interactions, and van der Waals forces (Talmage and Cann, 1961). The initial reaction between antigen and antibody appears to occur rather quickly. Secondary events–i.e., precipitation or cell lysis–may take hours to appear, however.

One class of antigen-antibody reaction of great importance in immunologic injury is that involving the fixation of complement (C′). The lysis of erythrocytes by hemolytic antibody is the best example of this process. This occurs according to the following scheme:

$$E + Ab \longrightarrow EA$$
$$EA + C' \longrightarrow E^*$$

EA is an erythrocyte that is now activated by the combination of antibody through the primary interaction of antibody and antigen. E* represents the lysed erythrocytes from which hemoglobin has escaped after the membrane has been damaged by the secondary reaction involving C′. Complement is a complex of nine proteins present in the serum, and the secondary reaction of EA + C′ is a complicated reaction of many stages which finally lead to the disruption of the erythrocytic membrane (Müller-Eberhard, 1968) (see Chapter 2).

C. Deficiencies of the Immune Response

Before considering the mechanisms by which injury can be mediated by immunological phenomena, it seems useful to consider briefly those diseases that appear as a result of a faulty development of immune responses. These are due primarily to the lack of the protective action of immunologic reactions. The development of immunologic responsiveness can be affected by genetic defects that lead to various deficiencies in the natural or acquired immune mechanisms. Since defense mechanisms develop in sequential steps, it is logical that various deficiencies of these mechanisms can result, depending on the stage of development at which the genetic defect has taken place (Cooper *et al.*, 1968; Sell, 1972).

There are, on the one hand, pure defects involving the phagocytic function, the immunoglobulin synthetic function, or the appearance of cellular immunity. On the other hand, there are mixed defects in which two or more of these mechanisms may be deficient (Table 5-1). Some of these defects also involve deficiencies of complement components or of enzymes needed to activate them.

Table 5-1 Immunologic Deficiency Defects

1. Defects of the phagocytic system
Chronic granulomatous disease
Splenic insufficiency
2. Defects of immunoglobulin synthesis
Congenital hypogammaglobulinemia
Acquired hypogammaglobulinemia
3. Defects of cellular immunity
A. With slight immunoglobulin synthesis deficiency
Thymic dysplasia
Thymic aplasia
B. With severe immunoglobulin synthesis deficiency
Thymic alymphoplasia
Swiss agammaglobulinemia
Wiskott-Aldrich syndrome
Ataxia-telangiectasia

1. Defects of the phagocytic system

Chronic granulomatous disease is the first example of a defect of phagocytosis. This disease, seen in children, is characterized by microabscesses and granulomas containing plasma cells and macrophages. The polymorphonuclear leukocytes in patients with this disease will ingest bacteria or particulate matter normally, but after ingestion, killing and digestion does not occur. The normal lysosomal process of microbial digestion (see Chapter 2) is deficient in chronic granulomatous disease, apparently because an oxidase for reduced nicotinamide adenine dinucleotide (NADH) is lacking. In this disease the inborn error is thus manifested in normal degranulation of the polymorphonuclear leukocytes with no killing and digestion. This defect is a sex-linked recessive character appearing only in males, with the carrier female having somewhat decreased leukocytic activity (see Chapters 3 and 4).

Another syndrome which fits this category of diseases is splenic insufficiency, manifested as decreased resistance to infection. This is a poorly understood condition that depends on the absence of the spleen but is related to the age at which the spleen is removed and to the disease for which the spleen has been removed. In fact, in some children who have had splenectomy for rupture of the spleen or for hematologic disorders (like idiopathic thrombocytopenia), there is no splenic insufficiency; whereas in children who have had splenectomy for lipid storage diseases, splenic insufficiency results.

2. Defects of immunoglobulin synthesis

These are disorders due to lack of B cells and are exemplified by congenital and acquired hypogammaglobulinemias. Congenital hypogammaglobulinemia is very clearly a sex-linked inherited disorder limited to boys and manifested in childhood by multiple infections resistant to therapy, particularly pneumonia, otitis media, sinusitis, and sepsis. There are no plasma cells in the bone marrow, lymph nodes, or any other organs, with a resulting lack of immunoglobulin synthesis manifested in very low IgG and in absent IgM and IgA. Lymphocytes are always present in normal number, although lymph nodes may be hypoplastic; the thymus appears to be normal. Acquired hypogammaglobulinemia occurs in association with a variety of diseases, especially those associated with the lymphoreticular system.

3. Defects of cellular immunity

These are disorders of T lymphocytes, and fall into two classes: those that are purely defects of cellular immunity, with little or no immunoglobulin-synthesis deficiency, and those that have a concomitant immunoglobulin-synthesis deficiency.

The first group comprises thymic dysplasia and thymic aplasia. Patients with thymic dysplasia have either normal or slightly low levels of immunoglobulins. The number of circulating lymphocytes may be normal or low, but there is depletion of the lymphoid tissue. Plasma cells are present in normal quantity. The clinical course of this disease is characterized by a lack of delayed hypersensitivity responses. This is not inherited as a sex-linked recessive disease, since both males and females are affected and since there are normal siblings where a male and a female in the same family have been affected. Thymic aplasia is a disorder resulting from lack of embryological development of the thymus and parathyroid glands. The symptoms are similar to those of thymic dysplasia but much more severe. There has been some success in treating this disease with fetal thymus grafts.

The combined defects of cellular immunity and immunoglobulin synthesis are represented primarily by thymic alymphoplasia and Swiss agammaglobulinemia. These diseases are manifested as total immunological incompetence: no delayed hypersensitivity, no homograft rejection, and no humoral antibody formation. Although the diseases are similar, they have distinct manners of inheritance: thymic alymphoplasia as a sex-linked recessive defect, and Swiss agammaglobulinemia as an autosomal recessive. Some have therefore considered the two diseases as one, with a mixed inheritance pattern. Children with these diseases fail to thrive and have chronic pulmonary infections, moniliasis, vaccinia following vaccination, and *pneumocystis carinii* pneumonia; they die very early. There is an absence of lymphocytes in the lymph nodes, which are very small and have a poorly developed architecture. The thymus is small with no lymphocytes, and no plasma cells can be demonstrated. Variants exist in which some plasma cells are present and little immunoglobulin is formed. An example of such a variant is Wiskott-Aldrich syndrome in which eczema, thrombocytopenia, and recurrent infection are common. The thymus is hypoplastic; there is depression of delayed hypersensitivity; and peripheral lymphocytes are sparse. IgM may be depressed while the IgA is increased. Ataxia telangiectasia, also a hereditary disease, is another example. The thymus shows lymphopenia; there is no delayed hypersensitivity present; IgA is very low, but IgG is present in secretions to replace IgA; and plasma IgG is essentially normal. Combined defects appear to derive from lack of development of lymphocyte lines from stem cells.

As is apparent from this brief description, understanding of immunologic deficiencies is still quite incomplete. As understanding of developmental immunology becomes more complete, the relation between the various steps that occur during immunological ontogenesis, and the pathologic entities which are seen when this ontogenesis is disturbed will be clarified (Janeway, 1968).

D. Immunologic Injury

Understanding of immunologic injury has progressed greatly in the last few years, thanks particularly to the establishment of experimental models that have clarified many phenomena of importance in the production of immunologic diseases. Nevertheless, because of the complexity of these syndromes that may depend on multiple mechanisms of injury, the pathogenesis of many of these diseases remains unclear.

For the sake of clarity, it seems convenient to present first what is known of the various mechanisms by which immune phenomena may cause pathologic manifestations, and then discuss some of the complex diseases observed in clinical practice. This will by no means be an exhaustive treatise on immunopathology but will for the main part stress simple pathogenetic mechanisms, with the understanding that at times more than one of these may participate to cause disease.

1. Differentiation between cell-mediated and serum-mediated hypersensitivities

Historically, hypersensitive responses to antigens were differentiated on the basis of time elapsed between administration of antigen and the appearance of the allergic response. Some of these reactions appeared in as little as thirty minutes to a few hours, and others took forty-eight hours or longer to become apparent. Thus, the expressions *immediate* and *delayed hypersensitivity* came into use. A more exact differentiation is now used, based on the mechanism by which the hypersensitivity is mediated. Immediate hypersensitivities or, for the purposes of this discussion, humoral hypersensitivities, are mediated by a serum immunoglobulin (primarily IgE in the case of anaphylaxis, and IgM or IgG in the case of Arthus reactions) synthesized by plasma cells (the progeny of B cells). If these globulins from a hypersensitive individual are injected into a normal individual,

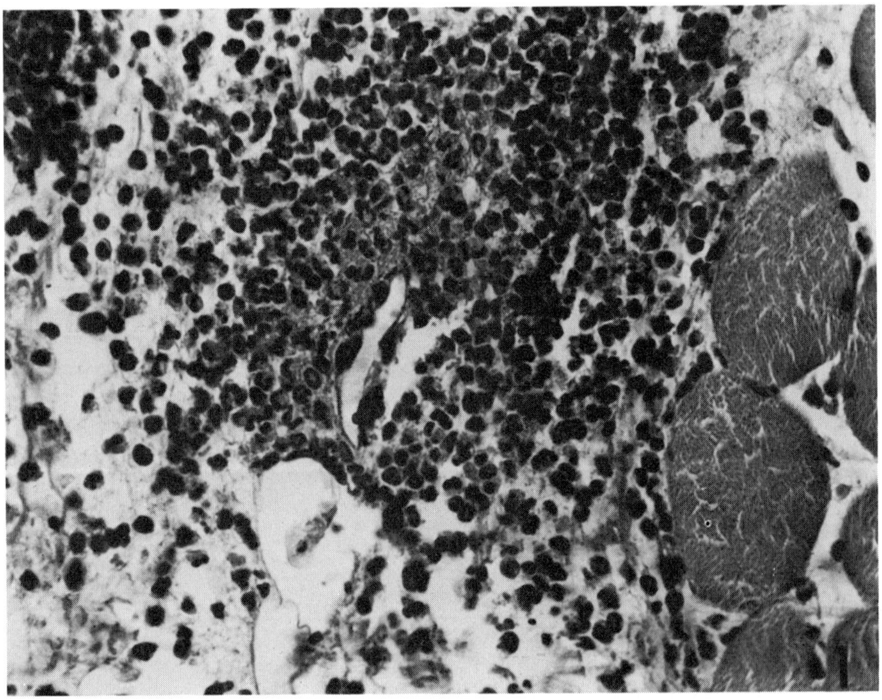

Figure 5-1. Characteristic infiltrate of immediate hypersensitivity consisting of polymorphonuclear leukocytes. (Courtesy of P. Ward)

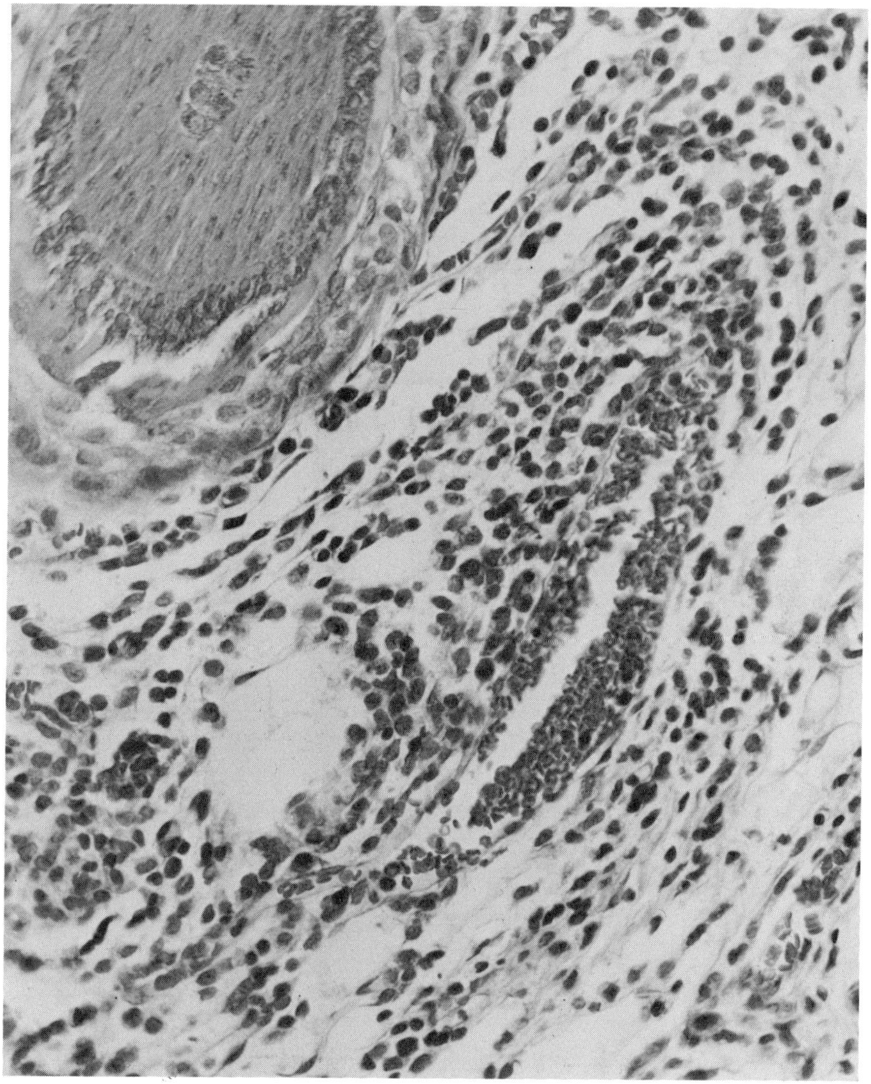

Figure 5-2. Perivascular infiltrate, containing lymphocytes and macrophages, typical of delayed hypersensitivity responses. (Courtesy of J. Feldman)

he will become temporarily hypersensitive to the specific agent to which the donor was sensitive (Prausnitz and Kustner, translated 1962). The delayed hypersensitivities, on the other hand, cannot be transferred by serum proteins, but can be transferred by lymphoid cells (the progeny of T cells) (Chase, 1946). Obviously, the terms *humoral* and *cellular hypersensitivity* are derived from the method by which transfer can be achieved.

Hypersensitivities may also be differentiated histologically (Turk, 1967). In general, the inflammatory exudate in immediate reactions is composed of polymorphonuclear leukocytes (Fig. 5-1). In contrast, the delayed response is characterized by a perivascular infiltrate rich in mononuclear cells (lymphocytes and macrophages) (Fig. 5-2). Perhaps these cell types reflect nothing more than the difference between chronic and acute inflammatory reactions.

Another major difference between delayed and immediate hypersensitivities is in the pharmacologic mediators that take part in the reaction. In many immediate reactions the antigen-antibody complex causes host cells to release histamine or other vasoactive substances that affect smooth muscle or the autonomic nervous system. In contrast, these agents have not been found to play a role in delayed hypersensitivity.

2. Classification of mechanisms of immunologic injury

There are four mechanisms by which immunologic injury is mediated. These have been the object of extensive research in the past ten to fifteen years.

On the basis of their characteristics these mechanisms may be divided into the two categories outlined above: humoral or serum-mediated injury in which the antibody is in one of the serum-protein fractions; and cellular or cell-mediated injury in which no measurable antibody has been identified thus far, but in which responsibility for the injury can be assigned to cells of the small lymphocyte type (Table 5-2).

a. Direct injury by circulating antibodies—cell lysis

When an antibody directed against cell surface antigens–usually IgM or IgG–reacts with that antigen and complement, a series of enzymes is activated and the cell wall is punctured with release of intracellular contents (Humphrey and Dourmashkin, 1969).

Lysis of cells after reaction of a cellular antigenic determinant with antibody and complement may be protective in some cases and injurious in others. If the cell lysed is an invading microorganism or a neoplastic cell, lysis is obviously pro-

Table 5-2 Mechanisms of Immunological Injury

	CELL LYSIS	SERUM-MEDIATED HYPERSENSITIVITY (IMMEDIATE)		CELL-MEDIATED HYPERSENSITIVITY (DELAYED)
		ANAPHYLAXIS–ALLERGY	ARTHUS	
Predominant antibody involved	IgG, IgM	IgE ($7S\gamma_1$ in guinea pig)	IgG	?
Predominant cell type involved	0	Mast cell	Polymorphonuclear leukocyte	Small lymphocyte
Complement	+	0	+	0
Mediators	0	Histamine, serotonin, slow-reacting substance, kinins	Lysosomal enzymes	Lymphokines
Principal type of injury	Cell destruction	Smooth muscle contraction	Basement membrane damage	Cell destruction (chronic inflammation)

tective to the host. On the other hand, if the cell is the host's erythrocyte, this reaction clearly is harmful.

The mechanism of lysis of erythrocytes by antibody has been carefully studied. For lysis to occur, antibody and complement are necessary; if complement is not present the antibody will agglutinate but will not lyse the cells. The end result of the interaction of antigenic determinants, antibody, and the eleven components of complement is the appearance of small holes, about 80-100 Å in diameter in the cell membrane, which in turn lead to loss of intracellular contents. Red-cell lysis by antibody and complement occurs typically in the case of mismatched transfusions when transfused cells are lysed by the antibodies present in the plasma of the recipient.

b. Indirect injury due to circulating antibodies—immediate hypersensitivity

Certain individuals, on first exposure to an antigen, react by becoming "sensitized" instead of merely immune. When such an individual is exposed a second time to the same antigen, the hypersensitivity reaction between antigen and immunoglobulin leads to release of pharmacologic agents from disrupted basophils and mast cells. These agents cause increased vascular permeability and smooth-muscle contraction. Since this occurs within a few minutes after antigen administration to the hypersensitive individual, it has been called an immediate hypersensitivity. When passively transferred, the antibody is capable of sensitizing the tissues of a previously unsensitized individual.

Histamine is the most important pharmacologic agent involved. The symptoms of many types of hypersensitivities can be mimicked by injection of histamine, and in the hypersensitive individual, a reaction can be ablated by antihistaminic drugs. When tissues taken from hypersensitive individuals are exposed to antigen *in vitro,* histamine is released. Recent studies have implicated other pharmacologic agents as well, however. These are: (1) "slow reacting substance," a material of unknown composition that can cause relatively slow contraction of smooth muscle; (2) bradykinin, a basic polypeptide that can cause contraction of smooth muscle, mediates increased vascular permeability, and is leukotaxic (see Chapter 3); and (3) serotonin (5-hydroxytryptamine), which causes broncho-constriction in the guinea pig, cat, and dog (Austen and Humphrey, 1963; Patterson, 1969). Some components of complement are also involved in these reactions.

In some cases of serum-mediated immediate hypersensitivity, the globulins involved (*reagins*) are somewhat different from other immunoglobulins and belong to the IgE class. They are heat labile, cannot be detected by conventional *in vitro* immunologic techniques, have an unusual affinity for skin and mucous membranes, and tend to become fixed to basophils and mast cells. The lack of a suitable tool for *in vitro* measurement of these antibodies has hampered research in immediate hypersensitivities. It has been suggested that they constitute an "abnormal" class, resulting from the splitting of normal immunoglobulins in such a way as to produce a cell-fixing antibody (Ishizaka and Ishizaka, 1968).

The cellular events leading to cell damage by these immunoglobulins are not completely understood. The IgE becomes fixed to specific receptors on the mast-cell surface in a particular conformational state; antigen then appears to bridge two combining sites on two antibody molecules. Degranulation then occurs, with the release of histamine and other pharmacologically active substances, and the complex of symptoms results from the action of these substances. In addition, aggregates of antigen and antibody are sometimes seen obstructing the pulmonary alveolar capillaries.

Anaphylaxis is an important example of immediate hypersensitivity. This occurs when antigen is administered parenterally to a sensitized host; pharmacologic agents are liberated throughout the body with a variety of serious consequences. In the guinea pig, the smooth muscle of the bronchi and bronchioles is the primary shock organ; contraction of these muscles renders the animal unable to exhale, and death is caused by suffocation. In the dog, the liver is primarily affected, with pooling of enormous quantities of circulating blood. In man, anaphylaxis is manifested by laryngeal edema, bronchospasm, and pulmonary edema, frequently leading to death.

The atopic hypersensitivities (commonly referred to as *allergies*), restricted almost entirely to man, are another important group of serum-mediated hypersensitivities, exemplified by hay fever. In this case, local administration of the antigen leads to local phenomena, such as edema of the mucosa of the nasal passages.

Not all individuals exposed to antigen develop hypersensitivity. On the other hand, most individuals who are allergic to one antigen are allergic to several antigens. Frequently several members of the same family are atopic. Thus, predisposition to atopic hypersensitivity is thought by some to be hereditary; but the evidence supporting this suggestion is circumstantial, and no known genetic mechanism is compatible with the existing data.

Atopic allergies are often treated by multiple injections of minute quantities of the offending allergen. Antigen administered in this fashion apparently induces a different type of antibody, known as the *blocking* antibody, which competes with the reagins upon natural exposure to the allergen. If the titer of blocking antibody is high enough, all antigen will be absorbed, and release of the pharmacologic agents will not occur. This process is not as simple as it seems; circulating antibody titers, for instance, give no clue to an individual's responsiveness or lack of responsiveness to a given allergen (Peterson, 1968).

c. Immune complex formation—Arthus reaction

Antigens and antibodies, usually of the IgG type, may combine in sensitized individuals as antigen-antibody complexes that attach to vascular basement membranes, fix complement, and initiate an acute inflammatory reaction with necrosis (Cochrane, 1968).

The pathogenesis of injury due to immune-complex formation is best exemplified by the Arthus phenomenon. Experimentally, the Arthus reaction is produced by injecting an antigen into the skin of an animal previously immunized to that antigen. Within thirty minutes to an hour the injected area becomes hemorrhagic, and if the reaction is severe, necrotic. This reaction is caused by the precipitation of antigen, antibody, and complement (the *immune complex*) in and around capillaries. The complement present in these precipitates acts as a chemotactic agent and attracts polymorphonuclear leukocytes, which are essen-

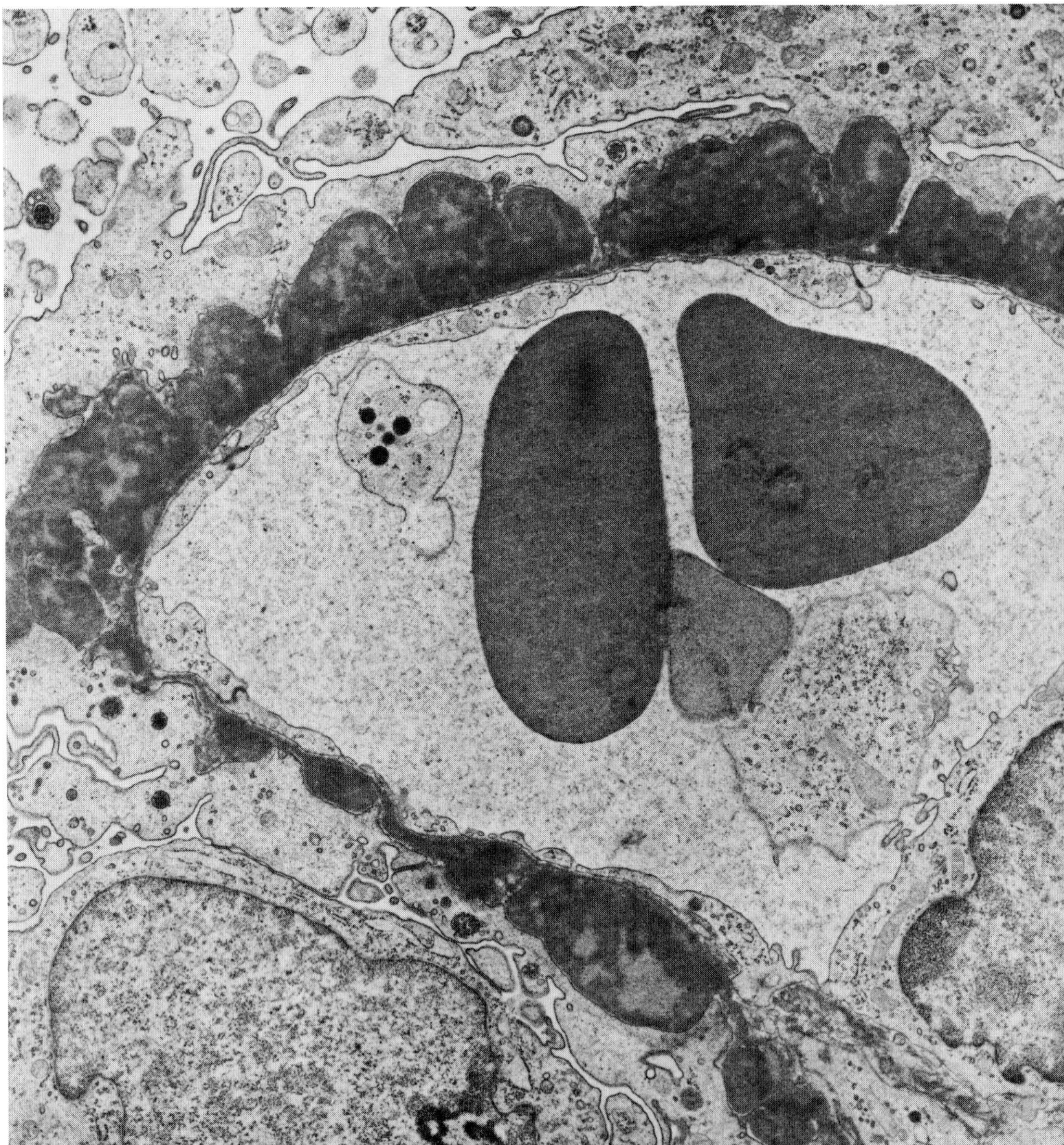

tial to the reaction. A classical, acute inflammatory reaction ensues, the area becomes edematous, and thrombi may form in the vessels; there is destruction of vascular walls and resulting hemorrhage and necrosis. The polymorphonuclear leukocytes contribute to the tissue destruction by releasing cathepsins (see Chapter 3).

By electron-microscopic observation, precipitates of antigen and antibody can be found in the vascular lumen, in the wall of the small vessels between the basement membrane and the endothelium, and in the perivascular spaces (Fig. 5-3). Thus, the Arthus reaction is essentially an acute inflammatory reaction related to deposition of immune complexes and release of enzymes from polymorphonuclear leukocytes.

The mechanism of injury described for the Arthus reaction is not only a laboratory finding but is present in human diseases in the form of serum sickness. This may be encountered in man after therapy involving administration of immune serum from another animal species and is characterized by precipitation of antigen-antibody complement complexes. The reaction may occur immediately after treatment if the patient was previously sensitive to the antigen, or it may be delayed for a week or more until the patient begins to produce antibodies; enough antigen may persist to form antigen-antibody complexes.

Although serum sickness is not a homogeneous entity, many of the symptoms caused by this mechanism are similar to those seen in the Arthus reaction. Patients with serum sickness develop inflammation associated with immune complex deposits in various organs (joints, lymph node, and kidney). This condition can be reproduced experimentally by injecting foreign protein intravenously into an immune animal. Soluble antigen-antibody complexes circulate in the bloodstream, bind complement, and are deposited in vascular lumina. Ultrastructural studies of the kidneys of rabbits during this time have demonstrated proliferation and swelling of the glomerular endothelium, often occluding the lumen.

d. Cell-mediated immunity—delayed hypersensitivity

Administration of certain antigens will lead to a series of cellular reactions resulting in the production of specifically reactive lymphocytes. These in turn will produce injury by means of a poorly known mechanism which may in part depend on cell-bound, non-circulating substances, when these lymphocytes accumulate at the site of the reaction. The term *delayed hypersensitivity* has been used to

Figure 5-3. Section of a loop of glomerular capillary, showing the heavy deposition of electron-opaque material on the basement membrane; this material can be shown to contain antigen and antibody. (Courtesy of J. Feldman)

identify this type of reaction, since it usually takes several days for it to become apparent (Turk, 1967).

As indicated earlier, delayed hypersensitivity is not dependent on humoral antibodies. It is believed to be an immunological phenomenon because of the following characteristics that are recognized as earmarks of immunological processes: an interval of several days is required between the immunizing injection and the appearance of a positive reaction to the test injection; the reaction is specific for the immunizing antigen; the reaction is mediated by cells of the lymphoid series. The most important consideration, however, for classifying delayed hypersensitivity as an immunological process is that it exhibits an essential characteristic of immune reactions: immunologic memory.

The prototype of delayed hypersensitivity is the tuberculin reaction, a reaction to the proteins of the tubercle bacillus. If one has been sufficiently exposed to *Mycobacterium tuberculosis* and is given an intradermal injection of tuberculin (an extract of the bacterium), the injection site becomes erythematous, indurated, and sometimes necrotic after about twenty-four hours. Histologically, the reaction site is infiltrated first with a small number of polymorphonuclear leukocytes, and later with lymphocytes and histiocytes. The hallmark of this reaction is perivascular accumulation of these mononuclear cells (See Fig. 5-2). The formation of these *granulomas* is typical of many delayed hypersensitivity reactions. A more complete description of granulomatous inflammation can be found in Chapter 3.

In man only, delayed hypersensitivity can be transferred with extracts of peripheral blood leukocytes; intact cells are not needed. Moreover, when delayed hypersensitivity is transferred by means of intact cells, only a small percentage of the transferred cells appear to participate in the reaction (Najarian and Feldman, 1961). Thus, the reaction may be initiated by only a few cells or their products. The cellular component that transfers delayed hypersensitivity in man has been called *transfer factor*. It has not yet been purified, but has been partially characterized. It is a stable substance unaffected by heating to 37° C for six hours or five months' storage at 20° C, and unaffected by treatment with DNase, RNase, or trypsin (Lawrence, 1959a). It is a dialyzable material with a molecular weight of less than 10,000 (Lawrence, 1963). When the transfer factor is administered to a normal recipient, he becomes hypersensitive within twenty-four hours. In contrast to the situation in passively transferred humoral or immediate hypersensitivity, the recipient of transfer factor may remain sensitive for as long as two years (Lawrence, 1959b). This long duration of hypersensitivity suggests that the transfer is not merely passive, since, if it were, the hypersensitivity in the recipient would decline in a few weeks–the length of time it takes for transferred antibody to be metabolized. Notwithstanding resistance of transfer factor to RNase treatment, these data on duration of transferred hypersensitivity have caused some investigators to suggest that transfer factor is a low-molecular-weight RNA. Possibly the transfer occurs by a mechanism analogous to bacterial transformation. Thus, the host cells would carry the information for the hypersensitivity, and the individual would remain sensitive for long periods of time. These studies on transfer factor fail to explain the mechanisms of the delayed response.

In vitro studies have shown that the antigen has marked effects on lymphoid cells taken from a hypersensitive animal. Depending on the concentration of the antigen, either cell death or cell proliferation may be observed. These reactions are specific for the antigen to which the individual is hypersensitive, and cannot be elicited in cells derived from a normal person.

Accepting, then, that antigen affects the sensitized cell, how does this antigen-cell interaction cause a lesion? One can only conjecture, but an attractive possibility is that some of the antigen injected into the skin diffuses from the site, retaining hypersensitive lymphocytes that generate mediators. These mediators, in turn, may attract non-specific monocytes and lead to release of toxic products from the monocytes. A substance that increases capillary permeability has recently been described in monocytes of hypersensitive animals (Willoughby and Spector, 1964). A recent book (Bloom and Glade, 1971) describes other possible mediators of this reaction.

Delayed hypersensitivity has important clinical implications. For example, the pathogenesis of tuberculosis appears to involve this mechanism. The tuberculosis organism itself is innocuous; it does not produce toxins, and it grows slowly. Pathogenicity is related to its ability to induce hypersensitivity in the host, which in turn results in an inflammatory lesion around the organism, just as the protein extract of the organism produces a lesion in the skin of the sensitized host. In fact, the lung lesion may be reproduced by placing proteins extracted from *M. tuberculosis* in the lungs of a tuberculin-sensitive animal (Crowle, 1962).

The delayed reaction is useful also in diagnosing the organism responsible for a particular disease. For example, *Mycobacterium tuberculosis* and *Histoplasma capsulatum*—two unrelated organisms—cause diseases that lead to remarkably similar symptoms, both characterized by delayed hypersensitivity. Extracts from each of the possible organisms can be given intradermally; the one corresponding to the infecting organism will produce the total skin reaction of delayed hypersensitivity.

The contact hypersensitivities, induced and elicited by application of the allergen to the skin, are a group of delayed hypersensitivities caused by extremely low-molecular-weight antigens. The molecular weight of many contact antigens is so low one would not expect them to be antigens. For example, some individuals become allergic to elemental gold or nickel and others to aniline dyes. Another example is poison ivy. These allergens are not complete antigens, but they do have the capacity to combine as haptens with skin proteins and thus become large enough to be complete antigens. Possibly the hapten-protein interaction changes the tertiary structures of the skin protein, to make this altered protein antigenic as well. In other respects, contact hypersensitivity is a typical delayed hypersensitivity. It is transferable by cells but not by serum; the reaction takes hours to develop; the inflammatory exudate consists primarily of mononuclear cells.

E. Immunologic Diseases

The processes described in the preceding section illustrate some of the basic mechanisms by which antigen-antibody reactions cause injury, producing pathologic manifestations either by primary action on cells or by the release of pharmacologic agents. Many disease entities that arise by these mechanisms have been described in humans and in experimental animals. These can be subdivided into three main categories: heterologous immunologic diseases if the antigens causing them are exogenous; auto-immune diseases if there is evidence that the causative antigens are autologous or endogenous; and finally, diseases dependent on complex immunological phenomena. These latter include the *collagen diseases,* so designated because of the localization of the secondary inflammatory reactions in the connective tissue.

1. Heterologous immunologic diseases

The allergic diseases, discussed in a previous section, constitute an important group of immunologic diseases due to external antigens. Other diseases with an immunologic component, poorly understood, are triggered by an external antigen. Examples are acute post-streptococcal glomerulonephritis and rheumatic fever, in which the kidney and the heart are the primary target organs of immunologic damage, leading to cardiac or renal failure. Other organs may be involved, though less severely.

These diseases occur after an infection with Group A streptococcus, and high titers of antibody to the streptococcus are usually present. The lesions seen in the myocardium of patients with rheumatic fever and in the kidney of those with glomerulonephritis have some similarities to those of serum sickness. Immune complexes, containing complement, are usually present in the glomeruli in acute glomerulonephritis; gamma globulins tend to deposit around vessels in rheumatic fever.

The steps in the development of immunologic tissue injury following streptococcal infection are not known. It has been suggested that the streptococcus is capable of (1) altering host tissue so as to render it antigenic, or (2) inducing the production of antibody that cross-reacts with host tissue (myocardium or glomerular basement membrane). In either case, the presence of antibodies capable of reacting with normal tissue components may lead to tissue injury.

Another group of diseases related to external antigens occurs after the administration of certain drugs. The no longer used drug Sedormid, for instance, is capable of sensitizing platelets, which are then susceptible to attack by antibodies that fix complement with lysis of the platelets. This occurs because Sedormid is a hapten; when combined with proteins of the platelet membrane, it is antigenic. The result is that the patient becomes deficient in platelets and may bleed quite severely from minor injuries. Similar mechanisms produce a variety of antibodies directed against other cells of the body.

2. Auto-immune diseases

Antibodies reactive with "self" antigens may arise by several means: (1) endogenous antigens can be altered in such a way as to be recognized as non-"self" by the immune mechanism, and the antibody is formed in response to what now appears to be a "foreign" antigen; (2) endogeneous substances such as thyroglobulin, which are inaccessible to the antibody-forming tissue, are normally never recognized as "self," although low levels of antibody to thyroglobulin may be present without injury. If large amounts of such a sequestered antigen reach the immunologically competent tissue–e.g., as a result of injury to the thyroid–antibody production to the antigen is induced; (3) a heritable alteration of the antibody-forming cells may result in abrogation of the property of self-recognition, although no data exist in support of this hypothesis. Cells thus altered and their progeny will be capable of producing antibodies to normal self-constituents, and a disease process will result. It is not yet known which of these explanations is correct; in fact, all may be incorrect.

It is important to realize that if one finds antibodies against an organ, this does not necessarily indicate auto-immune disease. In myocardial infarction, for instance, when heart muscle is severely injured, antibodies to heart-muscle protein frequently occur, but it is clear that they are not the cause of myocardial infarction. One must distinguish whether the antibody is a primary cause of the disease or the result of some damage not of immunological nature.

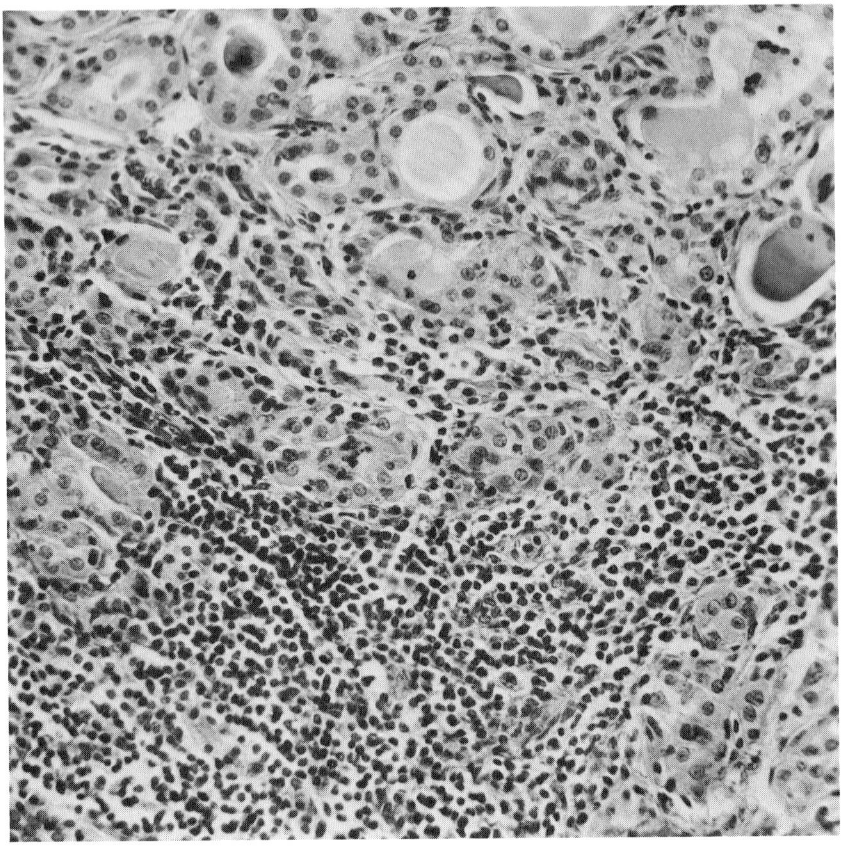

Figure 5-4. A section of thyroid from a patient with Hashimoto's thyroiditis, showing the typical lymphocytic infiltrate and some still fairly normal thyroid follicles.

For a disease to be defined as auto-immune, the following conditions should be satisfied: (1) the demonstration in the area of injury of antibodies to host tissue, or lymphoid cells capable of reacting with or attaching to host tissue or cells; (2) transfer of the disease with the patient's serum or lymphocytes; and (3) production of the disease experimentally by immunization or sensitization with the specific tissue antigen. These criteria are satisfied infrequently in human pathology.

A group of auto-immune diseases are the so-called auto-immune hematologic disorders, e.g., auto-immune hemolytic anemia. In these the circulating blood cells and the fixed bone-marrow cells are the target cells of circulating antibodies. The disease can be transferred passively by transferring circulating antibodies. They are detectable on the cells and in the serum. Antibodies can be of two varieties: incomplete (warm) antibodies, which react at 37° C and are usually 7S immunoglobulins; and complete (cold) antibodies, which react at 2 to

5° C and are found in the 19S macroglobulin fraction. The antibodies are specific, and the antigen is usually found in the Rh group of antigens. The sensitization mechanism is not very clear but may involve any of the mechanisms previously mentioned. The destruction of red cells by lysis or hemagglutination and erythrophagocytosis in the spleen leads to chronic insufficiency of circulating red cells, known as *anemia*.

Hashimoto's thyroiditis, or auto-immune thyroiditis, is another example of auto-immune disease. The antigen appears to be thyroglobulin or another of the constituents of colloid. Patients with this disease have circulating complement that fixes antibodies to thyroid, and lymphoid cells that destroy the thyroid *in vivo* by direct invasion and attach to thyroid epithelium in tissue culture. Histologically, one observes lymphocytic infiltration of the thyroid with destruction of the epithelium (Fig. 5-4). Eventually, progressive loss of thyroid leads to functional inadequacy or hypothyroidism.

There are many other diseases that may have an auto-immune component. In cases where the cause of a disease is obscure, it is easy to ascribe an auto-immune etiology, particularly if one observes auto-antibodies, elevated levels of circulating immunoglobulins, large numbers of plasma cells in the tissue, and a destructive disease characterized by dense lymphocytic infiltration, or if one demonstrates complement or antibody in the affected tissue by immunofluorescent or other techniques. In most cases, however, rigorous demonstration of an auto-immune etiology is lacking. In the two diseases cited, auto-immunity appears to be clearly implicated.

3. Diseases due to complex immunologic phenomena

These diseases are also known as *collagen diseases,* and comprise lupus erythematosus, rheumatoid arthritis, dermatomyositis, polyarteritis, scleroderma, and similar disorders. In these, one can demonstrate affinity of the gamma globulin and lymphocytes of the host for tissue constituents. At least some of the damage is produced by antibodies associated with these constituents. The affinity can be demonstrated by serologic techniques, such as complement fixation, hemagglutination, and antiglobulin consumption, by fluorescent antibody techniques, or by the culturing of lymphocytes in mixed cultures.

An important example of these diseases is lupus erythematosus, characterized by pathologic changes occurring in the vasculature and connective tissue of many organs and leading to a spectrum of symptoms. A wide variety of auto-antibodies to nuclear and cytoplasmic constituents has been identified in the serum of patients with this disease, but the exact relation of these to the pathogene-

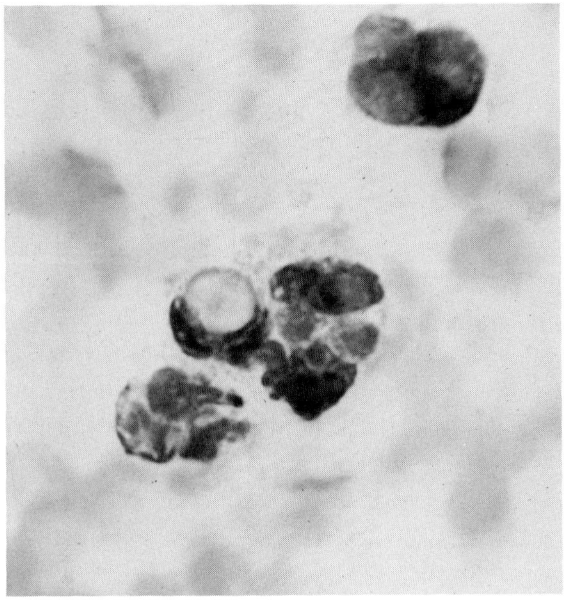

Figure 5-5. Characteristic LE cell in blood smear of a patient with systemic lupus.

sis of the disease remains obscure for the most part. In spite of the fact that so many different auto-antigens are present, passive transfer of serum does not cause disease in the recipient. Antigen-antibody complexes also appear to play some role in the pathogenesis of this disease.

One aspect of the disease clearly does have an immunologic pathogenesis and leads to severe disability. This is the deposition of immune complexes in the renal glomeruli, leading to immune-complex nephritis that may be progressive and ultimately lethal.

Advantage has been taken of the presence of certain 7S antibodies directed against nuclear components in devising a diagnostic test. When serum from a patient with lupus erythematosus is incubated *in vitro* with white blood cells from his own or other blood, an "LE cell" forms (Fig. 5-5). This phenomenon results when a damaged nucleus interacts with antibody and is then phagocytosed by an intact phagocytic cell, usually a neutrophil. This mechanism seems, however, to have little if any relation to the production of disease.

Auto-antibodies can be demonstrated in a number of other collagen diseases. In these other diseases, however, the relation of auto-antibodies to the pathogenesis of the lesions is even less clear. In rheumatoid arthritis, for instance, a complex mechanism for the formation of auto-antibodies exists. Aggregated 7S globulin of indeterminate origin becomes antigenic, and both 19S and 7S antibodies, known as *rheumatoid factor,* are formed to this aggregate and can be demonstrated in the serum of patients with well-developed rheumatoid arthritis. Antibodies similar to but not identical with gamma globulin can be found in the sera of patients with other, unrelated diseases such as bacterial endocarditis, tuberculosis, syphilis–all characterized by prolonged, continuous exposure to an external antigen, and in some individuals who are repeatedly immunized to the same antigen.

Manifestations of rheumatoid arthritis cannot be induced by passive transfer of antibodies, however, and there is no other evidence at present that these antibodies are responsible for the chronic progressive destruction of articular surfaces which characterizes rheumatoid arthritis. Some have pointed to the lymphoid aggregates and occasional granulomas seen in this disease as evidence of the role of cellular hypersensitivity in the pathogenesis; proof of this is also lacking.

4. Experimental models

Experimental models exist for the study of auto-immune disease involving either circulating antibodies or cell-mediated immunity. The usual method of production of these diseases is to inject autologous, homologous, or heterologous tissues in conjunction with Freund's adjuvant. Both circulating and cell-bound antibodies will result. For maximal usefulness of the model, the pathologic manifestations should appear in the tissue corresponding to that which is used as antigen, and the damage should be comparable to what is caused by similar diseases in humans. Diseases produced in this fashion are very numerous. Those that have been most thoroughly studied are thyroiditis, glomerulonephritis, and experimental allergic encephalomyelitis. Attempts have been made to produce uveitis, orchitis, adrenalitis, atrophic gastritis, and so on.

Thyroiditis, corresponding to Hashimoto's thyroiditis in humans, has been produced in rats, guinea pigs, rabbits, and dogs by using thyroglobulin and epithelial thyroid antigens as the inducing agent. Cell-bound immunity has been demonstrated, and usually the severity of the disease correlates with this. Circulating antibody has also been shown to exist, however, and the disease can be transferred with serum. The typical mononuclear infiltration and destruction of the thyroid present in the clinical disease is also seen experimentally.

Several animal models for glomerulonephritis have been developed. Models exist for immune-complex nephritis, in which sustained levels of circulating immune complexes are achieved utilizing various antigens. The diseases are very similar to human immune-complex disease, as seen in post-streptococcal glomerulonephritis, or lupus glomerulonephritis. A model for another type of glomerulonephritis with formation of anti-basement-membrane antibody has also been achieved by immunizing animals with basement membranes prepared from other species. This condition, which can be transferred to non-immunized homologous animals with serum from immunized animals, is similar to that seen in Goodpasture's syndrome in human beings.

The experimental allergic encephalomyelitis produced primarily in monkeys, but also in dogs, rabbits, guinea pigs, rats, and mice, has also been seen in human subjects who have been given rabies vaccine prepared by growing the virus in rabbit spinal cord. The antigen contained in the vaccine is associated with myelin in the white matter of the rabbit central nervous system. Circulating antibodies to myelin are quite prominent, are toxic to the central nervous system cells in tissue cultures, and destroy myelin. Cellular sensitivity has also been shown to exist, and the disease can be transferred with lymphocytes. The pathologic changes are characteristic, consisting of demyelination with a concomitant inflammatory process, both acute and chronic, and production of gliosis during repair. The axons are not affected by the pathologic process. It is still not clear what the human counterpart of this experimental auto-immune disease is. The encephalomyelitides, which are seen after viral infections, and multiple sclerosis have been suggested, but no clear-cut evidence can be offered.

The importance of auto-immune reactions in human pathology has been well documented by laboratory experiments. The foregoing discussion has revealed, however, that basic concepts of auto-immune disease are still in need of much clarification. In many cases the pathogenesis is still in doubt, the antigens are not clearly known, and even the auto-immune nature of the disease may be questionable, since the original etiologic agent may be something other than an antigen. Be that as it may, in cases where a reasonably clear endogenous antigenic component, an exogenous cross-reacting antigenic component, or a combination of the two, can be demonstrated, and where a reasonable pathogenetic mechanism can be delineated, one is usually justified in calling the pathologic entities auto-immune diseases.

F. Organ Transplantation

The study of tolerance and of its counterpart–rejection–has occupied immunologists for a long time, since it was hoped that through an understanding of these phenomena the use of organ transplantation in humans could become feasible. Although great advances have been made toward elucidating the mechanisms regulating histocompatibility, the ultimate goal of transplantation without rejection still eludes the physician. Progress in surgical techniques has essentially eliminated the purely technical obstacles to transplant surgery and has made even more pressing the need for a deeper understanding of histocompatibility and of immunosuppression in order to achieve a very low degree of homograft rejection (Merrill, 1967).

Many of the characteristics of this reaction have been determined by using skin grafts on inbred mouse strains. When a skin graft is placed on a mouse of a strain different from the strain of the skin donor, initially the graft will appear to take. That is, it will begin to heal, become vascularized, and appear to become part of the skin of the recipient. After several days, immunization has been achieved, mononuclear cells invade the graft bed, thrombosis and failure of the blood supply occur, and eventually the graft is sloughed. If a second graft from the same donor is placed on the recipient, the events of graft rejection will be qualitatively unchanged but greatly accelerated. Thus, the first graft immunizes the recipient (Wilson and Billingham, 1967).

Homotransplantation reactions are typically placed in the category of delayed hypersensitivity inasmuch as passive immunity (accelerated graft rejection) is accomplished by transfer of lymphoid cells but not, except under unusual circumstances, after transfer of serum. Accelerated graft rejection has also occurred, however, when the transferred lymphoid cells are contained within diffusion chambers. These chambers are built so as to prohibit the movement of cells out of them, but soluble material diffuses freely. Thus, graft rejection appears to be mediated primarily by cellular mechanisms. Nevertheless, it may also be facilitated by humoral mechanisms.

Humoral antibodies are clearly involved in one uncommon type of graft rejection, the so-called "white graft" reaction. The rejection events are different from those described above in that the graft is not vascularized, and sloughing occurs very rapidly. The white-graft reaction occurs in animals having humoral antibody to the graft and is transferable by serum. Thus, the white-graft reaction is probably mediated by humoral antibodies.

Complete success in homotransplantation is assured only if the donor and recipient are genetically identical. If only those antigens already present in the recipient are administered with the graft, an immune response will not be elicited. Transplantation is therefore possible between identical twins and between experimental animals of the same inbred strain, but in mice a change at only one genetic locus is sufficient to cause rejection. In spite of this, a considerable degree of success has been attained in human homotransplantation with drugs that suppress the immune response. Unfortunately, treatment with these drugs does not completely eliminate the rejection response, and it also decreases the patient's resistance to infectious agents. It is encouraging, however, that the recent development of a variety of methods of suppressing the immune response has allowed the physician more flexibility. One hopes for eventual selective ability to inhibit transplantation rejection with minimal interference with other immune mechanisms.

References

Abramoff, P., and La Via, M. F. (1970), Biology of the Immune Response, McGraw-Hill, New York.

Ackerman, G. A. (1967), Developmental relationship between the appearance of lymphocytes and lymphopoietic activity in the thymus and lymph nodes of the fetal cat, Anat. Rec., *158*:387.

Austen, K. F., and Humphrey, J. H. (1963), *In vitro* studies of the mechanism of anaphylaxis, Adv. Immunol., *3*:3.

Bloom, B. R. (1971), *In vitro* approaches to the mechanism of cell mediated immune reactions, Adv. Immunol., *13*:101.

Bloom, B. R., and Glade, P. R. (1971), *In vitro* methods in cell-mediated immunity, Academic Press, New York.

Cannon, J. A., Terasaki, P. I., and Longmire, W. P., Jr. (1958), Unexpected manifestations of induced tolerance to skin homografts in the chicken, Ann. N. Y. Acad. Sci., *73*:862.

Chase, M. W. (1946), The cellular transfer of cutaneous hypersensitivity, J. Bact., *51*:643.

Cochrane, C. G. (1968), Immunologic tissue injury mediated by neutrophilic leukocytes, Adv. Immunol., *9*:97.

Cooper, M. D., Perey, D. Y., Peterson, R. D. A., Gabrielson, A. E., and Good, R. A. (1968), The two-component concept of the lymphoid system, *in* Immunologic Deficiency Diseases of Man, R. A. Good, Ed., The National Foundation–March of Dimes, New York.

Crowle, A. J. (1962), Delayed Hypersensitivity in Health and Disease, p. 18, Charles C Thomas Co., Springfield, Ill.

Edelman, G. M., and Gall, W. E. (1969), The antibody problem, Ann. Rev. Biochem., *38*:415.

Fowler, R., Jr., Schubert, W. K., and West, C. D. (1960), Acquired partial tolerance to homologous skin grafts in the human infant at birth, Ann. N. Y. Acad. Sci., *87*:403.

Gell, P. G. H., and Benacerraf, B. (1961), Delayed hypersensitivity to simple protein antigens, Adv. Immunol., *1*:319.

Humphrey, J. H., and Dourmashkin, R. R. (1969), The lesions in cell membranes caused by complement, Adv. Immunol., *11*:75.

Ishizaka, K., and Ishizaka, T. (1968), Human reaginic antibodies and immunoglobulin E., J. Allergy, *42*:330.
Janeway, C. A. (1968), Syndromes of diminished resistance to infection, J. Pediat., *72*:885.
Katz, D. A., and Benacerraf, B. (1972), The regulatory influence of activated T cells on B cell responses to antigen, Adv. Immunol., *15*:2.
Koch, F., Schultze, H. E., and Schwick, G. (1959), Macroglobulin determination in the blood of healthy children during the first year of life, Arch. Kinderheilk., *3*:199.
Landsteiner, K. (1936), The Specificity of Serological Reactions, Charles C Thomas Co., Springfield, Ill.
Lawrence, H. S. (1959a), Cellular and Humoral Aspects of the Hypersensitive States, p. 279, Harper and Hoeber, New York.
Lawrence, H. S. (1959b), Homograft sensitivity. An expression of the immunologic origins and consequences of individuality, Physiol. Rev., *39*:811.
Lawrence, H. S. (1963a), General perspectives, *in* Cell Bound Antibodies, p. 3. B. Amos and H. Koprowski, Eds., Wistar Inst. Press, Philadelphia.
Lawrence, H. S. (1963b), Transfer of immunological information in humans with dialysates of leukocyte extracts, Trans. Assoc. Am. Phys., *76*:84.
Mackay, I. R., and Burnett, F. M. (1965), Autoimmunity: experimental and clinical aspects, Ann. N. Y. Acad. Sci., *124*:Parts I and II.
Mage, R. G., and Kabat, E. A. (1963), Immunological studies on dextrans, J. Immunol., *91*:633.
Maurer, P. H., Gerulat, B. F., and Pinchuck, P. (1963), Antigenicity of polypeptides (poly-a-amino acids). V. Studies in rabbits, J. Immunol., *90*:381.
Medawar, P. (1957), The Uniqueness of the Individual, Basic Books, New York.
Merrill, J. P. (1967), Human tissue transplantation, Adv. Immunol., *7*:275.
Müller-Eberhard, H. J. (1968), Chemistry and reaction mechanisms of complement, Adv. Immunol., *8*:1.
Najarian, J. S., and Feldman, J. D. (1961), Passive transfer of tuberculin sensitivity by initiated thymidine labeled lymphoid cells, J. Exp. Med., *114*:779.
Patterson, R. (1969), Laboratory models of reaginic allergy, Progress in Allergy, *13*:332.
Peterson, R. D. A. (1968), Allergy: Status and perspectives, J. Ped., *73*:436.
Prausnitz, C., and Kustner, H. (1962), Studies on hypersensitivity, *in* Clinical Aspects of Immunology, translation, p. 808, P. G. H. Gell and R. R. A. Coombs, Eds., F. A. Davis Co., Philadelphia.
Schinckel, P. G., and Ferguson, K. A. (1953), Skin transplantation in the foetal lamb, Aust. J. Biol. Sci., *6*:533.
Sell, S. (1972), Immunology, Immunopathology, and Immunity, Harper & Row, New York.
Shaffer, J. H., Lo Grippo, G. A., and Chase, M. W. (1959), Mechanisms of Hypersensitivity, Little, Brown and Co., Boston.
Silverstein, A. M., Uhr, J. W., Kraner, K. L., and Lukes, P. J. (1963), Fetal response to antigenic stimulus. II. Antibody production by the fetal lamb, J. Exp. Med., *117*:799.

Smith, R. T., Good, R. A., and Miescher, P. A. (1966), Phylogeny of Immunity, University of Florida Press, Gainesville.

Smith, R. T., Good, R. A., and Miescher, P. A. (1967), Ontogeny of Immunity, University of Florida Press, Gainesville.

Talmage, D. W., and Cann, J. R. (1961), The Chemistry of Immunity in Health and Disease, Charles C Thomas Co., Springfield, Ill.

Turk, J. L. (1967), Cytology of the induction of hypersensitivity, Brit. Med. Bul., *23*:3.

Unanue, E. R. (1972), The regulatory role of macrophages in antigenic stimulation, Adv. Immunol., *15*:95.

Willoughby, D. A., and Spector, W. G. (1964), The lymph node permeability factor: a possible mediator of the delayed hypersensitivity reaction, Ann. N. Y. Acad. Sci., *116*:874.

Wilson, D. B., and Billingham, R. E. (1967), Lymphocytes and transplantation immunity, Adv. Immunol., *7*:189.

Wolfe, H. R., Mueller, A. P., Neess, J., and Tempelis, C. (1957), Precipitin production in chickens. XVI. The relationship of age to antibody production, J. Immunol., *79*:142.

6

NEOPLASIA

Richmond T. Prehn, M.D.

A. Components of the Physiology of Neoplasia

1. Somatic cell variation

Higher animals are composed of vast numbers of interacting and often highly specialized cells, e.g., liver cells, epidermal cells, myocytes, and nerve cells. Each cell type behaves like a separate species in that each reproduces its own kind. No way has yet been found to induce a liver cell to produce, by mitosis, anything but another liver cell. Nevertheless, it is the present belief that there are no genetic differences among cell types, but that they are merely pseudospecies. The non-genetic changes during ontogeny that result in these different pseudospecies of specialized cells are termed *epigenetic* changes. This ontological process of cellular pseudospeciation is called *differentiation* (Harris, 1964).

There is a further aspect of differentiation: namely, the further specializations that occur within each cellular pseudospecies of the adult animal. For example, the epidermal cell population of the skin is not homogeneous but consists of basal cells and cells in various stages of keratinization. The mitotic activity of the epidermal pseudospecies is usually confined to the cells on the basement membrane, the basal cells. Mitosis of these cells produces more basal cells as well as cells which lose the capacity to divide but acquire the specialized capacity to produce keratin. Since the keratin-producing progeny cannot divide, no new pseudospecies is formed. The cells that retain the capacity to divide, and therefore to continue the cellular pseudospecies, are commonly termed *stem cells*. Normal differentiation thus may include loss of the capability to divide, as in the case of keratinizing cells of the epidermis, neurons of the adult central nervous system, and the multinucleated contractile cells of striated muscle.

The mechanisms that regulate normal differentiation are largely unknown. It is evident that cell-to-cell interactions often trigger the modifications of gene expression that occur. These interactions may be mediated at the cell surface. Repression of certain nuclear genes and activation of others may result–i.e., the transcription of particular genic messages to RNA may be started or stopped. Alternatively or additionally, translation of particular messages from RNA into protein may be initiated or halted. In any event, the end result is that in the differentiated cell only a small part of the genome is expressed in the cellular phenotype. What distinguishes a liver cell from a kidney cell is that small, only partially overlapping portions of their common genomes are expressed (Harris, 1964).

Differentiation is ordinarily quite stable. It is heritable through many cell generations. Most differentiated cells, however, retain a restricted range of variability, being able to undergo certain changes of phenotype in response to environmental stimuli. A common example is *squamous metaplasia* in the bronchus, in which basal cells differentiate into squamous cells instead of the usual columnar cells. It is commonly observed as a consequence of cigarette smoking or vitamin A deficiency. Since it is apparently a reversible condition, it is not usually considered a new differentiation but is termed a *modulation*. It is probably more dependent upon a continued environmental stimulus than upon a change in cellular heredity (Harris, 1964).

In mammalian systems differentiation usually implies an increased specialization accompanied by a restriction of the cell's potentialities to perform other functions or to give rise to other cell types. Increased specialization, however, does not necessarily and inevitably imply a restriction of totipotency. This is illustrated in its most extreme form in plant materials. Here a highly specialized cell from a mature plant can sometimes regenerate the entire organism–it has retained all the totipotency of the seed itself. Thus, the term *differentiation* is used somewhat ambiguously in mammalian systems to refer to either or both of two properties that are not necessarily correlated (Harris, 1964).

Although epigenetic mechanisms probably account for most and perhaps all of normal differentiation, there is another form of somatic cell variation. This is somatic mutation. It is not known whether any normal processes are dependent upon it.

Neoplasia, as we shall see, is a form of abnormal somatic cell variation, due to somatic mutation and/or aberrant and defective differentiation; the result is a pathologic form of hyperplasia.

2. Hyperplasia

Not only do cellular interactions play important and poorly understood roles in regulating differentiation, but they are also vital to the regulation of tissue and organ mass. An increase in the size of an adult tissue or organ due to an increase in the number of cells is termed *hyperplasia*. Hyperplasia can be arbitrarily divided into two different but often overlapping types: (1) physiologic; and (2) pathologic or neoplastic. Physiologic hyperplasia is a normal reaction of a tissue to a variety of environmental stimuli. Perhaps the most commonly observed example is the thickening of the epidermis that occurs in response to trauma. This particular example has been analyzed in greater detail than most and deserves discussion as a general prototype.

It has been observed that any circumstance that kills and/or removes cells in the superficial epidermal layers results in an increase in mitotic activity in the basal layer. Increase of cell production in the basal layer leads to a restitution of the superficial layers, and this more than restores the original state. This restitution and overshoot is termed *compensatory hyperplasia*. If the stimulus that originally initiated the process is not recurrent, the mitotic activity in the basal layer eventually subsides and the hyperplasia disappears. Physiologic hyperplasia is thus dependent upon continued application of the external stimulus.

It is, of course, axiomatic that in any tissue at mass equilibrium the rate of formation of new cells must be exactly balanced by the rate of cell death. In a tissue like the epidermis this means that, on the average, exactly half the progeny resulting from mitosis in the basal layer must follow the pathway of cellular differentiation that leads to keratin formation and to eventual cell death. Hyperplasia will be self-limiting only when this ratio is maintained or restored.

The observation that removal of the superficial layers results in mitotic activity in the basal layer led to the hypothesis that the superficial layers were inhibitory to the basal. It has now been demonstrated that the keratinizing layers produce a mitotic inhibitor. The inhibitor has been partially purified and called a *chalone* (Bullough *et al.*, 1967). It does not appear to be specific to the animal species. One can, however, anticipate that different chalones probably occur in different tissues.

Chalones are chemical inhibitors that operate at short range, i.e., near their points of origin. Longer range regulatory substances, both stimulatory and inhibitory, have been identified in some tissues. The hormones, somatotropin, gonadotrophin, and estrogen are good examples. Also, there are very short-range regulatory effects at the level of cell-to-cell contact, called *contact inhibition of mitosis* (Harris, 1964). Thus it is clear that there are many interacting mechanisms and controls of cell growth and division.

Neoplastic hyperplasia differs from the physiologic type just described, in that it involves a change in the intrinsic cellular heredity. This intrinsic cellular change produces a race of cells less subject to the normal tissue regulatory mechanisms. In the skin, for example, this may mean that neoplastic cells produce less chalone and/or are less sensitive to the inhibitory effects of chalone. In this race of cells, cellular maturation or differentiation is defective; somewhat less than 50 per cent of the daughter cells in the basal layer are set on the pathway to keratinization. Of course, a fall in the proportion of differentiated cells implies a fall in the level of the chalone, though this may not always be the case. Some neoplastic hyperplasias have a lower than normal mitotic rate, but the tissue continues to expand because of the imbalance in the ratio between stem-cell renewal and differentiation. The molecular reasons for this imbalance are unknown.

B. Characteristics of Tumors

1. Definition

Neoplasia may be defined as *that form of hyperplasia which is caused, at least in part, by an intrinsic heritable abnormality in the involved cells.* Although it is difficult to define a condition before it is fully understood, this definition successfully excludes those conditions not usually regarded as neoplastic, while it encompasses all that are.

It is apparent that this definition includes two portions. The first, that neoplasia is a form of pathological hyperplasia, needs no justification. The second, relating to a heritable cell variation, requires evidence derived from experiments of the following kind in animals. Animal neoplasms can be transplanted from animal to animal by the inoculation of living neoplastic cells. This can be done serially *ad infinitum,* provided that immunity to the foreign neoplastic cells is eliminated by some technique. It can be shown with the aid of chromosomal or antigenic markers that the cells of the new neoplasms arising in the recipient animals are usually the progeny of the transplanted cells rather than of cells of the recipient. In man the process of metastasis supplies somewhat similar evidence; neoplastic cells are carried by the bloodstream or by lymphatics to sites distant from their place of origin. Here they set up neoplasms of the parental cell type. Recently, the inadvertent transplantation of neoplasia during kidney transplantations has also provided evidence of the heritable nature of the disease at the cell level.

From what has been said, it is obvious that neoplasia is a disease characterized by abnormal cell behavior and abnormal interactions among cells. The cells of a neoplasm do not behave in the highly integrated, interdependent manner of normal metazoan cell populations. Thus, neoplasia can perhaps be looked upon as an imperfect cellular reversion to a more primitive, ancestral cell type, in which some of the regulatory mechanisms that normally operate among metazoan cells are defective or absent. This seeming atavism results in abnormalities of function, growth, and territorial behavior. Before going on to discuss in greater detail the characteristics of neoplastic cells, however, it is necessary to consider briefly the conditions of pseudoneoplasia that may closely mimic actual neoplasia.

2. Mimicry of neoplasia

It is not sufficient that a definition of neoplastic hyperplasia specify a change in cellular heredity; it must further specify that this change is present in those cells directly involved in the hyperplasia. Otherwise, some diseases closely related to neoplasia, but not usually regarded as true neoplasms, would not be definitionally excluded. An excellent example of such a disease that mimics neoplasia is pernicious or Addisonian anemia. This disease is characterized by a massive hyperplasia of immature erythroid cells in the bone marrow. Anemia, seen in the peripheral blood, results from the failure of these cells to mature. The ratio of proliferating stem cells to maturing non-reproductive cells has been altered. And yet, although the condition is due to an alteration in cellular heredity, the lesion exists, not in the cells of the hematopoietic system undergoing the hyperplasia, but rather in cells of the stomach which normally provide a factor necessary for the absorption of vitamin B-12. This vitamin in turn is required for the maturation or differentiation of erythrocytes. Pernicious anemia is thus a disease very similar in most characteristics to a true neoplasm. It is, furthermore, a disease that can be corrected by the injection of a cell-maturing factor.

Chronic physiologic hyperplasia may simulate neoplasia in almost all its histologic features. The distinction may be difficult even for an experienced pathologist. The two types of hyperplasia, neoplastic and physiologic, are often present simultaneously in varying degree in one and the same lesion. Cells with a heritable abnormality are often capable of responding to some extent to an environmental stimulus.

3. The growth curve

It is often thought that tumor growth is simply exponential. There is, however, considerable evidence that this is not strictly the case. With most experimen-

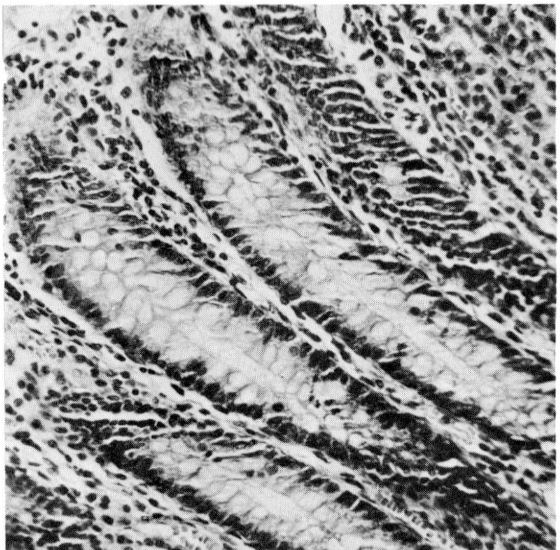

a

Figure 6-1. Photomicrographs of tumors of the colon.

a. This tissue from a benign adenomatous polyp is virtually indistinguishable from normal colonic mucosa. The lamina propria consists of appropriate quantities of connective tissue and various mononuclear cells, and the epithelium of the crypt is regular with normal mucous production in the apical portion of the cells. A few mitoses are seen.

b. In this section from a moderately well differentiated adenocarcinoma, the epithelium is lined up to form glandular spaces with the stroma approximating the appearance of lamina propria. The nuclei of the cancerous epithelium are very

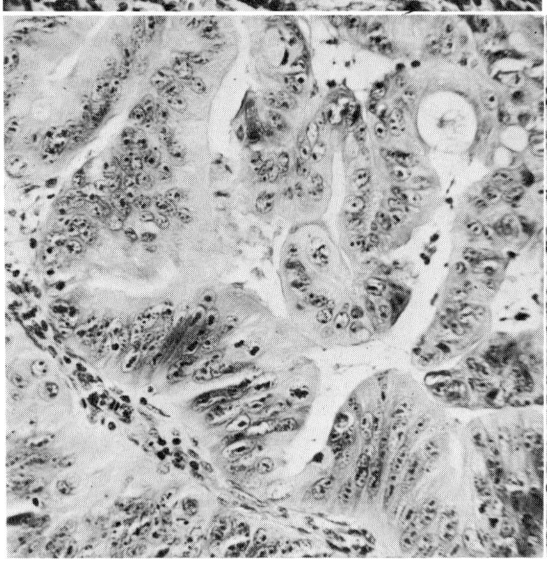

b

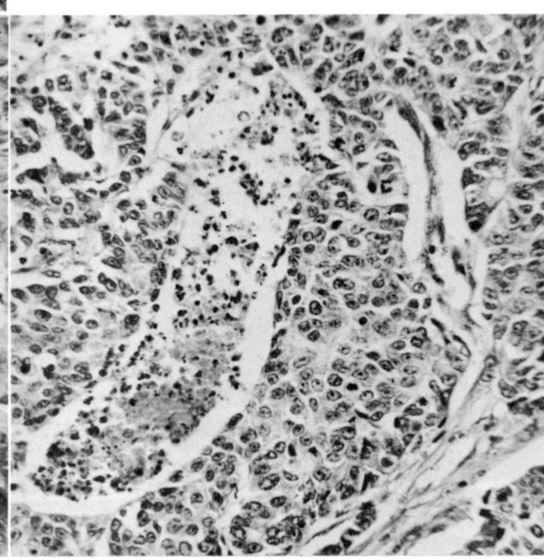

c

irregular in size and shape, and staining qualities. Mitoses are quite numerous. The amount of mucus production is greatly decreased, and the cells are in a considerable degree of disarray with respect to the stroma and the lumen of the "gland."

c. In this example of a rather poorly differentiated adenocarcinoma of the colon, it is difficult to identify a glandular lumen, and the cancerous epithelium does not line up at all but tends to form masses of cancer cells. Some fibrous stroma is still present. In the center the cancerous tissue has become necrotic, presumably because of lack of blood supply, and a mass of dead cells can be seen.

tal tumors it can be demonstrated that the rate of tumor growth decreases with time (Laird, 1965). Complex mathematical functions have been presented by several workers to describe this relation. These curves imply that even the most malignant and fast-growing tumors would eventually reach plateaus of little further growth if the animals lived long enough. Unfortunately, death usually occurs while the tumors are still in the almost purely exponential portions of their growth curves. With more benign tumors, a plateau is often reached within the life span of the animal, and unless further neoplastic progression occurs, the lesion may remain virtually stationary in size. The reasons for this type of behavior are not known.

The fact that immunity may alter tumor growth rates will be discussed in a subsequent section. Nevertheless, it may be appropriate, in connection with tumor growth curves, to point out at this time that in one experimental tumor system, two populations of tumor stem cells have been demonstrated. One of these was non-replicating. If immunity was blocked, part of the non-replicating subpopulation of stem cells underwent mitosis (DeCosse and Gelfant, 1968). It would seem that an immune reaction—at least in the systems studied—was capable of reversibly blocking mitosis in a small but variable percentage of the tumor-cell population. It may be that a mechanism such as this can contribute to the complexity of tumor growth curves.

4. Benign and malignant

Neoplasia may involve any vertebrate tissue or organ whose cells are capable of division. The cellular defect may be very mild, the cells hardly varying from their normal counterpart, or it may be so severe that the normal differentiated counterpart is utterly unrecognizable in the distorted cells of the neoplasm. This continuum of differing degrees of aberration is customarily divided into two or sometimes three categories.

Those neoplasms that are highly differentiated and thus differ only minimally in morphology and behavior from their tissue of origin are generally termed *benign,* even though they may rarely prove fatal (Fig. 6-1a). These lesions are usually relatively slow-growing, and the individual cells may in extreme cases be morphologically indistinguishable from the corresponding normal cells. They remain localized and inflict damage by spatial encroachment on normal tissues.

At the other extreme, those neoplasms showing marked cellular atypia and marked deficiency of differentiation (anaplasia) are termed *malignant,* even though cures may sometimes be effected (Fig. 6-1b, c). A *cancer* is a malignant neoplasm. Cancers of ectodermal or endodermal derivation are usually called *carcinomas,* while those of mesodermal origin are, with few exceptions, termed *sarcomas.* The cells of a malignant lesion are usually aneuploid and have a variety of chromosomal abnormalities. There is often much pleomorphism (variation from cell to cell in morphology). Multiple nucleoli are common and the cells are usually larger than normal, with large nuclei and large nuclear-cytoplasmic size ratios. There is often a deficiency of rough endoplasmic reticulum with an increase in the number of free ribosomes. Mitoses are often numerous in tissue sections and are frequently abnormal. The malignant cell's most important characteristic, however, is a tendency to lose to a variable extent its normal adhesiveness to its neighbors. Cell-to-cell contact is decreased and ionic communication between cells is diminished. The cells acquire an increased propensity for ameboid migration away from their site of origin. This tendency is seen in the entry of neoplastic cells into lymphatics, blood vessels, or the pleural or peritoneal cavities. In this manner they may be widely disseminated and may establish new and distant secondary sites of neoplastic growth. It is this process, called *metastasis,* that so often defeats attempts at curative surgical excision. Because of its overriding clinical importance, it is the capacity to metastasize, whether it is realized or potential, that is the hallmark of malignancy.

Between these two extremes is a group of lesions that exhibit the cytologic and morphologic characteristics of malignancy but lack any evidence of invasive tendencies. Such a lesion is commonly called a *carcinoma in situ* (Fig. 6-2).

The existence of carcinoma *in situ* demonstrates dramatically that there is no certain correspondence between the cytologic features usually associated with malignancy and the actual propensity to metastasize. Nonetheless, the experienced pathologist can usually arrive at a reasonable estimate of malignant potential by studying cytologic and, especially, histologic evidence. There is no single criterion for this difficult judgment.

It has been a useful practice in the evaluation of malignant neoplasia to assign histologic grades. For this purpose the grading system introduced by Broders is most commonly used. In this system the lesions are rated on a scale of 1 to 4,

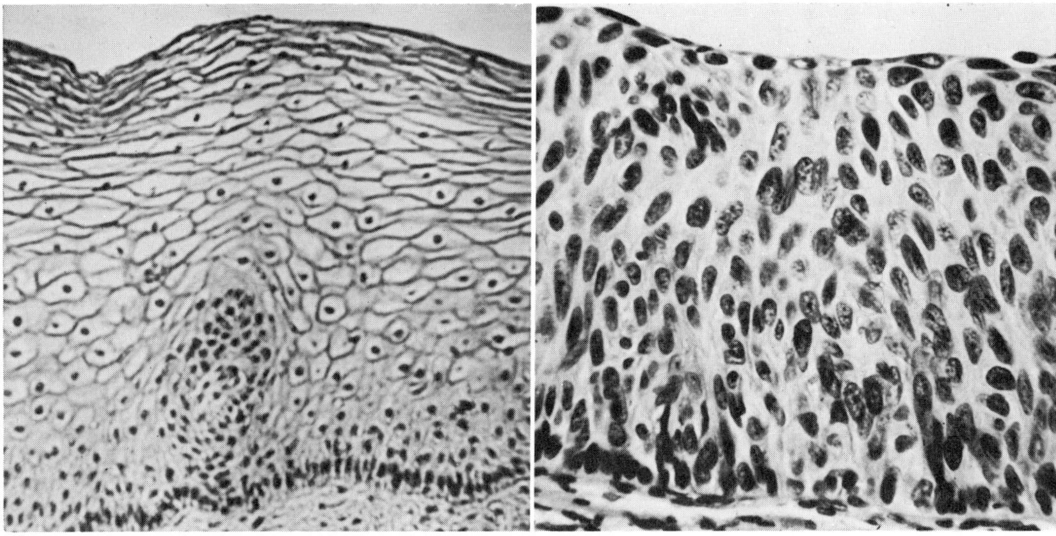

b

Figure 6-2. **a.** Normal cervical epithelium. The basal cells are lined up regularly against the lamina propria, and the orderly maturation of cells with formation of parakeratin is apparent. As the cells mature they become flattened and the cytoplasmic contents stain poorly.

b. Carcinoma *in situ* of the uterine cervix. The cells are in considerable disarray. The basal layer is uneven. No maturation of cells is apparent and there is a great deal of nuclear variability.

according to the percentage of undifferentiated cells: the most differentiated type of lesion is rated 1 and the completely anaplastic is lesion 4. These grades have been shown to have a statistically significant relation to prognosis in a variety of types of malignancies.

Smears of fixed and stained, exfoliated epithelial cells are useful diagnostic tools, especially in assessing the uterine cervix. In the system of Papanicolaou, the smears are rated on a scale of O to V, according to the cell or clump of cells that appears most malignant. Class V is considered certain carcinoma and class O is completely normal (Papanicolaou, 1958).

5. Metastasis

Despite the fact that the pathologist is often asked, as a matter of grave urgency, to identify neoplasms on the basis of histologic or cytologic criteria as be-

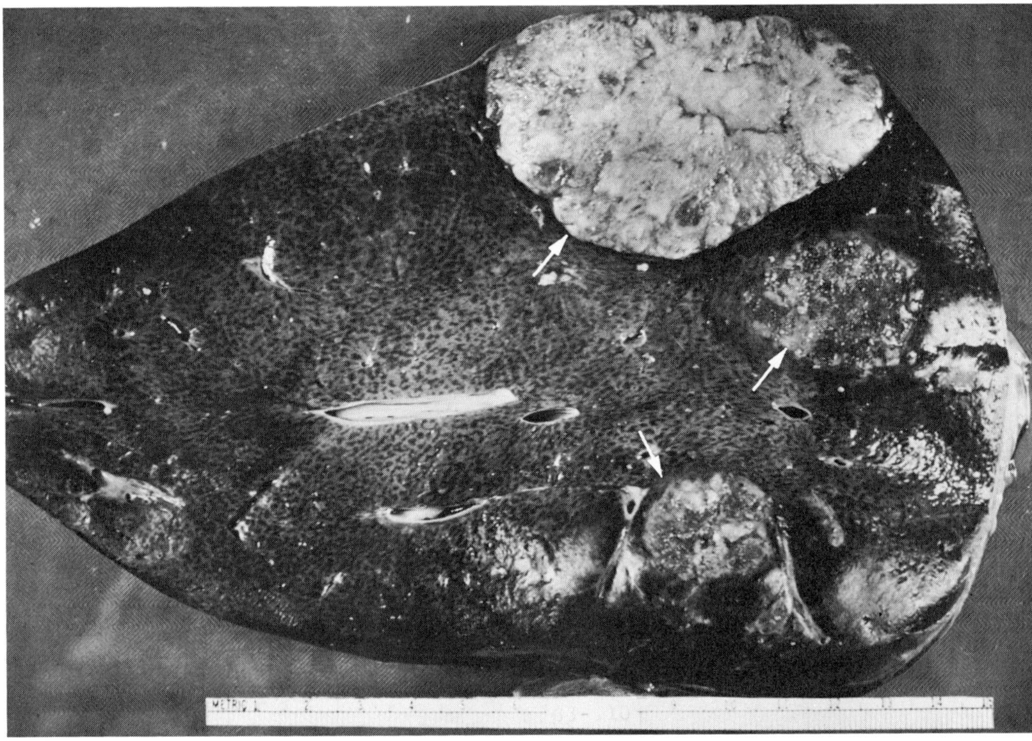

Figure 6-3. A cross section of liver from a patient with metastatic carcinoma from the colon. The vascular pattern in the liver is accentuated. The rounded masses (arrows) constitute nests of carcinoma cells arising from metastases distributed to the liver through the portal venous system.

nign or malignant, it must be emphasized that these categories are arbitrary, that there is no sharp biological dividing line between them. The tendency to metastasize, like so many biological functions, is a probability function and not an absolute quality.

The process of metastasis, which is so important in prognosis, is not well understood. Before metastasis can occur, however, the neoplastic cells must invade the surrounding normal tissues. Initially at least, the normal tissues are apparently inhibitory to both the growth and migration of small foci of neoplastic cells. With time the characteristics of the cells change, so that this inhibition breaks down and the neoplastic focus can grow and/or spread. The nature of this inhibition is not understood but is undoubtedly complex. It is known to involve cell-to-cell contact processes as well as inhibitors capable of acting over short distances.

Characteristically, the cells of the malignant lesion are less adhesive, one to another, than are normal cells. This is associated with a decreased calcium content in the plasma membrane. Some malignant cells produce hyaluronidase, which may assist the process of invasion. Also, the cells acquire a more negative surface charge, and this may help to reduce aggregation.

Most individual neoplastic cells that enter the bloodstream die without forming a new nidus of malignant disease (Ziedman, 1965). In order for a metastasis to be established, circulating neoplastic cells must adhere to the vascular endothelium, a process determined by a number of factors such as cell or clump size, diameter of the capillary, and "stickiness" of the capillary wall. The latter property is dependent in part on clotting factors in the blood.

Metastases do not arise with a random distribution throughout the body (Fig. 6-3). Each type and location of malignant lesion has characteristic patterns and routes of most probable metastasis. These patterns are in part determined by purely mechanical factors such as the location of the primary lesion and the extent of the capillary bed in various organs. Many neoplasms have a tendency to lung metastasis because the pulmonary capillary bed serves as the first capillary filter through which the neoplastic cells pass after entering the circulation (Southam *et al.,* 1967).

In addition to these purely mechanical considerations, some patterns are explicable only on the basis of a more receptive "soil" at certain sites for a particular neoplasm (Southam *et al.,* 1967). Since the chemical and physical environment varies from organ to organ, it would indeed be surprising if this were not the case.

It has been pointed out that many neoplasms spread by direct extension or metastasis through the lymphatic channels. The role of the lymph nodes has been a subject of much debate (Crile, 1968). The frequency of metastasis in the regional lymph nodes has cast doubt upon the hypothesis that they are defensive bastions. On the other hand, it may be argued that the tumor grows in and replaces a lymph node only after the node's hypothetical defensive potential is exhausted. More will be said of this subject in the discussion of immunity. For the present, it should be noted that the existence of gross or histologic tumor in a regional lymph node is usually a grave prognostic sign indicating shorter patient survival. There are two reasons for this relation: lymph node metastasis may indicate the more aggressive or malignant neoplasm; and it indicates a lesion that has already started to spread and may be widely disseminated.

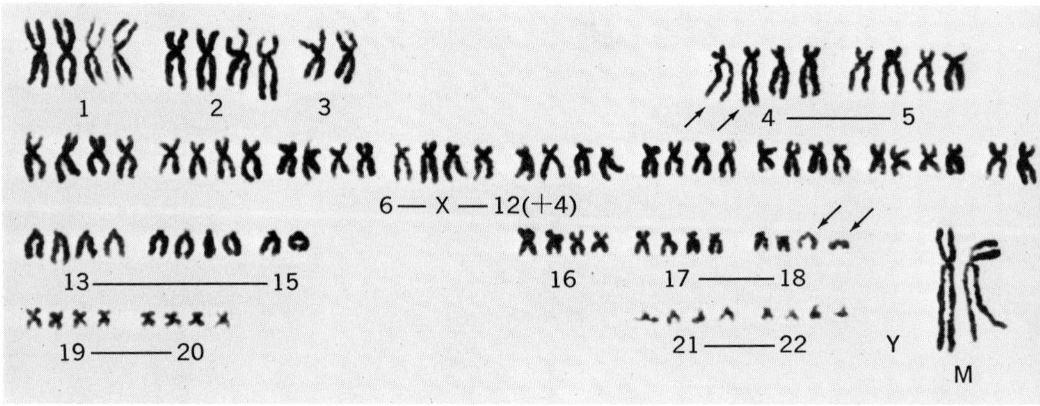

Figure 6-4. Karyotype from a lymph node cell in a patient with lymphoma. The cell is tetraploid with a total of 92 chromosomes. One extra abnormal chromosome is present as a pair (M). In addition, there are four additional chromosomes in group 6-12, loss of two no. 3 chromosomes, two group 13-15 chromosomes and two y chromosomes, and abnormalities of chromosomes in the 4-5 group and 17-18 group (arrows). Cells from some cancers show much more bizarre karyotypes than these. (Courtesy of Kajii, Neu, and Gardner, 1968)

C. Biology of the Neoplastic Cell

1. Chromosomal alterations

Since the neoplastic cell has a heritable defect, a study of the karyotypes of various tumors might reveal a distinctive lesion that directly results from or is the cause of the basic defect. With one remarkable exception, this does not appear to be the case.

It is true that virtually all malignant (and many benign) neoplasms show karyotypic abnormalities (Fig. 6-4). These cover a wide spectrum, including deletions, translocations, and more complex rearrangements in both aneuploid and euploid cells. No particular abnormality, with the one exception, seems to be associated with a particular type of neoplasm. Most neoplasms are aneuploid. Often more than one modal chromosome number is exhibited in a single lesion, although usually one mode predominates. A variety of abnormal chromosomes are frequently present. Occasional neoplasms, however, even some malignant ones, have perfectly normal chromosome complements, both by number and by quality, so far as present techniques reveal (Nowell, 1965).

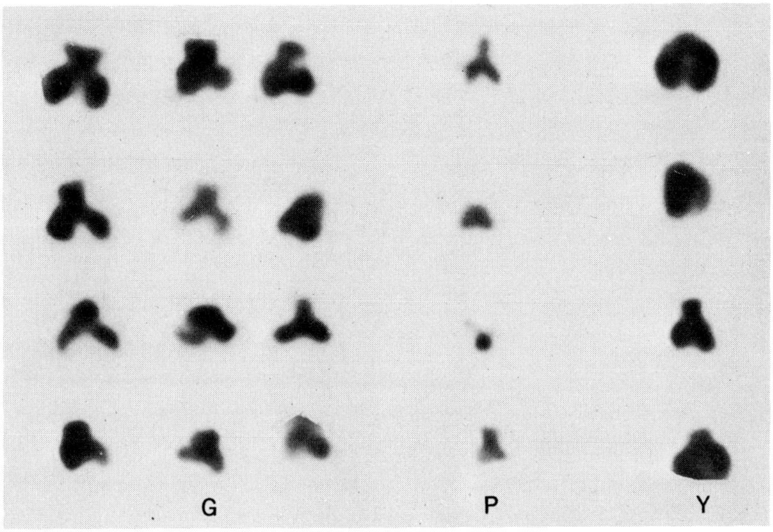

Figure 6-5. The Philadelphia chromosome. Normal chromosomes from groups G and Y are compared with Philadelphia chromosomes from various patients with chronic granulocytic leukemia. (Courtesy of Richard L. Neu)

The only exception we know of at present in which a specific chromosomal anomaly characterizes a particular type of neoplasm was discovered by Nowell and Hungerford. They found that in cases of chronic granulocytic leukemia, the neoplastic cells characteristically possess a small abnormal chromosome, the Philadelphia chromosome (Ph^1), apparently derived from a G group chromosome through loss of approximately half of the longer arm (Fig. 6-5). This abnormality is limited to the leukemic cells and persists throughout the course of the disease, although additional karyotypic changes may be seen in the terminal phase. It has not been observed in other forms of leukemia nor in non-leukemic individuals. The significance of this chromosomal anomaly in chronic granulocytic leukemia remains unknown (Nowell, 1965).

In summary, although most neoplasms show chromosomal anomalies of one type or another, the usual lack of specific anomalies suggests that those that do exist may be a secondary result of mitotic events occurring during neoplastic growth. Thus they probably have little etiologic significance but great importance in the process of neoplastic progression. In particular, changes in gene balance due to varying states of aneuploidy probably have profound effects on cell behavior (Hitosumachi *et al.,* 1971).

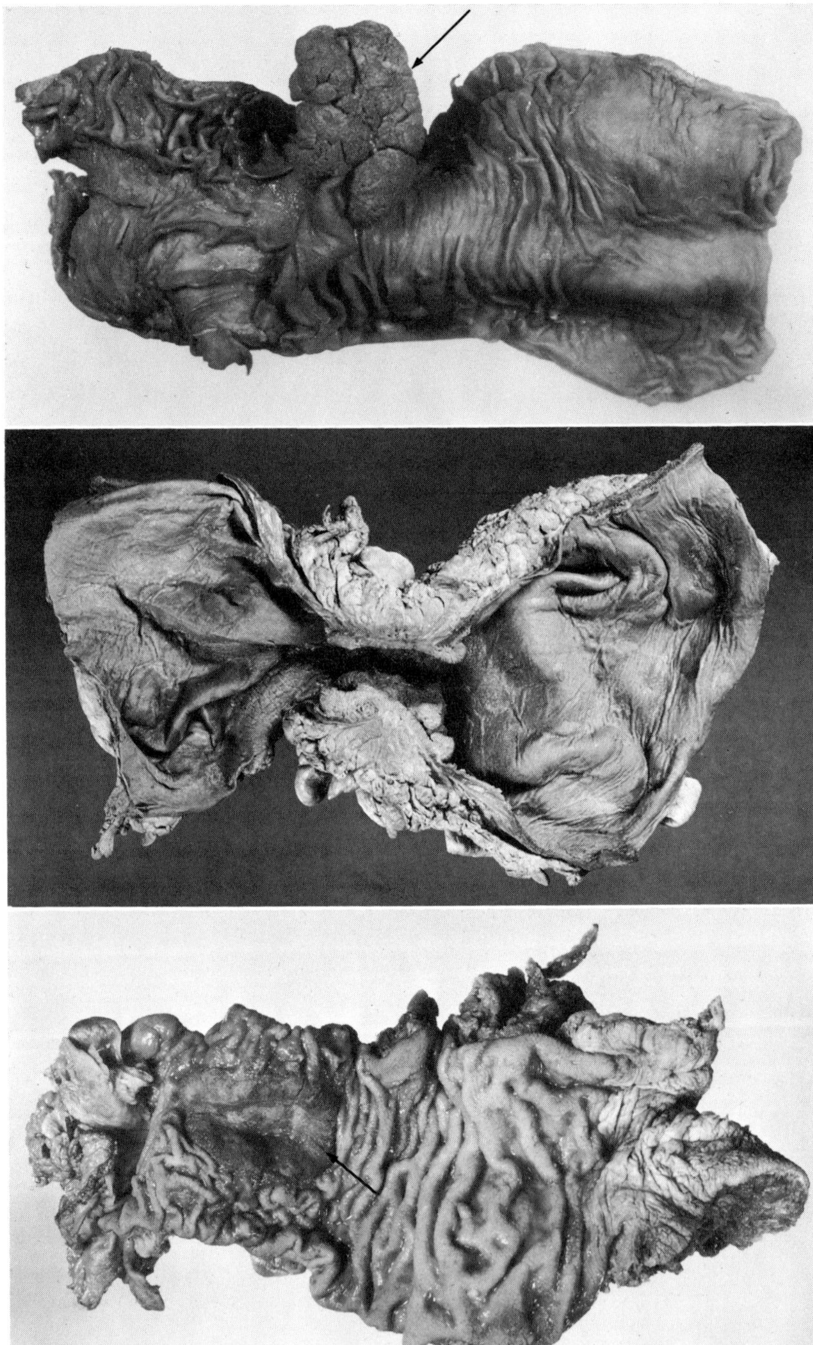

a

b

c

2. Neoplastic progression

It seems probable that no malignant neoplasm develops from the normal precursor tissue without intervening benign steps. The number of intervening steps is not definitely known and may be variable. Certainly, the length of time required to change patterns of differentiation and growth from normal to frankly malignant is highly variable. In some cases a benign neoplasm may develop which may never progress into a malignancy within the lifetime of the host animal. In other cases transitory changes may occur in the progenitor cells which cannot be detected with our present tools until frank malignancy has appeared. It is probably safe to conclude that benign, but aberrant, phases precede the development of frank malignancy in most and perhaps all cases (Fig. 6-6a).

The change in the biologic attributes of the cells of a neoplasm over a period of time is termed *neoplastic progression.* Of course, most neoplasms are growing and spreading, but neither of these changes is an intrinsic part of progression—only the cellular changes per se are encompassed by the term (Foulds, 1954).

Just as the neoplasm begins as a result of heritable alterations in the involved cells, so too all the varying attributes—morphological, biochemical, and behavioral—that in aggregate distinguish malignant from benign cells, are probably the result of progressive heritable alterations (Klein and Klein, 1957; Law, 1952; Patterson *et al.,* 1969). There is a tendency for these varied attributes to behave in the manner of "randomly assorting" genetic characters. It is probable that in no two malignant neoplasms are the varied attributes assembled in identical proportions (Fig. 6-6b, c). Not only do neoplasms vary greatly from one to another, but even within a single lesion the variation from area to area may be great (Henderson and Rous, 1962). Therefore, when a neoplasm is graded histologically, the assessment must be made upon the basis of the most anaplastic microscopic field that can be found, for fields of this sort determine the malignant potential of the tumor.

Figure 6-6. a. An adenoma measuring approximately 2 cm in diameter (arrow) is attached to the mucosa of the large bowel by a stalk. Histologically, a section of this polypoid adenoma would be expected to bear resemblance to Figure 6-1a.

b. and **c.** Photographs of two carcinomas of the colon demonstrating varying growth patterns. In Figure 6-6b the tumor has taken on a "napkin ring" appearance. The tumor has completely encircled the bowel and caused stenosis with partial reduction of the lumen. In Figure 6-6c the tumor is an ulcerating tumor and has formed a small crater (arrows). Either of these tumors could give rise to metastatic lesions similar to those seen in Figure 6-3.

The remarkable variation from area to area often seen in a single neoplasm may be a clonal phenomenon–i.e., each variant area may represent the progeny of a single deviant cell resulting from a relatively rare change analogous to, if not identical with, somatic mutation. It is possible, although it has been rigorously established in very few experimental systems, that all neoplastic progression may occur because of the random, chance appearance of clones of deviant cells and their subsequent amplification through the processes of natural selection (Klein and Klein, 1957).

If neoplastic progression occurs by the selection of randomly appearing, ever more deviant cells, is reverse progression (or perhaps it should be called retrogression) possible by a similar mechanism? It seems reasonable to suppose that a neoplastic cell population capable of giving rise to more malignant variants might also occasionally produce more normal variants. Variants of the latter type could not be observed unless the environment was such that they were not at their usual selective disadvantage. At present, this is little more than a speculation. Some few neoplasms, however, such as the Crown Gall of plants and the neuroblastoma of childhood, seem able to resolve by becoming more normal or more differentiated. Perhaps this can be considered a form of reverse progression.

3. Biochemical features of progression

It is virtually axiomatic that the heritable alteration that produces a neoplastic cell has a biochemical basis. This biochemical basis has not yet been discovered, although a number of hypotheses have been put forth.

The neoplastic cell possesses a number of characteristic biochemical features. Of most importance is *biochemical convergence,* extensively documented by Greenstein (Knox, 1967). The cells of each normal tissue type have a characteristic pattern of enzyme activity. Certain enzymes very active in kidney tissue have a low titer in liver and vice versa. In the neoplastic cell these patterns tend to become less characteristic of the normal tissues of origin. A very malignant kidney cell neoplasm may be, in pattern of enzyme activity, more like a very malignant hepatocellular carcinoma than it is like normal kidney. There is a tendency for the varied normal patterns of enzyme activity to converge toward a common pattern in the more malignant lesions. This is simply the biochemical counterpart of the morphologic changes known as *anaplasia,* which may prevent recognition of the site of origin of a neoplasm by its histologic features. The characteristic special features of a tissue give both morphologic and biochemical individuality. In the undifferentiated neoplasms these characteristics are much diminished.

Energy metabolism in relation to biochemical convergence has been investigated extensively since the observations of Warburg and his associates in the 1920's (Knox, 1967). Warburg established that the malignant cell has the capacity to produce large quantities of lactic acid from glucose and that this capacity is not markedly reduced in the presence of oxygen–i.e., the malignant cell exhibits an abnormally weak Pasteur effect. This high aerobic and anaerobic glycolysis was thought to be a characteristic of malignancies; yet a number of exceptions, especially in well-differentiated neoplasms, has been described. A high anaerobic metabolism (usual range of 15–40 μl of lactic acid equivalent per milligram dry tissue per hour) is observed in most malignancies. With the exception of embryonic, placental, retinal, and cerebral cortical tissues, most normal tissues exhibit an anerobic, glycolytic metabolism of only 10–20 per cent of that of most malignant neoplasms. In the presence of oxygen, glycolysis is reduced in malignant tissue to approximately 50 per cent of that observed anaerobically, while in most normal tissues glycolysis is nearly abolished in the presence of oxygen.

Warburg and his followers have argued that the degree of malignancy may be correlated with an increase in fermentation and a decrease in respiration, and that a defect in respiration is the root cause of the increased fermentation. Other investigators believe it would be accurate to state that the anaerobic glycolysis of malignancies is so high that a normal respiration and a normal Pasteur effect are incapable of reducing glycolysis to normal low levels. Despite much work by many investigators, the energy metabolism of neoplasia is still an area of considerable controversy primarily over two points: the role, if any, of defects in the respiratory apparatus in producing the usually high glycolytic activity of poorly differentiated neoplasms, and the basic significance of these metabolic abnormalities in the etiology of neoplasia.

A third biochemical characteristic of neoplasms has been described by Potter (1968). Using a series of rat hepatomas or hepatocellular carcinomas, he found that each neoplasm had a pattern of enzyme activity different from normal liver and characteristic of that individual lesion. The striking discovery was that the level of activity of any particular enzyme was much more invariable in the neoplasm, in the face of diurnal cycles or environmental stresses of various types, than in normal liver. The normal liver could adapt its enzyme levels to suit conditions; the neoplasms had less flexibility. All of the different stable levels of various enzymes in the various neoplasms were encompassed by the range of levels that could be produced in normal liver–but the levels in normal liver were much more easily varied. Pitot (1968) has advanced data to suggest that the varied levels of enzyme activity may be due not to variations in production of specific messenger RNA's, but to alterations in their stabilities or in the efficiency of translation of the particular message into protein. It seems that a crucial step in enzyme synthesis–probably that of translation–tends in the neoplasm to lose its normal regulatory flexibility.

In the previous sections it has been noted that neoplasms, once formed, tend to lose their specialized, differentiated characteristics. In terms of enzyme levels, however, the cells of the neoplasm seem to be more rigid, less adaptable, and thus perhaps in a sense more specialized than are the normal cells of origin.

4. Inappropriate cell products

Malignant neoplasms, as we have seen, exhibit a loss or diminution of specialized products or functions. Thus a highly malignant carcinoma of the epidermis may make little or no keratin, or a rhabdomyosarcoma may make little myosin. In recent years, however, it has become apparent that many neoplasms may acquire to some extent the capacity to make products typical of a completely different organ or tissue. For example, some bronchogenic carcinomas make insulin. Inappropriate hormone production has been described in a variety of other neoplasms (Lebovitz, 1965). The organ-specific cellular antigens identified by heteroantibody may also be inappropriate (Olenov and Fel, 1968). Tumor cells are characteristically deficient in these normal antigens, but often there is also an apparent replacement with other antigens. A kidney carcinoma, for example, may be found to possess antigens characteristic of liver. In addition to acquiring inappropriate antigens characteristic of another organ, tumor cells acquire antigens that are not found in any other adult tissue. (These tumor-specific antigens will be discussed in some detail in the section on *Immunity*). Thus, in malignancy, differentiation is not only deficient but it may be abnormal as to type. It has been pointed out that each somatic cell, of whatever organ, supposedly possesses all of the genetic information contained in the egg cell itself. In malignancy, some of that information that is normally inactive is utilized in bizarre and unpredictable ways.

5. Dependency

Neoplasia may occur in organs or tissues that are undergoing physiologic hyperplasia. The early neoplasm, arising in such an area, is often composed of very benign cells that deviate only minimally from their normal counterparts. Like their normal counterparts but perhaps to a lesser degree, they may require a continued exogenous stimulus to continue the hyperplasia. It should be recalled that the definition of neoplastic hyperplasia emphasized that the condition must be due, *at least in part,* to a heritable defect in the cells. In many early lesions that have undergone little progression, the heritable alteration is insufficient to maintain the hyperplastic state in the absence of a stimulus to ordinary physiologic hyperplasia. These lesions, although neoplastic, are thus *dependent* upon the exogenous stimulus. An excellent example is provided by some carcinomas of the breast (Boyland, 1961). Normal breast epithelium undergoes physiologic hyperplasia in rhythmic fashion during the estrus or menstrual cycle. Estrogens are particularly important as a hormonal stimulus. It is not surprising, therefore, that many breast carcinomas, especially relatively early in their natural histories, are dependent upon estrogen for their continued growth. They will undergo regression if this hormone is removed by ovariectomy, but with further progression the carcinomas lose this dependency. Similarly, ovarian neoplasms may be dependent upon gonadotrophins, thyroid neoplasms upon thyrotropin, and so on. Although the term *dependency* is usually applied only to hormonal dependency, other types not so easily recognized undoubtedly exist in a variety of early neoplasms (Boyland, 1961).

A somewhat different form of dependency found in some neoplasms is of particular current interest because of its possible importance in therapy. This is dependence upon asparagine. Most normal cells require little or no exogenous asparagine for their growth and well-being. Some neoplastic cells, however, cannot grow without an exogenous supply. Such neoplasms may be treated by systemic administration of the enzyme asparaginase. This can effectively deprive the neoplastic cells of their required asparagine supply without harming most normal cells. It remains to be determined how many human neoplasms will prove to be dependent upon asparagine and for how long (Boyse *et al.,* 1967).

6. Growth in vitro

Neoplastic cells have certain behavioral characteristics *in vitro* that tend to distinguish them from their normal precursors. Most of these characteristics are the *in vitro* counterparts of behavioral features seen *in vivo,* but they are sufficiently distinctive to require special note. As is the case with *in vivo* characteristics, no single *in vitro* property is an absolute criterion either for neoplasia or for degree of malignancy.

One fairly general property of neoplastic cells is decrease of so-called contact inhibition of movement (Fig. 6-7). Many types of normal cells tend to be inhibited in their tendency to overlap other cells of the same type. They therefore tend to form monolayers over the bottom of a culture dish. Neoplastic cells are less inhibited by cell-to-cell contact and tend to crawl over one another to produce

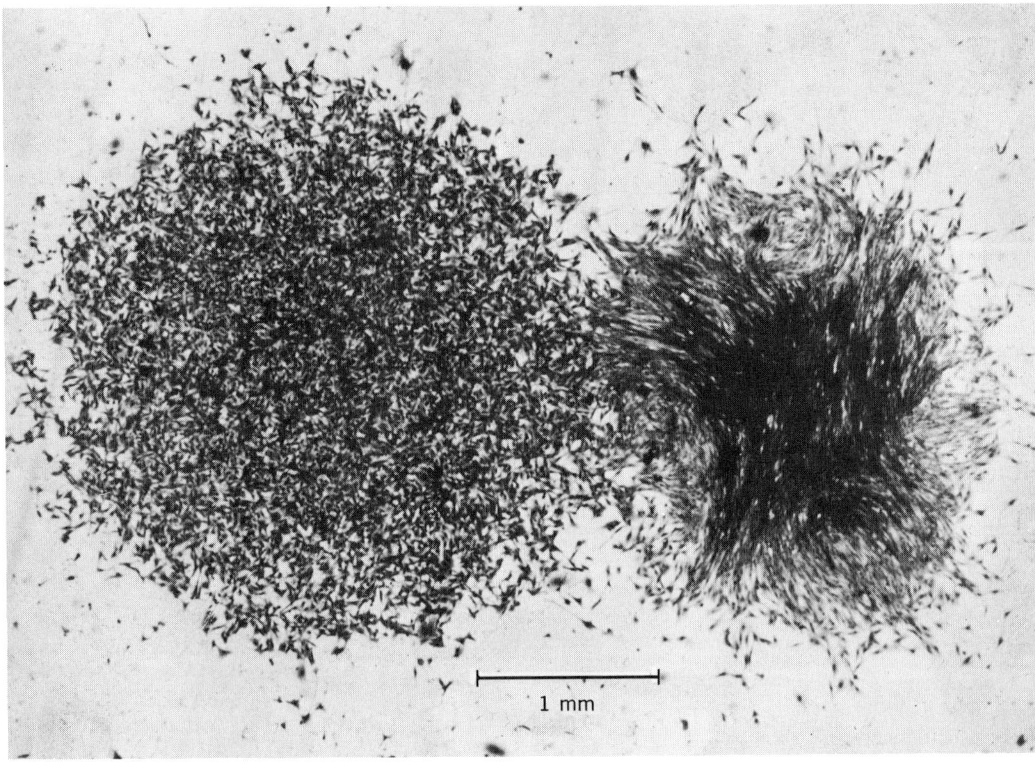

Figure 6-7. Hamster fibroblast cells in culture. The colony on the right has the normal configuration with cells lined up in parallel sheafs. On the left is a colony of malignant cells derived from the same explant after transformation by Rous sarcoma virus; the cells have a haphazard orientation and grow more widely. (Courtesy of MacPherson, 1965)

layers of randomly oriented cells. This property has been used to detect colonies of neoplastically transformed cells in cultures (Castor, 1968).

Another *in vitro* property which tends to distinguish the neoplastic cell from its normal counterpart is the ability to grow in very soft agar. Most normal cells, with the exception of hematopoietic cells, seem to require a firm substrate upon which to initiate growth. Many but not all neoplastic cells are able to initiate growth without a solid substrate (Stoker, 1968).

Perhaps the most important distinguishing characteristic is that neoplastic cells will proliferate *ad infinitum* under proper culture conditions. Normal cell strains, in contrast, appear to have a finite life span characteristic of the cell type and species. This very important attribute does not seem to be a function of the culture conditions but rather an innate property of the cells themselves (Hayflick and Moorhead, 1961).

This finite life span of races of normal cells can also be demonstrated *in vivo*. Hematopoietic tissues can be serially transplanted in mice if the recipient mice have been depleted of blood-forming cells by lethal doses of X-irradiation. The transplanted bone-marrow cells will proliferate and replenish the marrow and spleen of the recipient. Serial transplantation can in this way be accomplished four to six times, but the cells will not multiply further. In contrast, leukemic cells exhibit no such exhaustion.

Likewise, a small fragment of mouse mammary ductal epithelium can be transplanted in suitably prepared recipient mice and proliferate into a normal-appearing ductal tree. This can be done serially but apparently only for a limited time before the cells lose their growth potential. Mammary carcinoma, on the other hand, can be transplanted indefinitely.

Thus, both *in vitro* and *in vivo* neoplastic cell lines seem to be immortal while normal somatic cell strains have a limited potential, perhaps related to the normal life span of the animal.

D. Host Reactions

1. The stroma

The growth of most neoplasms is dependent upon an adequate, supporting connective-tissue stroma and blood supply (Fig. 6-8). These are normal tissues of the host that are induced to proliferate by the neoplasm. Most neoplasms cannot grow faster than the supporting vascular system. Many malignancies undergo extensive necrosis because they outgrow their blood supply or because the mechanical pressure of the tumor interferes with blood flow. The factors involved in the elicitation of a stroma and blood supply by the neoplasm are not known but may be similar to those operative in normal tissues. Recently a chemical substance called *angiogenesis factor* has been isolated from tumor tissue. It is capable of producing dramatic capillary proliferation (Gimbrone *et al.*, 1972). Among experimental animal tumors there is great variation in the speed with which newly transplanted tumor fragments elicit a blood supply (Day, 1964); presumably this is due to variations in the release of the angiogenesis factor.

The vascular system in malignancies is often abnormal. Rather than by a typical capillary bed, the tumor is sometimes supplied by a system of large thin-walled vascular sinuses. Blood flow is typically sluggish, and gas exchange is inefficient. (Perhaps this is why neoplasms tend to develop a high anaerobic gly-

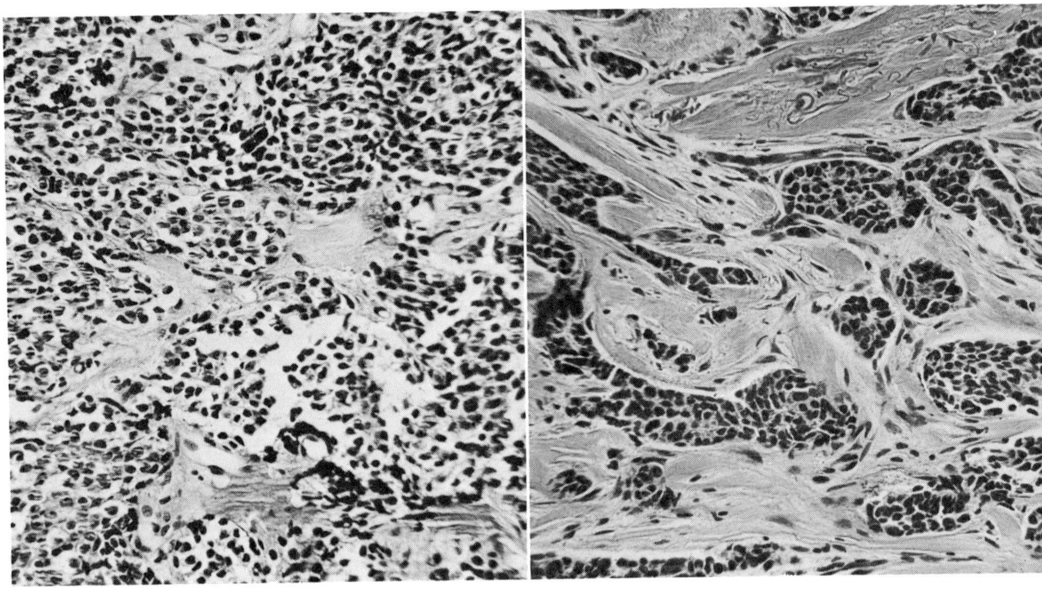

a

Figure 6-8. **a.** Metastatic carcinoma of the prostate. The cells with dense small nuclei, mainly scattered in nests, are the carcinoma cells. Intermingled with these are delicate bands of fibrous stroma, which tend to separate the individual nests of tumor cells. Similar stroma is seen in Figure 6-1. In this stroma runs the vascular network that feeds and drains the tumor.

b. In this example of scirrhous adenocarcinoma of the breast, the stroma is very dense, with large quantities of collagen. The cancerous epithelium is reduced to relatively small nests scattered in the stroma.

colysis.) The pH of the intercellular milieu is abnormally low. The vascular sinuses are fragile, and anoxia due to a temporary fall in blood pressure can produce extensive intratumoral hemorrhage.

Although most malignancies are supplied with a blood vascular network, induced stroma frequently lacks nerves and lymphatics. Still, there appears to be a variation from tumor to tumor, some tumors being supplied with nerves or lymphatics or both. Also, the fact that the so-called nerve growth factor was first isolated from mouse sarcomata indicates that at least some tumors may stimulate nerve growth.

Certain malignancies, particularly scirrhous carcinomas of the human breast, stimulate an extensive desmoplastic reaction. Indeed, the fibrous connective tissue may constitute a much larger part of the gross tumor than do the neoplastic cells

(Fig. 6-8b). Again, the chemical or physiologic basis of this reaction is not known.

Perhaps related to the qualitative abnormalities of the blood vascular supply is a characteristic abnormality in the inflammatory process. It has been observed in a number of experimental animal tumors that stimuli, such as foreign bodies placed within the neoplasms, fail to produce inflammation (Mahoney and Leighton, 1962). This interesting abnormality has not been further investigated, and its basis is completely unknown. It may be a very important factor in the tendency of some tumors to become infected with bacterial agents and to harbor these agents chronically.

2. Physiologic effects

The most important physiologic effect of malignant neoplasia on the host animal is the production of cachexia. In the human being, weight loss is often one of the most prominent symptoms of malignant disease. While it is found that the energy requirements of a tumor-bearing animal are greater than normal and that at the same time its dietary intake is usually reduced, these facts do not seem to account completely for the cachexia. A tumor appears to be a "nitrogen trap." A high nitrogen consumption in the diet appears beneficial in counteracting the effects of the neoplasm, which can be considered as a large parasite diverting amino acids from the metabolic pool for its own use.

Many malignancies have other widespread effects on the host animal apart from those of purely mechanical nature. One quite general effect in experimental animals is depression of liver catalase activity. This is not usually seen in human cancer, probably because the human neoplasms seldom reach the proportionate sizes seen in rodents. Anemia is a frequent feature of neoplastic disease even in the absence of bone-marrow replacement by the tumor. Not much is known about the basis of these effects, although some workers have described possible toxic agents released by the tumor and have given these the name *toxohormone* (Nakahara, 1960).

3. Immunity

Many neoplastic cells are so sufficiently different in their surface characteristics from any normal cell that they are regarded as foreign by the host's immunologic mechanism. Thus, the level of host immunity is of vital importance in the biology of neoplasia. It is only recently that a mass of experimental data has overthrown the widely held view that immunity against neoplasia is theoretically impossible—the view that the neoplastic cell, as part of the "self," could not be the target of an immune reaction. It is now commonly believed—although perhaps incorrectly—that most incipient neoplasms may be suppressed by an immune reaction before they reach macroscopic size. Clinical neoplasia, as seen by the physician, would then represent the remaining small minority of lesions that for one reason or another escape this defense (Klein, 1968a, 1968b).

The evidence for the importance of immunity is mainly of two types: (1) the demonstration that animals can be immunized, using tumor tissue as antigen, so that the growth of tumor transplants is markedly inhibited or prevented; and (2) the correlation between altered immunologic reactivity and the incidence of neoplasia under the altered conditions.

Experiments to demonstrate the antigenicity of tumor tissue and the antitumor effects of induced immunity are usually performed in inbred mice. Since all the mice of a particular inbred strain are virtually identical genetically, it is possible to transplant normal or neoplastic tissues from one animal to another without encountering any immunity of the homograft type—i.e., immunity aroused by antigenic differences among the animals. Consequently, when an animal of such an inbred strain is inoculated with a suspension of killed tumor cells obtained from another animal of that same strain, the immunity to a subsequent inoculation of living tumor cells must be directed against tumor-specific antigens—i.e., antigens peculiar to the tumor and not shared with the normal tissues of the animal in which the tumor originated. This type of experiment is most conveniently carried out by transplanting tumor tissue from one mouse to another within the inbred strain. By means of immunization, however, immunity can be increased in the very animal in which the tumor first appeared, thus obviating even the slightest possibility that the immunity might not be directed against tumor-specific antigens. The growth of a neoplasm in its primary host may not always stimulate the maximum possible immunity in that animal (Klein, 1968a, 1968b).

The tumor-specific antigens that induce immunity to tumor growth are apparently located on the cell surface. They seem very similar to the homograft antigens that distinguish different, non-inbred animals of the same species. Thus far, their exact chemical nature is unknown, since efforts to extract them from the cell result in diminished antigenicity.

Tumor antigens frequently are characteristic of a specific tumor, and cross-immunity often cannot be demonstrated between two similar tumors, even when the tumors are produced by the same stimulus in the same animal. This is particularly true of tumors produced by chemical or physical agents. By contrast, many neoplasms produced by a given virus will cross with other tumors produced by the same virus. This makes it theoretically possible to immunize against tumors caused by a particular virus (Klein, 1968a, 1968b; Prehn, 1968). In the human there seems to be a greater probability of cross-reactivity among different tumors of the same histological type than is the case among rodent neoplasms.

Antigenic strength on the tumor cell surface varies greatly. Thus, some experimentally induced tumors immunize against themselves very well, others only slightly, if at all. In general, it seems that those neoplasms induced rapidly after an oncogenic stimulus, whether chemical, physical, or viral, tend to be highly antigenic in contrast to those with long latent periods. Some etiologic agents, however, tend to produce more or less antigenic neoplasms independent of variations in latent period. Within a single neoplasm there may be variation in antigenic titer among the cells, perhaps as a result of covering of antigenic sites by sialo-mucins. Consequently, immunoselection during tumor growth may gradually produce a progressively less antigenic neoplasm. While immunoselection has been convincingly demonstrated among chemically induced neoplasms, some viral neoplasms may be relatively resistant to this process.

Unfortunately, those animal neoplasms that occur spontaneously in low incidence seem to have little or no antigenicity. Perhaps it is owing to this fact that they escaped an immune reaction and were not suppressed in their incipiency. Neoplasms induced rapidly by chemicals or viruses escape not only because of their rapid growth but because the chemical oncogens, and perhaps some viral oncogens as well, seriously depress immune reactivity. (This subject will be discussed again in the section on etiology.) Furthermore, some neoplasms may induce a state of partial specific immunologic tolerance to the tumor cell antigens.

The immunity that is aroused by the tumor-specific antigens is mediated by lymphocytes and is thus analogous to delayed hypersensitivity. Except in the case of lymphomas, there is little evidence that circulating antibody participates in the suppression of tumor cells. In fact, there is much evidence that high levels of antibody may often make a tumor grow better. Somehow, the humoral antibody protects the tumor cells from the lymphocyte-mediated type of immune reaction, a process called *tumor enhancement.* Some tumors are much more enhanceable than others. For this reason, if for no other, attempts at immunotherapy of tumors in man must be approached with the greatest circumspection.

Although all the foregoing evidence concerning the antigenicity of neoplastic cells comes from animal studies, there is some evidence to suggest that human neoplasms have similar properties. Probably most suggestive is the histologic evidence. Many human neoplasms show a heavy lymphoid infiltration in and around the lesion. This is apt to be most prominent, especially in the skin neoplasia, at about the time in tumor progression when invasion of surrounding tissues is commencing. Later lesions usually show a less prominent lymphoid reaction. This lymphoid reaction is very suggestive of the type of reaction seen in experimental neoplasms that have aroused an immune reaction. In human breast carcinoma there is convincing evidence that a heavy lymphocytic reaction is associated with a relatively favorable prognosis. Evidence of a so-called sinus histiocytosis in the regional lymph nodes also suggests a good prognosis. Sinus histiocytosis probably reflects prolonged reaction to an antigenic stimulus.

Direct experimental evidence of tumor antigenicity in man is meager, though there have been a number of suggestive reports. The ethical difficulties in experimental manipulation severely limit progress in this area. Recently, however, this has been circumvented by a variety of *in vitro* techniques. It has been possible by immunofluorescence techniques to demonstrate an apparently common tumor antigen among cases of human melanosarcoma (Morton *et al.,* 1968). Another technique involves growing both tumor and lymphoid cells from the same patient in tissue culture. By this means an immune reaction of the lymphocytes, directed against a number of different tumors, can be demonstrated, while homologous (i.e., foreign) lymphoid cells usually fail to react or at least show a slower response (Hellstrom *et al.,* 1968).

The second basic approach to the study of the importance of immunity–namely, the correlation between alterations in immune capacity and susceptibility to neoplasia–has been explored extensively in mice and to some extent in man. In mice, immune capability can be reduced by neonatal thymectomy. Adult thymectomy combined with radiation can also produce immunologic deficiency. Either procedure may lead to increased susceptibility to tumorigenesis.

In addition to showing that a decreased immune capacity increases susceptibility to oncogenesis, it has also been possible to demonstrate the converse: to increase resistance by nonspecific stimulation of immune mechanisms. Administration of a derivative of B.C.G. has been shown to stimulate a variety of immune responses in mice and to inhibit mouse mammary tumor formation and skin papilloma development.

In the human, it has been observed that a variety of clinical syndromes known to be associated with diminished immunologic capacity have predisposed to neoplasia, usually some form of lymphoma. Most striking is the development of neoplasia in kidney transplant recipients who have been maintained for long periods on immunosuppressive drugs.

A final link between alteration in immunocompetence and the development of neoplasia is suggested by the fact that the increasing incidence of neoplasia with advancing age is paralleled by age-associated lymphoid atrophy and a decline in general immunocompetence.

Although the immune response is usually considered a defensive reaction, probably it also plays a role in the production of some neoplasms. This paradoxical probability will be discussed in subsequent sections of this chapter.

E. Etiologic Mechanisms

1. Threshold concepts

Since the fundamental molecular defect in the cancer cell is not yet known, a discussion of etiology must be confined to mere descriptions of environmental and genetic factors and to speculations concerning the precise details of how they work. Research on etiology has suffered, not from a dearth of etiologic factors, but from a plethora. Commonly, very diverse factors have an additive effect in tumor production, so that it is incorrect to speak of the cause of any cancer. *Cancer is a multifactorial disease* (Heston, 1945).

This multifactorial etiology has perhaps been most clearly elucidated in the study of breast cancer of the mouse. The general principle applies, however, in varying degree to all neoplasms.

Historically, breast cancer in the mouse was considered a genetic disease because, by selective breeding, it was possible to obtain inbred strains with varying incidences of the disease, from virtually 0 to 100 per cent. In the 1930's, however, a series of studies at the Jackson Memorial Laboratory at Bar Harbor, Maine, under the general direction of C. C. Little, established that an "extrachromosomal factor" was also involved. In these experiments, reciprocal crosses between low and high tumor strains were bred, and then the mammary tumor incidences in the resulting two series of F_1 hybrids were compared. It was found that F_1 mice derived from the cross between high-tumor-strain females and low-tumor-strain males had a much higher tumor incidence than F_1 mice derived from the reciprocal cross between low-tumor-strain females and high-tumor-strain males. Since the genotypes of the F_1 mice of both series were identical, some nongenetic or extrachromosomal factor associated with a high-tumor-strain mother must have been involved. Three possibilities, not mutually exclusive, were considered:

1. the factor could be transmitted in the ovum of the high-tumor-strain female;
2. it could be transmitted across the placenta to the young;
3. it was present in and transmitted by the milk.

A further series of experiments using foster nursing established that the extrachromosomal factor was in the milk. If mice nursed upon high-tumor-strain mothers, their mammary tumor incidence in later life was high; conversely, the incidence was low if *all* the nursing was on a low-tumor-strain mother. Subsequent studies showed that the factor was an RNA-containing virus. Despite the importance of this virus, however, the genotype of the nursing mouse remained of great importance.

In the male mouse the mammary gland is rudimentary. Despite a favorable genotype and the presence of the milk agent, mammary cancer in the male is very rare. It can, however, be brought up to the same level as in the female by the chronic administration of estrogens or prolactin. Conversely, the female ovariectomized in early life usually fails to develop tumors. Thus, not only are genotype and milk agent important, but estrogen also is an etiologic agent.

No one of these factors is of predominant importance in mouse breast cancer. Tumors occur in the absence of the milk agent if the hormonal stimulation and genotype are very favorable. In the presence of the milk agent, the other factors need be much less optimal. A variety of factors acting in conjunction must reach a certain threshold if a tumor is to occur.

It is possible that human breast cancer involves a milk agent, although this possibility has not been fully established. The importance of the mouse system lies rather in its demonstration of the threshold concept. In the discussion that follows, various specific etiologic agents will be described. Although the threshold principle may not be reiterated in each case, it should be remembered that no one of the agents discussed can be considered *the* cause of any one neoplasm.

2. Oncogenic viruses

It seems certain that very soon a human malignancy will, for the first time, be proven to have a viral etiology. There are two leading candidates—the Burkitt lymphoma, and carcinoma of the uterine cervix. The Burkitt lymphoma is predominantly a childhood disease prevalent in Central Africa. Its geographical distribution has strongly suggested transmission, possibly by an insect vector. Alternatively, malarial infection may alter the susceptibility to an oncogenic virus. Recently, immunologic studies have suggested a tumor antigen common to most cases and capable of inducing an antibody response. Herpes-type viruses have been implicated as the possible viral etiologic agents of both Burkitt's lymphoma and the supposedly quite unrelated disease, infectious mononucleosis (Henle *et al.,* 1968). The latter disease is a contagious, self-limiting, febrile illness often seen among young adults.

Whether Burkitt lymphoma and infectious mononucleosis are ever conclusively shown to have a common viral etiology, the fact that a single viral species can produce such very disparate types of disease is well established. Thus, Duran-Reynals (1950) showed that the Rous chicken sarcoma virus could produce either a hemorrhagic and inflammatory disease in young chickens or sarcomas in older ones, depending entirely upon the age and immunologic capacities of the birds at the time of virus injection. His work suggested that this particular oncogenic virus would produce tumors only if there was a moderate degree of immunologic resistance to the virus. If resistance were very low, the hemorrhagic disease occurred; if it were high, no infection was established or else the tumors were only transient (Duran-Reynals, 1950).

The other leading candidate for a viral etiology, carcinoma of the cervix, has long been thought to be correlated with coitus, and particularly coitus with uncircumcised males. Thus, the incidence of the disease is low among nuns and Jewish women. Only recently, epidemiologic studies have shown that it is not coitus *per se* that correlated with the incidence, but the number of *different* coital partners. The greater the number of different coital partners, the greater the possibility of carcinoma of the cervix. This fact strongly suggests that this disease is venereal and caused by an agent probably transmitted by some uncircumcised males. Again, a Herpes virus (not the same type found in so-called fever blisters) has been isolated from a high percentage of cases. Only time and more research will establish whether or not this is actually a causative agent.

In any case, it is virtually certain that many human neoplasms must have a viral cause. The viral etiology of many animal cancers has now been demonstrated, and it is inconceivable that man might be unique in this regard (Eckhart, 1968).

The known animal oncogenic viruses can be divided into two major categories, RNA viruses and DNA viruses. The names of some of these are listed in Table 6-1. Many more will undoubtedly be discovered. These viruses will not be discussed in detail, but rather a few examples will be discussed sufficiently to illustrate general principles.

The Rous sarcoma virus, which has already been mentioned, is the most thoroughly studied of the RNA viruses. In 1967, Peyton Rous of the Rockefeller University received the Nobel Prize, in large part for his discovery of this virus in 1910. As this long lag suggests, the viral theory of cancer is more popular now than it was then. At that time, in fact, there was much opposition to accepting a chicken tumor as a "true" cancer. The very fact that it was caused by a transmissible agent was considered proof of its dubious qualifications.

Like other RNA viruses, the Rous virus particle is completed by budding from the surface of an infected cell, the viral coat being formed in the cell wall. Evidence now suggests that some strains of the virus are ordinarily "defective" in that they are unable to form a protein coat and replicate without help from another closely related virus, a "helper" virus. The defective Rous virus can produce

Table 6-1 Best-Known Oncogenic Viruses

DNA	RNA
1. Polyoma	1. Murine leukemia viruses
2. Shope papilloma	2. Avian leukosis viruses
3. Simian virus 40	3. Rous sarcoma virus
4. Shope fibroma	4. Mouse mammary tumor viruses
5. Human adenoviruses (tumors in hamsters)	
6. Lucké frog kidney carcinoma	

neoplastic "transformation" of infected cells–i.e., it can somehow produce a neoplastic alteration–but it cannot replicate itself without help. The viral genome remains in the neoplastic but non-viral-releasing cells, as is proven by the fact that infectious virus can be "rescued" by superinfection with the helper (Rubin, 1964).

In the case of the DNA viruses, viral replication and release from infected cells is associated with cell lysis. Neoplastically transformed cells do not release virus. Why certain cells undergo only this abortive type of infection is unknown. Apparently, in some way the conditions in transformed infected cells are "defective" for viral replication (Dulbecco, 1966).

When cells in tissue culture are exposed to DNA viruses, it is found that only a small fraction of the cells actually undergo visible transformation. Also, this small fraction will not grow to produce a neoplasm when inoculated into appropriate animals. Further changes must first take place (a form of progression?) before the cells are sufficiently transformed. In all probability, the virus does no more than trigger the start of the process. Although a variety of studies demonstrates that virally coded messenger RNA is continually made in the transformed cells, the function of this RNA is unknown. Very early in cell infection, whether the infection be of a replicative and destructive or of an abortive and transforming type, a new antigen (so-called T or tumor antigen) is detectable in the nucleus of the cell. This antigen is probably coded for by the viral genome and thus serves as a marker for the continued presence of the virus. It is only later and presumably only in transformed cells that the "transplantation" antigen is formed on the cell surface. This latter antigen arouses host resistance to the tumor cells. Whether the genetic information specifying this antigen is contained in the viral or the cellular genome is not yet definitely known. Recent work, however, suggests that the surface antigen is probably specified by a cellular gene. The form of the viral DNA inside the transformed cell is also not clear, but it is probable that it is integrated into the cellular genome.

Whether viral information may be required to maintain the neoplastic state or is a mere trigger is a moot point. It has, however, been shown with the aid of temperature-dependent virus mutants that, at least in some cases, the neoplastic phenotype reverts to normal when the virus is inactivated by the appropriate temperature change.

It has already been pointed out that a number of host variables can determine the type of response to a virus. For example, it has been found that a number of human adenoviruses are capable of producing neoplasms in newborn hamsters. There is no evidence that these viruses are oncogenic in their natural host, man, although this remains a possibility. It is entirely possible that any virus could be oncogenic, given the right type of host cell and suitable conditions. Moreover, many supposedly non-oncogenic viruses can potentiate the action of chemical agents that are themselves only weakly oncogenic or that are applied in suboncogenic doses.

It might be thought that the problem of whether a particular animal tumor is of viral etiology could be simply solved by analysis of the surface transplantation antigens. This is not the case, however. Although the known virally induced tumors are typically characterized by cross-reacting surface antigens induced by that particular virus, tumors of non-viral etiology may acquire cross-reacting antigens by virtue of infection with a passenger virus–one that had nothing to do with the initial transformation. Furthermore, if a neoplasm is caused by a virus that is ubiquitous in the animal population so that all the animals are infected at an early age, they may be rendered immunologically tolerant to both viral antigens per se and to virally-induced cellular antigens. Under these conditions the cross-reacting surface antigen produced by the action of the virus will not produce an immune reaction in the animals and may be undetectable.

Whether a particular neoplasm involves a viral etiologic agent cannot be determined merely by the isolation of a virus from the lesion or its visualization by the electron microscope. Viruses are apparently quite ubiquitous in nature, and mere passenger viruses unrelated to a tumor's etiology are commonly present in tumor tissue. Conversely, failure to isolate or visualize a virus hardly argues at all against a viral etiology, since viruses may disappear temporarily or permanently in a number of experimental virus-induced tumors. Considering these difficulties and the lack of persistent virus production in neoplasms of known viral etiology, it is probably not surprising that, more than a half century after discovery of the first oncogenic virus, viral malignancy in man is yet to be definitely identified.

Recently it has been found that normal cells and oncogenic viruses contain enzymes able to produce the polymerization of DNA on an RNA template. These reverse transcriptases have not yet been identified in definitely non-oncogenic viruses. The transcriptases of the virus appear to be immunologically distinctive and thus may serve as "footprints" of viral etiology in tumor cells, even when no virus can be found by other methods.

3. Chemical agents

In the nearly two hundred years since the classical observation of Percival Pott that chimney sweeps were "peculiarly liable" to cancer of the scrotum, hundreds of chemical oncogens of a variety of types have been identified. Almost all of these have been found within the last half century. Although it was evident that the oncogenic factor in chimney sweeps' cancer was to be found in soot, this factor could not be isolated and identified for nearly a century and a half for the simple reason that, despite numerous attempts, tumors in experimental animals could not be produced with soots and coal tars. It was not until 1915, when Yamagiwa and Ichikawa had the patience to continue painting rabbits' ears with coal tar every two or three days for over a year, that cancers were induced. Once an assay was available, the crude material could be fractionated and the active chemicals identified. In 1930 Kennaway and his associates isolated and identified the first known chemical oncogen. This was dibenz(a,h)anthracene, a polycyclic aromatic hydrocarbon with the formula:

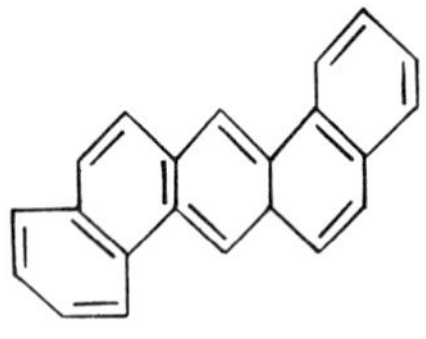

Numerous other somewhat similar agents were soon identified and made available for study. Some are remarkably powerful; microgram amounts are sufficient to produce skin cancers rapidly when applied topically to suitable animals. Chemically, these aromatic substances are fat-soluble. They often have a superficial resemblance to some of the steroids. For example, 3-methylcholanthrene, one of the most powerful, actually has some estrogenic activity. Whether or not these resemblances are of biologic significance is still not known. To this day, the aromatic polycyclic hydrocarbons are among the best studied but least understood of oncogenic agents.

These hydrocarbons are general oncogens in rodents—i.e., they can produce tumors locally in virtually any tissue to which they are applied or which they can reach. Adult liver is a notable exception, apparently because liver contains the necessary enzymes to convert the hydrocarbon to an inactive metabolite.

Some oncogens attack a much more restricted range of tissues and characteristically produce tumors at remote sites instead of the site of application. In general, if the chemical must be metabolized in a special way in order to serve as an oncogen, the range of susceptible target tissues may be reduced. A striking example concerns certain aromatic amines, especially 2-naphthylamine, which, when absorbed through the skin or inhaled by industrial workers in the dye industry, produce cancers primarily of the urinary bladder epithelium. Apparently, the aromatic amines are inactive as such and require conversion *in vivo* into a *proximate* oncogen. N-hydroxylation to the N-hydroxy derivative, which can be performed by bladder epithelium, has been shown to be a necessary metabolic step. Synthetically prepared N-hydroxy derivative is better able to produce tumors locally at a subcutaneous site of application than is the parent compound (Miller and Miller, 1969).

There is little point in discussing in detail the features of the vast variety of compounds that have some degree of oncogenic activity, although, as industrial hazards or contaminants of foodstuffs, many of them have considerable practical importance. It is almost certain that our environment, as it is progressively altered by technology, harbors more and more oncogens (Wogan, 1969).

Among the environmental oncogenic hazards, two have aroused sufficient interest in recent years to deserve special mention. In 1795 Soemmerring first noted the association between chronic pipe smoking and cancer of the lip, but only in the past two decades have the dangers of tobacco been widely recognized. The epidemiologic evidence now clearly implicates tobacco smoking, especially of cigarettes, in the causation of the growing pandemic of bronchogenic, squamous lung cancer. Tobacco probably plays a role also in the causation of cancer of the oral cavity and larynx, and possibly of the esophagus, kidney, and urinary bladder. The exact chemical oncogens in cigarettes and their interplay with other factors have not yet been elucidated.

Two widely separated epizootics in 1961 drew attention to another environmental oncogenic hazard. Hepatotoxicity due to ingestion of peanut meal killed thousands of turkey poults, ducklings, and chicks in England. Simultaneously, in the Pacific Northwest, trout hatcheries were plagued by an epidemic of hepatomas among the fish, which was also traced to the feed. It was soon determined that both conditions were due to contamination of the feed by the common fungus *Aspergillus flavus*. Four related compounds, all aflatoxins, were isolated from the contaminated feed. These, on a molar basis, are by far the most active known hepatocarcinogens, even more active than the aminoazo dyes that are the standard laboratory hepatocarcinogens. Recently there has been a suggestion that the prevalence of hepatocarcinoma in man in Uganda and of stomach carcinoma in the Orient may be associated with high aflatoxin levels in the native diets.

When an aromatic hydrocarbon oncogen such as 3-methylcholanthrene is applied to the skin of a mouse in a vehicle such as acetone or olive oil, it accumulates in the hair follicles and sebaceous glands and has a toxic and destructive action on these epidermal appendages. Even a year or more later, however, long after its dissipation, a second application of the compound will still produce an additive oncogenic effect. Successive doses are at least somewhat additive no matter how widely spaced, but there does appear to be a threshold dosage below which no toxicity is evident and no cumulative oncogenic effect is seen. It is apparent that each effective dosage of the oncogen produces some long-lasting effect in the treated skin. The skin may look grossly and histologically normal between applications, but with each successive exposure to the hydrocarbon the probability of cancer formation increases.

When a chemical of this sort is first painted on an area of skin, many of the cells are killed. Very rapidly thereafter, a transitory, compensatory hyperplasia occurs. There is virtually no evidence in favor of a more direct mechanism of the hyperplasia production. With each successive application the epithelial cells show a greater and greater resistance to the toxic effect of the chemical, but the hyperplasia becomes more prolonged and abnormal. Eventually carcinoma makes its appearance, usually in a quite localized focal area (Iversen and Evensen, 1962).

Against this picture of a gradual and progressive alteration is the evidence supporting the so-called two-stage theory (Boutwell, 1964). If mouse skin is treated with a suitable suboncogenic dosage of hydrocarbon, papillomas can be subsequently elicited by painting the same area with croton oil, a very weakly oncogenic but powerfully irritating substance. If the procedure is reversed, that is, if using the same dosages, the croton oil precedes the hydrocarbon, the papillomas are not produced. Berenblum (1970) suggests that these facts prove that the hydrocarbon and the croton oil act in qualitatively different ways. If this were not so, he argues, it would make no difference which one were applied first. He suggests that the hydrocarbon initiates and the croton oil promotes oncogenesis. According to this formulation, a complete oncogen like 3-methylcholanthrene can achieve both initiation and promotion, but in low dosage the initiating effect predominates. Croton oil, on the other hand, is predominantly a promoter, while ethylcarbamate (urethane), when applied to the skin, is a nearly pure initiator.

Initiation is apparently cumulative regardless of the intervals between initiating treatments; promotion is not. In the mouse, promoters must be applied at successive intervals of less than a week to be cumulative.

Berenblum (1970) postulates that the function of an initiator is to convert normal cells into latent tumor cells (mutation?). These then persist in the epithelium until exposed to the promoter. It is now quite clear that any procedure that causes transient hyperplasia, such as wound healing, can serve as a promoter. One final point needs to be made about the two-stage system in the skin: the papillomas produced are multiple, benign focal lesions that almost always regress. Very few progress to carcinomas. The regression is caused, at least in part, by an immune response mediated by lymphocytes. If more initiator and less promoter is applied, the number of papillomas decreases but the percentage that progresses to carcinoma increases. No dilution of dosage or alteration of schedule can enable one, using a complete carcinogen alone, to simulate the result achieved with the sequence of an initiator followed by a virtually pure promoter.

How applicable the two-stage theory is outside the skin system is not known. The facts involved are very important, no matter how disputed their interpretation or possibly limited their applicability, because they must necessarily have a bearing upon theories of carcinogenesis.

Despite the plethora of oncogenic agents, it may now be a worthwhile exercise to search for common chemical and biological properties that might be clues to the mechanisms of neoplastic transformation by chemical oncogens. First, we can list the common biologic features:

1. All the oncogens that have been tested are apparently cytotoxic to the target tissue when used in effective dosage, and apparently, for that reason, all produce hyperplasia.
2. Most of the "complete" hydrocarbon oncogens tested are more toxic to most normal cells than to most tumor cells (Vasiliev and Guelstein, 1963). This is not true of urethane, the seemingly pure initiator, or of certain alkylating agents. The exceptions are sufficiently numerous to cast doubt upon differential toxicity as an important general mechanism in chemical oncogenesis (Diamond, 1969).
3. Hydrocarbon oncogens and the azo dye and fluorenylamine hepatocarcinogens combine with a protein in the target tissue to produce physically similar conjugation products (i.e., the charge category is similar)—products that are diminished or absent in the resulting tumors. This may prove a general phenomenon of great importance.

Figure 6-9.

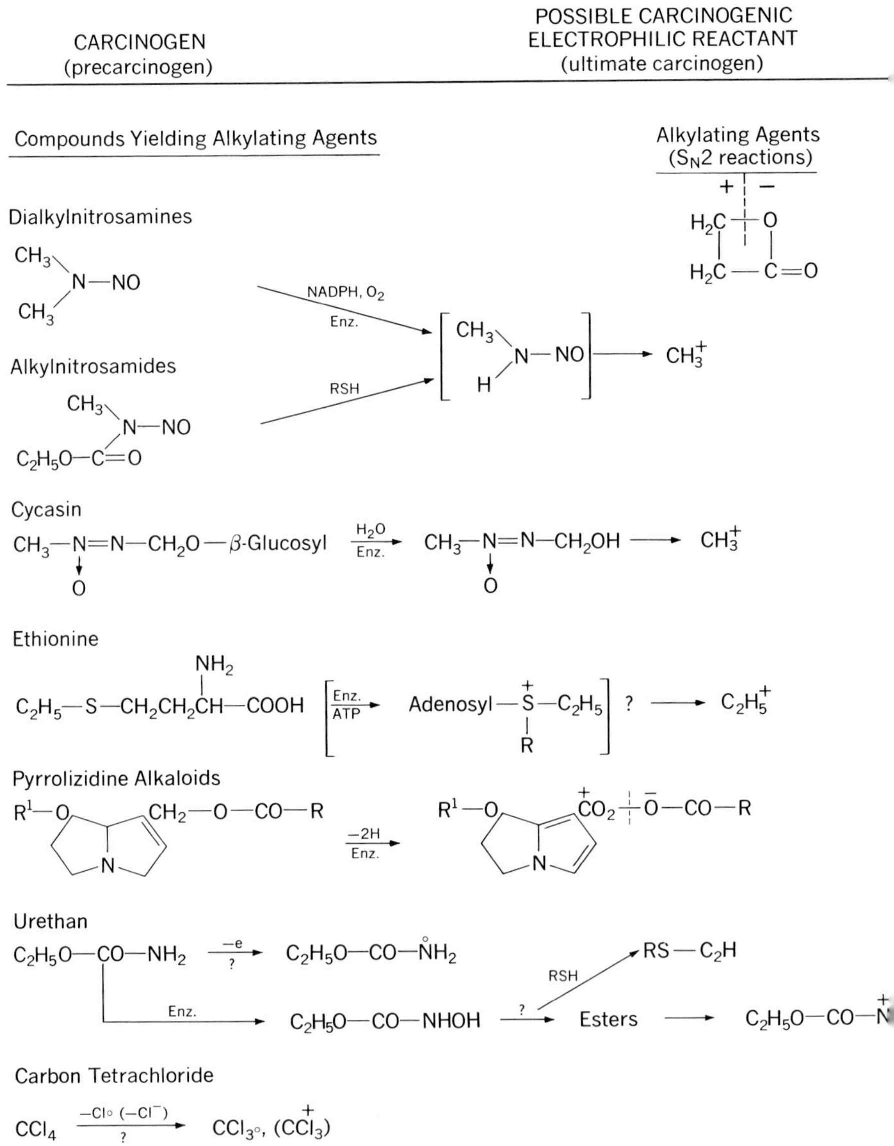
CARCINOGEN (precarcinogen)
POSSIBLE CARCINOGENIC ELECTROPHILIC REACTANT (ultimate carcinogen)
Compounds Yielding Alkylating Agents
Alkylating Agents (SN2 reactions)
Dialkylnitrosamines
NADPH, O2
Enz.
Alkylnitrosamides
RSH
Cycasin
CH3—N=N—CH2O—β-Glucosyl
H2O
Enz.
CH3—N=N—CH2OH
Ethionine
C2H5—S—CH2CH2CH—COOH
Enz.
ATP
Adenosyl—S—C2H5
Pyrrolizidine Alkaloids
R1—O
CH2—O—CO—R
−2H
Enz.
Urethan
C2H5O—CO—NH2
−e
C2H5O—CO—NH2
Enz.
C2H5O—CO—NHOH
RSH
RS—C2H
Esters
Carbon Tetrachloride
CCl4
−Cl∘ (−Cl−)
CCl3∘, (CCl3)

CARCINOGEN (precarcinogen)	POSSIBLE CARCINOGENIC ELECTROPHILIC REACTANT (ultimate carcinogen)

ompounds Yielding Arylating, Arylamidating, and Related Agents

romatic Amides and Amines

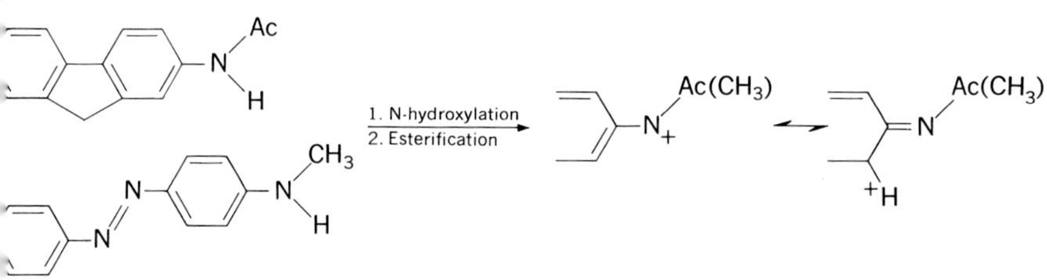

phenyl-N-nitroso Urea

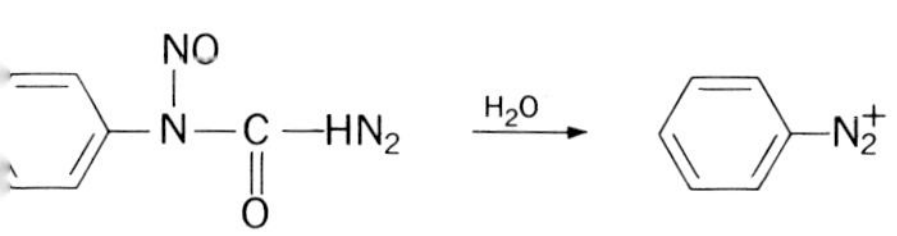

nitroquinoline-l-oxide

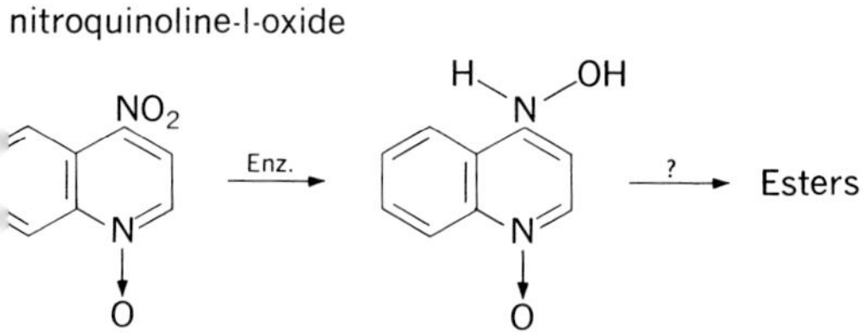

lycyclic Aromatic Hydrocarbons?

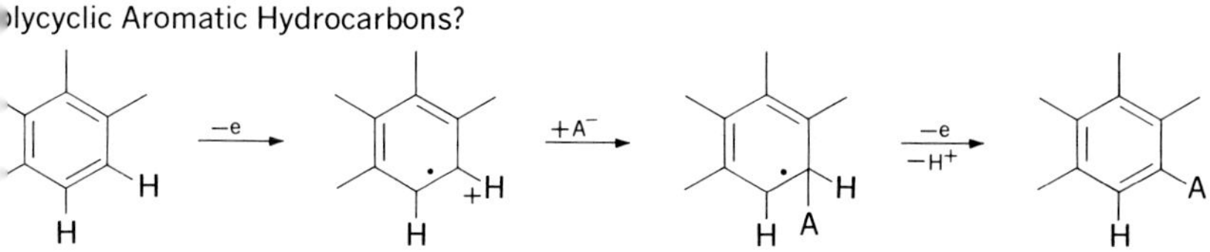

Radical cation

Carcinogenic Metals

Be^{++}, Cd^{++}, Co^{++}, Cr^{+++}, Pb^{++}, Ni^{++}

odified from Miller and Miller, 1969)

4. Many, but not all, chemical oncogens are mutagens. Moreover, not all mutagens are oncogenic. It could perhaps be argued that the exceptions are due to lack of a proper test system. Not even known mutagens are mutagenic under all conditions and in all biologic systems. Perhaps all proximal oncogens will be shown to be mutagens. At present, however, this correlation is not very good.
5. All oncogens thus far examined, when used in oncogenic dosage, interfere with normal immunologic reactions (Prehn, 1963). In this connection it should be remembered that most neoplasms are probably at least moderately antigenic.
6. Many (all?) chemical oncogens and radiation are capable of uncovering or activating latent oncogenic viruses.

As we look back over this list, it seems that #1, #5, and #6 are the properties that have thus far failed to show exceptions; #3 has probably not been widely enough investigated to permit confident generalization. In #1, the production of compensatory hyperplasia after toxicity, it is probably the hyperplasia per se that is important, since hyperplasia, as we shall see, also precedes oncogenesis by hormones. When hyperplasia occurs after hormone treatment, it is probably not a matter of compensation after toxicity. The importance of #5, interference with immune mechanisms, is further suggested by the fact that neoplasms produced by the chemical agents tend to be more antigenic than those produced by other modalities that may not seriously affect the normal immune reactivity. Thus, this property of the chemical oncogens may be an important facet of their activity. Number 6, the activation of viruses, cannot be ruled out as a general mechanism of action, but much further investigation is needed.

Recently some progress has been made toward elucidation of a common chemical mode of activity among the plethora of oncogenic compounds. Many oncogenic amides and amines have been found to undergo N-hydroxylation to a "proximal" oncogen, which is then converted to a highly unstable, reactive, electrophilic derivative. This derivative combines with nucleophilic groups in crucial cellular components, such as nucleic acids and proteins. Some suggested ultimate oncogenic electrophilic forms of various oncogens are given in Figure 6-9, modified from the Millers' work. Formulas in parentheses are conjectured (Miller and Miller, 1969).

The oncogenic polycyclic aromatic hydrocarbons form the only large group of chemical oncogens for which the nature of the probable reactive forms is still rather obscure. It seems probable, however, that the hydrocarbons also work via activation to electrophilic derivatives. It should be noted that the oncogenic hydrocarbons are relatively ineffective in primates. Thus, there may be profound species differences in the metabolism of these agents.

The knowledge of the ultimate reactive form of the various oncogens unfortunately does not delineate the target, which could still be either protein, RNA, or DNA, or even all three. More will be said on this subject when various theories of oncogenesis are discussed in a subsequent section.

4. Hormonal agents

Although many hormones serve as important factors that contribute to the oncogenic activities of various other agents, it is clear that hormonal imbalance can produce neoplasia in the absence of any known viral or chemical agent. This is perhaps best exemplified by the hormonal production of ovarian neoplasms in rodents.

This system, which was developed by the Biskinds, involves a surgical manipulation to provide chronic excessive gonadotrophin for the ovarian tissues (Biskind and Biskind, 1949). The technique was to ovariectomize young adult mice or rats and then to make an ovarian graft to the spleen. Under these conditions, the grafted ovarian tissue in the spleen became hyperplastic and, after many months, neoplastic. The tumors that developed were initially often dependent upon excessive gonadotrophin, but this dependence was usually rapidly lost by progression to more complete autonomy.

The mechanism of oncogenesis can be derived from the following facts:

1. The splenic transplant did not become tumorous if ovariectomy was incomplete.
2. Neoplasia was prevented also by implantation of ovarian tissue subcutaneously.
3. Hypophysectomy prevented the oncogenesis.
4. The pituitary also became hyperplastic and in some cases neoplastic.
5. Adhesions at the operative site between the spleen and body wall tended to prevent neoplastic transformation.

These and other facts support the theory that the neoplastic transformation in this system results from chronic stimulation of the transplanted ovarian tissue by excessive pituitary gonadotrophin. The feedback arc that normally regulates the production of pituitary gonadotrophin is broken by placing the only significant estrogen source in the hepatic portal system; the liver inactivates virtually all estrogen reaching it. Thus, in the experiment, estrogen from the intrasplenic transplant could not reach the pituitary. Without this estrogenic inhibition the pituitary produced excessive gonadotrophin, and the ovarian tissue was stimulated to hyperplasia.

This principle of hormonal oncogenesis is general. By chronic imbalance of the appropriate hormones, tumors have been produced in virtually all of the hormonally dependent organs. In all these organs, hormonally induced chronic hyperplasia may develop into neoplasia (Gardner, 1953).

5. Immunity as an oncogen

Immunity has thus far been considered only as an antineoplastic factor. This viewpoint is probably correct in general, but it is possible to produce lymphocytic neoplasms in mice by bringing about a chronic graft vs. host reaction. This can be done by inoculating F_1 mice with parental-strain homozygous spleen cells. The transplanted immunologic mechanism of the parental strain is capable of reacting against F_1 tissue, but for genetic reasons the F_1 cannot react against the transplant. Thus, the host is subject to prolonged immunologic assault. Under these conditions the host lymphocytes may develop a lymphoma. This reaction is poorly understood, but it has been shown that immune attack can produce chromosomal abnormalities in target cells without necessarily being lethal (Fialkow, 1967).

A further property of the immune response that may contribute to oncogenesis will be discussed in a subsequent section concerning speculative theories (Section F).

6. Physical agents

The oncogenic effect of *ionizing radiant energy,* particularly X-rays, was discovered by tragic experience shortly after the discovery of X-rays themselves. Among early radiologists there arose numerous cases of chronic ulceration followed by squamous-cell carcinomas of the hands or fingers, making the new agent's potentialities only too evident. X-irradiation was probably the first environmental oncogen to be clearly identified.

Many cases of neoplasia have been induced by the physician. Infants who received radiation to the neck for a rather nebulous condition, enlarged thymus, suffered in later life from an unusually high incidence of thyroid carcinoma. Patients with Marie-Strumpels syndrome, a severe rheumatoid arthritis of the spine, were in the past often treated with large doses of radiation with a resultant increased incidence of lymphoma. Even today there is mounting evidence that the small doses of radiation given in the course of diagnostic examination of the pelvis in complicated obstetrical cases can produce an increased incidence of leukemia later in the life of the children thus radiated *in utero* (Brues, 1954).

Radiant energy has been an industrial hazard, as witnessed by the osteogenic sarcomas that were produced following radium ingestion by watch-dial painters. It has also become a hazard of modern warfare, causing the increased rate of leukemia in the survivors of Hiroshima and Nagasaki.

In experimental systems irradiation can increase the incidence of neoplasms due primarily to other agents, but does not appear to be a very potent oncogen in its own right. The marrow and lymphoid systems seem most sensitive to its toxic effects, and it is in these tissues that neoplasia is most easily produced. In the mouse, X-irradiation can produce leukemias that are of virus etiology but would not have appeared had it not been for the action of the radiation. Perhaps the virus is activated by the radiation.

In many experimental systems it appears that the action of the X-rays is indirect–i.e., the tissues that eventually become neoplastic need not have been directly radiated. This is particularly well demonstrated in mouse thymic lymphomas. Most mouse leukemia has its origins in the thymus gland, and this is true of radiation-induced leukemia as well. Using inbred mice, with various genetic markers, it is possible to show that transplantation of a radiated thymus gland into a non-radiated recipient animal, induces neoplasia in the non-radiated lymphoid cells of that animal (Law and Potter, 1958).

The mechanisms by which ionizing radiation produces neoplasia are unknown. Of course, radiation is a known mutagen that can produce chromosomal aberrations; like chemical carcinogens, it depresses immune defenses, and it produces cell destruction and compensatory hyperplasia, especially in the marrow and lymphoid systems. Nevertheless, the intimate molecular events that produce neoplasia are just as obscure as in the case of chemical oncogenesis.

It is not really paradoxical that X-irradiation is also a very important therapeutic modality for various kinds of cancer. It can destroy cells, especially rapidly dividing cells. In the cancer patient this property is far more important than the possible risk of inducing a new neoplasm in normal cells that survive the treatment.

Radiant energy of yet another type is an important oncogen in man. It is quite clear that the vast majority of cases of skin cancer are the result of exposure to ultraviolet radiation. The oncogenic wavelengths are the same as those producing skin destruction and sunburn, approximately 2900-3200 A. It is clear that skin pigmentation is markedly protective, and for this reason the incidence of skin cancer is low in the more heavily pigmented races. The visible effects of aging in the skin are largely the result, not of senescence per se, but of exposure to ultraviolet light. In view of these facts and the ready availability of vitamin D from other sources, the "health" fad of suntanning has no rationale in the twentieth century. Ultraviolet light is toxic, accelerating both aging and oncogenesis in the skin. It should be avoided.

The effects of *mechanical trauma* on oncogenesis have already been dealt with to some extent in the consideration of the two-stage theory. There is no question but that mechanical trauma can contribute to the neoplastic process. Still, although chronic hyperplasia may in some circumstances be a complete oncogen, there is no evidence that acute trauma can do more than accelerate a process already under way. Clinical instances in which neoplasia has followed acute trauma are almost certainly due not to a causal relation, but rather to the fact that trauma may call the patient's attention to an incipient neoplasm.

There is one interesting form of physical oncogenesis in rodents and related animals that may have little counterpart in man. This can be called *smooth-surface sarcogenesis* and consists of the induction of sarcomas around smooth-surfaced films made of any material. The mechanism of the oncogenic effect of smooth films or foils is not known, but a few features have narrowed the possibilities. It is known that a rather acellular, fibrous capsule develops around a smooth film after the foreign-body reaction subsides. Neoplasia arises from cells inside this capsule on the surface of the film. These cells are very flattened and thin, and perhaps this physical fact contributes to transformation. It has been shown that the environment inside the fibrous capsule is unusually conducive to the growth of tumor implants. If a chronic granulomatous reaction is maintained about the film, as it is about a rough film, fibrous capsule formation is diminished and oncogenesis is reduced.

There is little evidence that films and foils produce similar effect in man. The subcutaneous tissues of the rodent seem unusually susceptible to oncogenesis.

Another possibly related form of oncogenesis should be mentioned here. It is virtually impossible, for unknown reasons, to keep rodent cells grown in tissue culture from becoming neoplastic and growing as tumor when returned to an *in vivo* environment (Sanford, 1965). Primate cells, in general, seem to be much more resistant to neoplastic transformation under these conditions. The smooth surface upon which the cultures are grown may contribute to the oncogenic process in the rodent cells, but this is sheer speculation.

7. Aging

Cancer, with few exceptions, is a disease intimately related to aging (Doll, 1964). In human populations the probability of developing carcinoma of the prostate rises exponentially to approach 100 per cent in the very aged. A somewhat similar relation is seen for gastric carcinoma, bronchogenic carcinoma, and carcinoma of the breast, though in these cases the curve is not quite so steep. In mammary cancer there is a distinct hump in the curve around the age of menopause.

There are, however, certain cancers that are peculiar to childhood. Most prominent among these are childhood leukemia, neuroblastoma, Wilm's tumor, and retinoblastoma.

The reasons for the fairly general relation between naturally occurring cancer and aging are not known, but they may be related to the possibility that the neoplastic cell may evolve by an accumulated series of random sequential alterations. In addition, the effectiveness of immunity decreases in old age.

8. Diet

There is an important and striking relation, especially in experimental animals, between nutrition and the incidence of neoplasia. It is a general phenomenon that chronic caloric restriction reduces the incidence and delays onset of neoplastic disease. In this there seems to be an association between the effects of caloric restriction on aging and the effects on neoplasia. Although caloric restriction (and lowered body weight) inhibits the cancer incidence, there is no evidence that starvation alters or slows the course of an already established neoplasm.

F. Speculative Theories of Oncogenesis

Most theories concerning the nature of the neoplastic cell fall into two different categories, though some are intermediate. The basic, unresolved question seems to be whether the neoplastic cell should be regarded as a form of somatic mutation or as a form of abnormal differentiation, more akin to the variation that permits cells of identical genotype to become liver cells or kidney cells. All the various etiologic factors that have been investigated, including the oncogenic viruses, can be accommodated under either theory. There is no logical necessity for a unitary hypothesis. Perhaps some neoplasms are of one type and some of another, and some may combine both elements. The difference between these two theories may actually not be very great. The term *somatic mutation* is often broadened for the purpose of this hypothesis to include any random heritable alteration, whether due to a change in a nuclear gene or not. Mutation-like processes in extragenic inheritance mechanisms thus qualify as somatic mutations. Many such systems are known at least in lower forms, and, in relation to cancer, have been assembled under the title of the *plasma gene theory* (Darlington, 1948). A real possibility along this line has been raised by the demonstration of the heritability of a surgically induced cell-surface change in paramecia (Sonneborn, 1964). If a random mutation-like change in the mammalian cell surface can also be heritable without gene mutation, one heuristically appealing hypothesis of neoplastic transformation is obviously available. If the hypothetical cell-surface changes are actually somewhat less random, however, they may serve as a mechanism of normal differentiation. In that event the two theories virtually merge.

It seems that one of the essential features distinguishing the two theories is really the question of the randomness of the change. Does the change originate in a single cell or in a few cells on a random basis or, conversely, as the result of simultaneous and predictable change in all or many cells in a certain area? This question cannot be answered, since only a limited amount of direct evidence is available. The histologic evidence suggests that a neoplasm often arises from an area, not from a randomly occurring abnormal progenitor. Conversely, the weight of experimental evidence tends to support the hypothesis of sporadic single-cell origin or at least origin from relatively few cells in a restricted area. It denies the general hypothesis that neoplastic growth ordinarily occurs by the continuous recruitment of newly transformed cells from the surrounding normal population, although this process does occur in some virus-induced tumors.

The histologic evidence to support the field theory comes from the observation that in many lesions, especially in skin and breast, there may be no recognizable dividing line between carcinoma and surrounding normal epithelial tissue. Instead there is often a gradation from areas of overt malignancy with the usual cytologic alterations through areas of less marked abnormality to areas of completely normal morphology. The appearance suggests the gradual conversion of cells from normal to malignant as the lesion expands. On the other hand, it is quite clear from transplantation experiments using cytologic, genetic, or antigenic markers, that most experimental animal tumors do not convert host cells to neoplastic cells. They behave as though derived from a single, abnormal ancestor. It will also be remembered that the usual explanation of the two-stage experiments is the production in the epithelium of randomly scattered, latent tumor cells.

Laboratory data have suggested a possible way to reconcile the histologic and experimental findings. It has been found that many carcinomas have the capacity to induce physiologic hyperplasia in a nearby normal epithelium (Argyris and Argyris, 1962). It has also been found that some epithelial neoplasms of the mouse breast regularly seem to contain a proportion of normal epithelial cells in some sort of symbiotic equilibrium with the neoplastic cells (Prehn, 1967). This normal component has apparently undergone an induced hyperplasia so that the cells are not distinguishable morphologically from neoplastic ones, but they have no heritable alteration. When separated from the neoplastic cells they revert to a normal morphology. Thus it is possible that neoplasia is essentially a clonal phenomenon which may, however, sometimes stimulate a diffuse arisal in an oncogenic field by inducing morphologic but not heritable alterations in the surrounding normal cells.

Perhaps a more important aspect of the original question is whether the varied changes seen in neoplastic cells represent altered patterns of normal gene expression or are the result of the acquisition of new genetic information, either by mutation or viral infection, not previously present in the ancestral cell line. Again, this is a question that cannot yet be answered with any certainty, and again, the theories are not mutually exclusive. Present evidence seems to favor the theory of altered patterns of normal gene expression rather than that of new genetic information.

Of course, it is becoming increasingly evident that many neoplasms have a viral etiology and that viral nucleic acid may be incorporated into the cellular genome. This would seem to be new genetic information. However, it is not yet established that continued presence and activity of the viral genes are necessary conditions of the neoplastic state. Perhaps they are only some kind of trigger mechanism. Nonetheless, it must be admitted that the evidence for continued viral-gene activity in the neoplastic cells, as shown with the temperature-sensitive mutants previously discussed and by the persistence of viral RNA, is at present the best argument in favor of the new genetic information hypothesis. Perhaps this will prove the better hypothesis for some virally-induced tumors.

There is a question whether or not the genetic information contained in the RNA of the RNA tumor viruses is really new information so far as the cell is concerned. One theory concerning latent viruses, the *oncogene theory,* proposes that all normal cells contain the necessary sequences of DNA to specify the RNA of the oncogenic virus (Huebner and Todaro, 1969). Thus, the virus information is considered to be locked within the normal cellular genome until derepressed by some environmental etiologic agent, viral or chemical.

Against the new genetic information theory, evidence has accumulated that neoplastic cells have no properties that are not found under other conditions in one or another line of normal cells. Neoplastic changes may be explained as stabilizations of abnormal patterns of expression in the normal genome. The recently acquired enzymatic evidence for this was discussed in the section on the biochemistry of the neoplastic cell (Pitot and Cho, 1965). The morphologic and behavioral features seem to be of a similar nature. Normal cells have the information necessary to undergo hyperplasia, but the neoplastic cell apparently becomes, to a varied degree, stabilized in that pattern of gene expression. Chronic physiologic hyperplasia may at times be difficult to distinguish morphologically from neoplasia and may even exhibit cytologic changes. Even invasiveness and the ability to metastasize cannot be considered evidence of new genetic information, since many non-neoplastic cells exhibit these qualities. Blood cells, for example, tend to be free-living and invasive. Bone-marrow cells can "metastasize" in experimental animals under suitable conditions. Endometriosis may represent metastasis of otherwise normal cells. Migration of normal cells is a frequent occurrence during embryogenesis, and probably no neoplasm exceeds in its growth rate that of the embryo. All these qualities in a neoplasm may be abnormal stabilizations of various patterns of expression of the perfectly normal cellular genome. The new antigens seen in neoplastic cells may all turn out, as some already have, to be normal gene products that are usually expressed only during ontogeny. As of this writing, there is no unequivocal evidence that any of the new antigens that play a role in the behavior of virally induced neoplastic cells are encoded by viral genes. All of them may represent specific alterations in the expression of the normal genome. Perhaps even the immortality of neoplastic cell lines could be looked upon as an abnormal stabilization of a normal life-giving pattern of gene expression.

If the basic alterations in the neoplastic cell need not involve changes in the genome, then theories concerning the mode of action of chemical agents need not involve reactions with DNA. An alternative but hypothetical way in which heritable alterations could be produced is through the direct arrangement of the patterns of lipoproteins on the cell surface. The basis for this hypothesis is the surgically induced heritable surface changes in paramecia already mentioned Sonneborn, 1964). Another hypothesis, based upon the theories of gene regulation

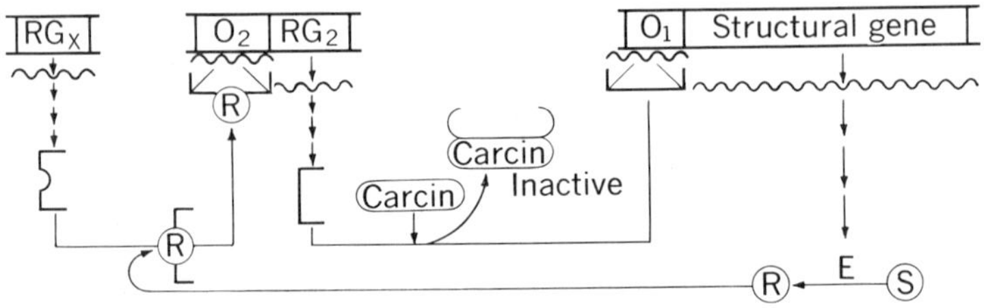

Modified product perpetuation circuit as a model for carcinogenesis. Carcin = carcinogen which combines with, and inactivates the product of, RG_2 which in turn allows synthesis of E, maintaining RG_2 in the inactive state.

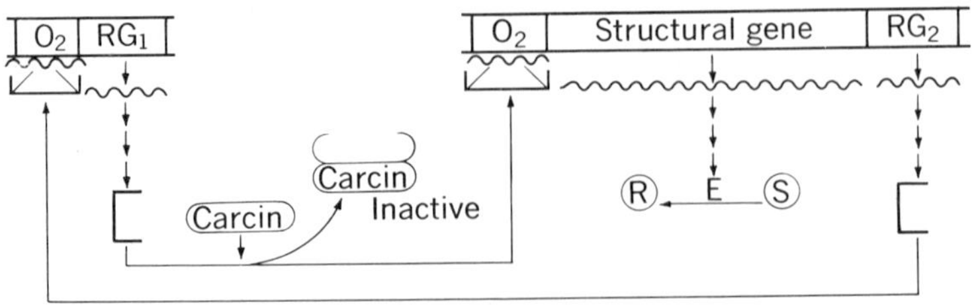

Product independent circuit.

Figure 6-10. Courtesy of Dr. H. C. Pitot

propounded by Jacob and Monod, has been put forward by Pitot and Heidelberger (Pitot and Cho, 1965). They suggest that the reaction of the oncogen with a repressor molecule could establish a self-perpetuating alteration in the regulation of an operator gene. Two such schemes are shown in Figure 6-10.

A third hypothesis of chemical oncogen action without the necessity of genic alteration can be called the *selectional hypothesis* (Prehn, 1964). It postulates that a variety of oncogen actions might alter the cellular environment so that spontaneously appearing neoplastic cells that would ordinarily lie latent or perish could proliferate to form a gross neoplasm. Among such actions might be interference with immune reactivity, greater toxicity to normal than to neoplastic cells, and production of extensive hyperplasia. It seems virtually certain that in most systems selective mechanisms are a necessary part of tumor production by a chemical agent. In some systems, in which the rate of spontaneous cellular variation may be high, selection might be a sufficient mechanism as well. Of course, selection would operate whether the basic neoplastic change were mutation-like or more akin to differentiation.

In view of the fact that immunoselection should reduce the antigenicity of tumors, the persistence of some degree of antigenicity even in long-transplanted neoplasms suggests that antigenicity is somehow an essential and intrinsic part of the neoplastic process. As cell-surface receptors of various types are probably important modulators of differentiation and tissue growth, it is possible that surface antigens represent an alteration in these receptors so that they no longer function properly in cell regulation. If these new antigens are a recapitulation of embryonic cell-surface features, they may simply be inappropriate as regulators in the adult, or they may be actively involved in the more embryonal type of regulation exhibited by tumors–i.e., anaplastic properties and lack of growth stabilization. One could anticipate that immunoselection would gradually reduce tumor antigenicity to a compromise level between the hypothetical benefits to the tumor of antigenic surface changes and the disadvantages of an immune reaction.

Tumor antigenicity may be even more directly related to the neoplastic state. As a result of recent observations, a theory of immunological stimulation of tumor growth has been proposed (Prehn, 1972). The theory is based on the observation that small numbers of specifically immune lymphoid cells may stimulate, rather than inhibit, the growth of target tumor cells. Thus, a weak immune response may actually promote tumor growth rather than inhibit it. Since all specific lymphoid reactions must be numerically weak before they become strong, the first result of the immune reaction will necessarily be the stimulation of the neoplastic target cells. Perhaps such an immune response is even a prerequisite for tumor growth.

Apparently, cell-fixed acquired immunity first arises in phylogeny in the early vertebrates–it seems to be a vertebrate adaptation. With the exception of Crown Gall and related diseases in plants, neoplasia may also be largely a vertebrate phenomenon, although this point is debatable. This phylogenetic coincidence of two major biologic traits has suggested to some investigators a causal relation between them. They have speculated that acquired cell-mediated immunity may have arisen specifically because of the need for some mechanism to inhibit neoplasia in vertebrate animals. In view of the immunological stimulation of neoplasia discussed above, it may be more likely that the paucity of neoplasms in invertebrates–if it actually exists–is directly due to the lack of an immune mechanism. Conversely, perhaps a genomic instability that made the immune mechanisms possible is itself the cause of the increased incidence of neoplasia among vertebrates. The latter hypothesis seems to be at variance with what has been said previously about abnormal stability in the expression of the neoplastic genome. This is not necessarily so. The individual neoplastic cell apparently shows abnormally great stability, failing to respond normally to environmental stresses; but the population may show great adaptive ability because of a high mitotic rate and an abnormally great variation from one cell to another. It is this adaptive ability of the neoplastic cell population as a whole that has thus far frustrated long-lasting chemotherapeutic or hormonal therapy.

The probability that neoplasia usually represents some abnormality in differentiation leads to the speculation that an etiologic factor might be found in a derangement of those tissue relations that are important in ontogeny. It is known that the development of many epithelial organs, such as the lung, kidney, and pancreas, are dependent upon a proper interaction with surrounding mesenchyme (Harris, 1964). The dependence of the epithelial component upon the connective-tissue component is not necessarily completely lost in the mature organ. Recently it has been suggested that a disruption of the dermal-epidermal junction by 3-methycholanthrene, as seen with the aid of the electron microscope, might be the primary lesion in skin oncogenesis (Tarin, 1968). Dawe (1966) has shown that polyoma virus will induce tumors in embryonic mouse salivary glands only if both epithelium and mesenchyme are present.

Consideration will now be given to one speculative theory. Not only is there a phylogenetic correlation between the development of the immune response and neoplasia, but a third major biologic trait also appears for the first time in vertebrates: the loss of regenerative ability. Again, the relation to neoplasia may be purely coincidental.

It is well known that many lower organisms possess remarkable regenerative capacities. The hydra, for example, can regenerate an entire organism from a small fragment, and regeneration in flat worms has been a classical object of study in developmental biology. As one ascends the phylogenetic tree, this regenerative capacity gradually becomes more restricted. In the vertebrates, limb and tail regeneration is found in some newts but not in the adult frog. In general, larval forms possess more regenerative capacity than adults–another example of ontogeny recapitulating phylogeny. Adult mammals–if one excepts the deer, whose antlers regenerate–possess very little regenerative ability, and what they do have is of a very restricted nature. To a considerable extent skin can be replaced, and the liver possesses the capacity to regain its original size after partial hepatectomy. In both these cases, however, the process seems to be the proliferation of surviving differentiated tissues, probably a very different process from the regeneration of an amputated newt limb. In the newt limb, dedifferentiation appears to take place in the stump, and the new limb is then formed by a process of redifferentiation, analogous to that which occurs in embryologic limb formation.

Regeneration of the newt limb is preceded by formation of a tumor-like mass of undifferentiated tissue, the blastema of regeneration. For a variety of reasons it is possible that a neoplasm may be a pathological counterpart of the regeneration blastema in an animal that has lost normal regenerative ability. Such a theory has the advantage, among others, of supplying a *raison d'être* for the existence of carcinoembryonic antigens in the tumor cells. In this formulation, neoplasia is again regarded as aberrant differentiation rather than somatic mutation. It raises the theoretical possibility of cure through differentiation, a process already known to occur in certain neoplasms arising from totipotent or near-totipotent tissues–for example, Crown Gall in plants, neuroblastoma in children, and ovarian teratoma in mice. Frequent temporary regressions and rarer spontaneous cures of even advanced cancers suggest that few, if any, neoplasms are completely independent of host homeostatic mechanisms. These mechanisms include not only immunity and various types of dependency, but perhaps also mechanisms by which the host may be able to induce tumor differentiation.

References

Andervont, H. B. (1945), The milk influence in the genesis of mammary tumors, *in* Mammary Tumors in Mice, F. R. Moultan, Ed., Publ. #22, p. 123, Am. Assoc. Adv. Sci., Washington.

Argyris, T. S., and Argyris, B. F. (1962), Differential response of skin epithelium to growth-promoting effects of subcutaneously transplated tumor, Cancer Res., *22*: 73.

Berenblum, I. (1970), The study of tumours in animals, *in* General Pathology, H. W. Florey, Ed., W. B. Saunders Co., Philadelphia.

Biskind, G. R., and Biskind, M. S. (1949), Experimental ovarian tumors in rats, Am. J. Clin. Path., *19*:501.

Boutwell, R. K. (1964), Some biological aspects of skin carcinogenesis, Prog. Exp. Tumor Res., *4*:207.

Boyland, E. (1961), Human hormone-dependent tumors, Prog. Exp. Tumor Res., *2*:146.

Boyse, E. A., *et al.* (1967), Suppression of murine leukemias by L-asparaginase. Incidence of sensitivity among leukemias of various types: comparative inhibitory activities of guinea pig serum *L-asparaginase* and *Escherichia coli L-asparaginase,* J. Exp. Med., *125*:17.

Brues, A. M. (1954), Ionizing radiations and cancer, Adv. Cancer Res., *2*:177.

Bullough, W. S., *et al.* (1967), The vertebrate epidermal chalone, Nature, *214*:578.

Castor, L. N. (1968), Contact regulation of cell division in an epithelial-like cell line, J. Cell. Physiol., *72*:161.

Crile, G., Jr. (1968), The natural history of metastases in lymph nodes, Am. J. Surg., *116*:1.

Darlington, C. D. (1948), The plasmagene theory of the origin of cancer, Brit. J. Cancer, *2*:118.

Dawe, C. J., Morgan, W. D., and Slatick, M. S. (1966), Influence of epithelio-mesenchymal interactions on tumor induction by polyoma virus, Int. J. Cancer, *1*:419-50.

Day, E. D. (1964), Vascular relationships of tumor and host, Prog. Exp. Tumor Res., *4*:58.

DeCosse, J. J., and Gelfant, S. (1968), Non-cycling tumor cells: mitogenic response to antilymphocyte serum, Science, *162*:698.

Diamond, L. (1969), The interaction of chemical carcinogens and cells *in vitro,* Prog. Exp. Tumor Res., *11*:364.

Doll, R. (1964), Epidemiological observations on susceptibility to cancer in man with special reference to age, Acta Unio Int. contra Cancrum, *20*:747.

Dulbecco, R. (1966), Mechanism of cell transformation by polyoma virus, Perspectives in Biol. and Med., Winter, vol. 9, p. 298.

Duran-Reynals, F. (1950), Neoplastic infection and cancer, Am. J. Med., *8*:490-511.

Eckhart, W. (1968), Transformation of animal cells by oncogenic DNA viruses, Physiol. Rev., *48*:513.

Fialkow, P. J. (1967), Hypothesis: immunologic oncogenesis, Blood, *30*:388.

Foulds, L. (1954), The experimental study of tumor progression: a review, Cancer Res., *14*:327.

Gardner, W. U. (1953), Hormonal aspects of experimental tumorigenesis, Adv. Cancer Res., *1*:173.

Gimbrone, M. A., Leapman, S. B., Cotran, R. S., and Folkman, J. (1972), Tumor dormancy *in vivo* by prevention of neovascularization, J. Exp. Med., *136*:261.

Harris, M. (1964), Cell Culture and Somatic Variation, Holt, Rinehart and Winston, New York.

Hayflick, L., and Moorhead, P. S. (1961), The serial cultivation of human diploid cell strains, Exp. Cell Res., *25*:585.

Hellstrom, I., Hellstrom, K. E., Pierce, G. E., and Yang, J. P. S. (1968), Cellular and humoral immunity to different types of human neoplasms, Nature, *220*:1352-54.

Henderson, J. S., and Rous, P. (1962), The plating of tumor components on the subcutaneous expanses of young mice. Findings with benign and malignant epidermal growths and with mammary carcinomas, J. Exp. Med., *115*:1211.

Henle, G., Henle, W., and Diehl, V. (1968), Relation of Burkitt's tumor-associated Herpes-type virus to infectious mononucleosis, Proc. Natl. Acad. Sci., U.S.A., *59*:94.

Heston, W. E. (1945), Genetics of mammary tumors in mice, *in* Mammary Tumors in Mice, F. R. Moultan, Ed., Pub. #22, p. 55, Am. Assoc. Adv. Sci., Washington.

Hitotsumachi, S., Rabinowitz, Z., and Sachs, L. (1971), Chromosomal control of reversion in transformed cells, Nature, *231*:511.

Huebner, R. J., and Todaro, G. J. (1969), Oncogens of RNA tumor viruses as determinants of cancer, Proc. Natl. Acad. Sci. U.S.A., *64*:1087.

Iverson, O. H., and Evensen, A. (1962), Experimental skin carcinogenesis in mice, Acta Path. Microbiol. Scand., Suppl. #156, Vol. 55.

Kajii, T., Neu, R. L., and Gardner, L. I. (1968), Chromosome abnormalities in lymph node cells from patient with familial lymphoma, Cancer, *22*:218.

Klein, G. (1968a), Tumor-specific transplantation antigens; G. H. A. Clowes Memorial Lecture, Cancer Res., *28*:625.

Klein, G. (1968b), Summary: Antigens of chemically induced tumors; and search for tumor-specific antigens in other human tumors, Cancer Res., *28*:1354.

Klein, G., and Klein, E. (1957), The evolution of independence from specific growth stimulation and inhibition in mammalian tumour-cell populations, Symp. Soc. Exp. Biol., *11*:305.

Knox, W. E. (1967), The enzymatic pattern of neoplastic tissue, Adv. Cancer Res., *10*:117.

Laird, A. K. (1965), Dynamics of tumor growth: Comparison of growth rates and extrapolation of growth curve to one cell, Brit. J. Cancer, *19*:278.

Law, L. W. (1952), Origin of the resistance of leukemia cells to folic acid antagonist, Nature, *169*:628.

Law, L. W., and Potter, M. (1958), Further evidence of indirect induction by x-radiation of lymphocytic neoplasms in mice, J. Natl. Cancer Inst., *20*:489.

Lebovitz, H. E. (1965), Endocrine-metabolic syndromes associated with neoplasms, *in* The Remote Effects of Cancer on the Nervous System, W. R. Brain and F. H. Norris, Eds., p. 105, Grune and Stratton, New York.

MacPherson, I. (1965), Reversion in hamster cells transformed by Rous sarcoma virus, Science, *148*:1731.

Mahoney, M. J., and Leighton, J. (1962), The inflammatory response to a foreign body within transplantable tumors, Cancer Res., *22*:334.

Miller, J. A., and Miller, E. C. (1969), The metabolic activation of carcinogenic aromatic amines and amides, Prog. Exp. Tumor Res., *11*:273.

Morton, D. L., Malmgren, R. A., Holmes, E. C., and Ketcham, A. S. (1968), Demonstration of antibodies against human malignant melanoma by immunofluorescence, Surgery, *64*:233-40.

Nakahara, W. (1960), A chemical basis for tumor-host relations, J. Natl. Cancer Inst., *24*:77.

Nowell, P. C. (1965), Chromosome changes in primary tumors, Prog. Exp. Tumor Res., *7*:83.

Olenov, J. M., and Fel, V. J. (1968), The antigenic structure of tumor cells as material for a study of tissue differentiation, J. Embryol. Exp. Morph., *19*:299.

Papanicolaou, G. N. (1958), Historical development of cytology as a tool in clinical medicine and in cancer research, Acta Unio Int. contra Cancrum, *14*:249.

Patterson, M. K., Jr., Maxwell, M. D., and Conway, E. (1969), Studies on asparagine requirement of the Jensen sarcoma and the derivation of its nutritional variant, Cancer Res., *29*:296.

Pitot, H. C. (1968), Some aspects of the developmental biology of neoplasia, Cancer Res., *28*:1880.

Pitot, H. C., and Cho, Y. S. (1965), Control mechanisms in the normal and neoplastic cell, Prog. Exp. Tumor Res., *7*:158.

Potter, V. R. (1968), Summary of discussion on neoplasms, Cancer Res., *28*:1901.

Prehn, R. T. (1963), Function of depressed immunologic reactivity during carcinogenesis, J. Natl. Cancer Inst., *31*:791.

Prehn, R. T. (1964), A clonal selection theory of chemical carcinogenesis, J. Natl. Cancer Inst., *32*:1.

Prehn, R. T. (1967), The significance of tumor-distinctive histocompatibility antigens, *in* Cross-reacting Antigens and Neo-antigens, p. 105, Williams & Wilkins Co., Baltimore.

Prehn, R. T. (1968), Tumor-specific antigens of putatively non-viral tumors, Cancer Res., *28*:1326.

Prehn, R. T. (1972), The immune reaction as a stimulator of tumor growth, Science, *176*:170.

Rubin, H. (1964), A defective cancer virus, Sci. Am., *210*:46.

Sanford, K. K. (1965), Malignant transformation of cells *in vitro,* Int. Rev. Cyt., *18*:249.

Sonneborn, T. M. (1964), The differentiation of cells, Proc. Natl. Acad. Sci., U.S.A., *51*:915.

Southam, C. M., Babcock, V. I., and Bailey, R. B. (1967), Selective localization of human cancer transplants in newborn rats, Transplantation, *5*:1.

Stoker, M., *et al.* (1968), Anchorage and growth regulation in normal and virus-transformed cells, Int. J. Cancer, *3*:683.

Tarin, D. (1968), Further electron microscopic studies on the mechanism of carcinogenesis: the specificity of the changes in the carcinogen-treated mouse skin, Int. J. Cancer, *3*:734.

Vasiliev, J. M., and Guelstein, V. I. (1963), Sensitivity of normal and neoplastic cells to the damaging action of carcinogenic substances: a review, J. Natl. Cancer Inst., *31*:1123.

Wogan, G. N. (1969), Naturally occurring carcinogens in foods, Prog. Exp. Tumor Res., *11*:134.

Zeidman, I. (1965), Fate of circulating tumor cells. 3. Comparison of metastatic growth produced by tumor cell emboli in veins and lymphatics, Cancer Res., *25*:324.

7

HEREDITY, DIFFERENTIATION, AND DEVELOPMENT

Robert H. Shikes, M.D.

A. Introduction

The biologic similarities common to all members of the human species are numerous and often quite obvious. Numerous, too, are the dissimilarities that distinguish individuals within the species. Individual variation in physiognomy, coloration, and physique enables us to recognize a friend in a crowd. Of medical significance are those differences that confer a biologic advantage or disadvantage upon the host.

Many of these differences are already present by the time of birth—i.e., they are inborn. The existence of inborn human variation has been recognized for at least as long as recorded history, and its nature and significance have provided a basis for much folklore as well as for scientific speculation and inquiry. For example, anatomists have for centuries assiduously recorded the multitude of variations in location, configuration, and vascular supply of human organs and structures; clinicians have long recognized the propensities of certain individuals to develop particular diseases.

Recent technical and conceptual advances in biochemistry, genetics, and molecular biology have expanded enormously our knowledge of inborn human variation. While many of these variations seem to have little or no effect upon the host, many others are associated with obviously deleterious effects in the fetus and newborn, or later, in the child and adult. These "birth defects" include the inherited disorders of metabolism, chromosomal disorders, and a variety of congenital malformations. In the United States alone, birth defects have been estimated to cause 500,000 fetal and 62,000 live-born deaths each year. Some 15 million Americans have various forms of disability due to one or more inborn variants (Apgar and Stickle, 1968).

Much of inborn human variation reflects individual differences in genotype. The anatomic, biochemical, and other properties by which we recognize and measure such genetically determined variants represent the phenotype. Other individual differences are not genetically determined but represent the consequences of environmental influences acting at other levels of biologic activity before birth.

B. Genetically Determined Biologic Variation

That a particular trait is genetically determined may be inferred from either of two observations:

1. Its occurrence within a family follows a pattern consistent with Mendelian genetics–i.e., it is inherited.
2. It is associated with a demonstrable chromosomal abnormality. Some of these are inherited; most, however, are acquired at some time during development.

Many of the inherited biologic variations are expressed as autosomal or sex-linked, and as dominant, recessive, or co-dominant traits. The heterozygote may show all, some, or none of the characteristic phenotypic manifestations. Some show differences in their degree of penetrance and/or expression; many are pleiotropic–i.e., they give rise to a variety of phenotypic alterations. Some individuals contain cells of two or more different genotypes (mosaicism); in these instances the phenotype depends not only upon the nature of the genotypic alteration but also upon how many and which of the individual cells are affected.

1. Protein polymorphism

It has been estimated that as many as 50,000 to 100,000 different species of protein molecules are present in the human organism (Pauling, 1964). Herein lies a vast reservoir of genetically determined heterogeneity in the form of protein polymorphism (Price, 1967; Harris, 1969). Each protein consists of one or more polypeptide chains characterized by a specific and unique sequence of amino acids. This sequence, in turn, is determined by a correspondingly specific sequence of nucleotides within the genome. Any alteration in nucleotide sequence, such as additions, deletions, or substitutions, is expected to result in a corresponding alteration in the polypeptide which it codes.

Theoretically, one can detect all the variations that exist in human proteins by sampling a large, representative population and by determining the amino-acid sequence of each individual protein. For many reasons such a study is at present impossible. Actually, most examples of protein polymorphism were discovered because of alterations in chemical and biologic activities of those proteins, resulting from changes in their primary structure. Thus, the substitution of one amino acid for another at a specific site may alter the configuration or electrical charge of the molecule in such a way as to confer upon it a different and unique electrophoretic mobility, antigenic specificity, or enzymatic activity. Finally, such a variation may result in abnormal host metabolism and disease.

The use of physical-chemical, biochemical, immunologic, and clinical screening has demonstrated protein polymorphism to be a widespread phenomenon in man. The serum protein, transferrin, is a case in point (Bearn and Parker, 1965). About 99 per cent of Caucasians have a transferrin that is electrophoretically homogeneous; in the remaining 1 per cent, transferrin is electrophoretically distinct from the "normal." Family studies demonstrate that this variant is inherited as a Mendelian co-dominant. Another electrophoretically distinct variant is found in 8 per cent of Navajo Indians and in 17 per cent of the Lacardan Indians of Central America. Altogether, eighteen different genetically determined electrophoretic variants of transferrin have been described in the human population, each variant presumably representing a different alteration in the genetic information that codes for this protein.

The search for protein polymorphism in the human population continues to yield an ever-increasing number of examples. In one study, Harris (1966) demonstrated protein polymorphism in several arbitrarily chosen enzymes in an unselected English population. One of these, erythrocyte acid phosphatase, occurred in five electrophoretically distinct and genetically determined varieties. A recent review (Childs and Der Kaloustian, 1968) cites eighty-four variants of hemoglobin, thirteen of haptoglobin, and twenty-five of glucose-6-phosphate dehydrogenase, as well as variants of lipoproteins, immunoglobulins, serum albumin, fibrinogen, and many enzymes.

The biologic significance of protein polymorphism is often unclear. The different forms of transferrin, for example, are equally active in their ability to bind and carry iron; none of the variants appear to confer any biologic advantage or disadvantage upon the host. Similarly, the various forms of erythrocyte acid phosphatase, although they appear to differ somewhat in their enzymatic activity, do not seem to have any significant effect upon the host.

2. Inherited disorders of metabolism

At the other end of the spectrum are those genetically determined variant proteins that have observable effects upon the host in the form of disease: the inherited disorders of metabolism.

Many of our present concepts relating to human genetic heterogeneity and disease are derived from the study of these disorders, and ultimately from the observations and insights of Sir Archibald Garrod (Childs, 1970). Sixty years ago this London physician introduced the one gene-one enzyme (or protein) concept and suggested the genetic basis for chemical individuality. He proposed that certain familial diseases were due to blocks at specific sites in metabolism, and that the metabolic block was determined by the loss of a specific enzyme. Such a block would result in the accumulation of substrate and substrate precursors and in a deficiency of product and product derivatives. Since the time of Garrod, a large number of diseases have been found which fulfill his criteria for inborn disorders of metabolism. Many of these are caused by a specific enzyme deficiency. Depending on the enzyme involved, such a deficiency may result in the impaired synthesis, degradation, mobilization, activation, secretion, absorption, excretion, or storage of one or more substrates or products. In addition to its direct effects, such a deficiency might have a variety of indirect consequences. These indirect effects can be seen in several of the enzyme-deficiency disorders.

In other cases the defect is manifested by the appearance of a protein that is altered because of a mutational event leading to a base change in the DNA and to an amino acid change in the resulting protein. This type of defect, which is at the basis of protein polymorphism, may in some cases result in more or less severe disease.

a. Sickle cell disease

Sickle cell anemia is the best characterized of these inherited disorders of metabolism. This disease is seen almost exclusively in Negroes; in the homozygous state, its major manifestation is severe anemia exacerbated by episodes of hemolysis. Erythrocytes from these patients assume a distinctive crescent or "sickled" appearance, particularly under conditions of relatively low oxygen tension. These erythrocytes contain hemoglobin S, a variant electrophoretically distinct from normal adult hemoglobin A. Amino acid sequencing has demonstrated a specific molecular lesion in hemoglobin S: the substitution of valine for glutamic acid at position #6 in the beta chain. Certain conformational and other physical-chemical alterations can be predicted to result from this particular amino acid substitution (Murayama, 1967), leading to stacking of hemoglobin molecules and distortion of the erythrocyte which causes the phenomenon of sickling (Fig. 2-32a). This process is facilitated by deoxygenation; hence it is in the small, peripheral blood vessels that the sequelae of sickling occur—hemolysis, stagnation of blood flow, and thrombosis. Anemia, hypoxia, tissue ischemia, and infarction follow and produce the constellation of clinical features characteristic of this disease.

Given this demonstrated amino acid substitution, one can infer the corresponding genomic lesion in terms of the genetic code. The codon for glutamic acid is UAG and that for valine is UUG. Thus, the substitution of a single base–uridine for adenine–can ultimately account for this disorder. Other single amino acid substitutions have been demonstrated in many other variant hemoglobins; most of these can be accounted for by a substitution of a single base. Some profoundly alter the properties of hemoglobin and cause disease; others appear to have little effect on either molecule or host (Ranney, 1970).

In addition to full-blown sickle cell anemia some patients carry the sickle cell trait. These subjects are usually heterozygous and they have only about 40 per cent hemoglobin S with partial sickling. Patients with this trait are resistant to malaria but susceptible to venous thrombosis under reduced oxygen tension. Among West Africans the trait is quite common, and this offers a biologic advantage to subjects living in an area where malaria is widely diffused. This may indeed be an example of a potentially harmful genetic change that may have developed in part as a defense mechanism.

b. Niemann-Pick disease

This disease is an autosomal recessive trait, seen in either sex and only in the homozygous state. It is a disorder of lipid metabolism, characterized by the intracellular accumulation of a specific complex lipid, sphingomyelin, in most tissues of affected children (Brady, 1966). The normal turnover of this important component of cell membranes is partially determined by sphingomyelinase, a lysosomal enzyme that acts at the initial step in its breakdown. This enzyme has been shown to be deficient in patients with Niemann-Pick disease, and, in its absence, substrate accumulates within lysosomes. Unable to digest sphingomyelin, large and abnormally structured lysosomal derivatives crowd out other cytoplasmic organelles within neurons, hepatocytes, blood-cell precursors in the bone marrow, and other cells (Fig. 7-1). Eventually this results in a multitude of clinical findings, including neurologic signs, hepatomegaly, and anemia.

Niemann-Pick disease is a prototype of many important inherited disorders of metabolism called "storage diseases," which are characterized by the accumulation of metabolites (Hers and Van Hoof, 1970). Other of these diseases are characterized by the accumulation of various lipids, glycogen, or mucopolysaccharides (Fig. 2-28c,d)

c. Phenylketonuria

This is a disorder of amino acid metabolism manifested early in life by mental retardation, large excesses of phenylalanine in the blood, and the excretion of large amounts of phenylpyruvic acid in the urine (Carpenter *et al.,* 1968). It is

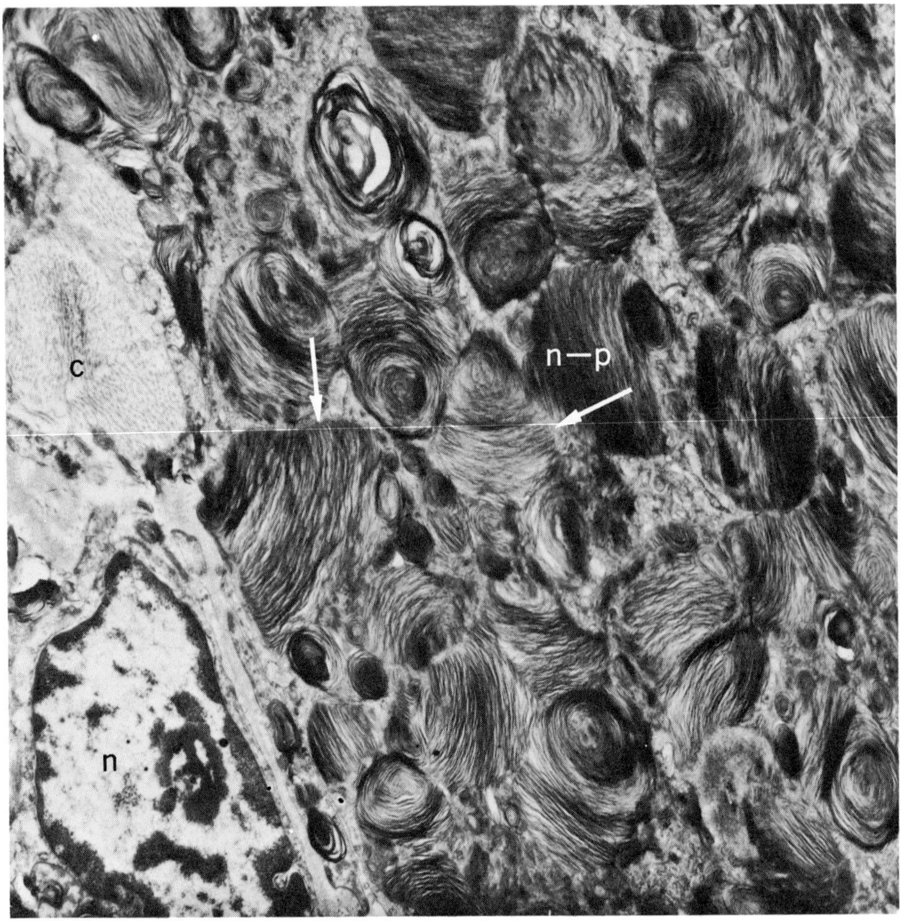

Figure 7-1. Electron-microscopic appearance of the lipid deposition in hepatic cell of a child with Nieman-Pick disease. N—nucleus, C—collagen, N-P—characteristic lipid deposits with whorling configuration (sphingomyelin deposited within lysosomes).

transmitted as an autosomal recessive trait. The deficient enzyme is phenylalanine hydroxylase, a liver enzyme that normally converts phenylalanine to tyrosine. When this major pathway of phenylalanine metabolism is blocked, the amino acid is channeled to an ordinarily minor alternate pathway, leading to phenylpyruvic acid and its derivatives. Phenylpyruvic acid can be detected in the urine by a single laboratory test that is now routinely done on most newborns; the early diagnosis of this disease is of particular importance, since the prompt withdrawal of dietary phenylalanine prevents the development of this form of mental retardation. The reason for the development of mental retardation is not clear, but it appears that the metabolic alteration impairs normal postnatal myelinization.

d. Galactosemia

In this disease a deficiency of galactose-1-phosphate uridyl transferase blocks the normal conversion of galactose to glucose (Hsia, 1967). Of particular importance is the failure to form UDP-galactose, an intermediate necessary for the incorporation of galactose into many large and important carbohydrate-containing molecules. The diversity of molecules so affected probably accounts for the pleiotropic effects of galactosemia, which include mental retardation, cataract formation, and cirrhosis. An autosomal recessive transmission is the trait in both this disease and the one immediately following.

e. Hereditary orotic aciduria

This is a disorder of pyrimidine metabolism characterized by the development, in infants, of megaloblastic anemia and developmental retardation (Smith *et al.,* 1966). In this disorder, two enzymes are deficient; these enzymes are responsible for sequential steps in the conversion of orotic acid to uridine monophosphate (UMP). UMP is an important precursor of RNA and of certain coenzymes. A good therapeutic response is achieved by dietary supplementation with uridine, thus by-passing the metabolic block.

f. Lesch-Nyhan syndrome

Lesch-Nyhan syndrome (Proceedings, 1968) is an X-linked recessive disorder and is observed only in males. The disease is manifest in childhood by mental and growth retardation, abnormal motor activity, and a peculiar behavioral pattern characterized by compulsive automutilation of fingers, toes, and lips. The deficient enzyme is hypoxanthine-guanine phosphoribosyl transferase. In its absence, hypoxanthine cannot be utilized in nucleotide synthesis, and there is a marked increase in the production of its catabolite uric acid. The increase in uric acid accounts for the gout seen in some of these patients; the other clinical manifestations cannot be explained on the basis of the known metabolic defect.

g. Miscellaneous disorders

Other inherited disorders of metabolism have been more or less well defined in terms of their clinical manifestations, patterns of inheritance, and specific metabolic and molecular alterations. In addition to the examples cited above, specific enzyme deficiencies have been demonstrated in various disorders involving carbohydrate, amino acid, lipid, purine, porphyrin, and hormone metabolism. Wilson's disease, an inherited disorder of copper metabolism, is associated with a deficiency of the serum protein, ceruloplasmin. The inherited disorders of coagulation are due to deficiencies of specific coagulation factors. The active transport of specific molecules across biological membranes appears to depend upon certain ill-defined "receptors" and "carriers"; abnormalities of such factors have been suggested in certain diseases with defective absorption, secretion, or excretion. Examples include some of the hereditary intestinal malabsorption syndromes and the renal aminoacidurias (Scriver, 1969b), and one form of hereditary hemolytic anemia may be due to a deficiency of erythrocyte Na-K dependent ATPase (Oski *et al.*, 1969).

The basic metabolic defect involved in a number of the inherited disorders of metabolism is completely unknown. An outstanding example is pancreatic cystic fibrosis, a fairly common disease. It has been suggested that some of the inherited disorders of connective tissue may be due to deficiencies of enzymes or other factors responsible for the synthesis or cross-linking of collagen or elastin; genetically determined alterations in the primary structure of these proteins may also occur. Some of the inherited disorders of metabolism may actually represent a variety of different biochemical lesions that give rise to a common clinical picture. Diabetes mellitus and gout are two examples; each will probably prove to consist of a group of genetically, etiologically, and pathogenetically distinct metabolic disorders. A small percentage of cases of gout is distinguished from the great majority by the genetically determined deficiency of a specific enzyme involved in purine metabolism (Kelley *et al.*, 1969).

Of major clinical significance are genetically determined individual differences in the response to drugs. Pharmacogenetics refers to the study of such variation in terms of response and the metabolism and excretion of various drugs and their bio-derivatives (LaDu, 1969). Use of the antimalarial primaquine causes hemolytic anemia in some persons; about 10 per cent of Negro males are at risk because of an X-linked defect. This unique response is associated with certain variants of erythrocyte glucose-6-phosphate dehydrogenase. Inherited variations in drug metabolizing enzymes have been demonstrated or implicated in untoward responses to a variety of drugs, e.g., isoniazid (antitubercular agent), succinylcholine (muscle relaxant), diphenylhydantoin (anticonvulsant), and dicumarol (anticoagulant).

h. Genetics and the immune response

Antibody specificity is at least partially due to variations in the primary structure of immunoglobulins; one theory of immunogenesis holds that some of this specificity is inborn and genetically determined. Examples of genetically determined individual variation within immunoglobulins have been demonstrated (Franklin, 1967). It is not yet known, however, whether such polymorphism is related to individual differences of response to antigenic stimulation, such as occurs in asthma and allergies. Inherited defects in antibody synthesis or cellular immunity account for some of the immune deficiency diseases (see Chapter 5). Genetically determined individual variations in cell-surface antigens have been extensively studied, particularly with regard to blood types and organ transplantation. Fetal-maternal immunologic incompatibility, most clearly demonstrated in erythroblastosis fetalis, may account for a significant portion of other forms of fetal wastage and disease (Brent, 1966).

i. Variations in the inherited disorders of metabolism

In addition to the "typical" examples, many of the inherited disorders of metabolism present a variety of clinically and/or biochemically "atypical" forms (LaDu, 1967). Each of the five enzyme-deficiency diseases we have discussed has shown one or more genetically determined variant form. Thus, cases of phenylketonuria have been described in which there has been little or no mental retardation, and various degrees of phenylalanine hydroxylase deficiency have been reported (Carpenter *et al.,* 1968). Such biochemical and clinical heterogeneity can be ascribed to the heterogeneity of genetically determined molecular alterations. Depending on the nature of the amino acid substitution and its location within the polypeptide chain, alterations in primary structure might have profound, minor, or no effects on the biologic activity of the protein, and result in severe disease, mild disease, or none at all.

Such a situation may be operative in the Duarte variant of galactose-1-phosphate uridyl transferase (Mathai and Beutler, 1966). Individuals homozygous for this variant show 50 per cent of normal enzyme activity and none of the stigmata of galactosemia. The variant is electrophoretically distinct from the normal enzyme and was incidentally discovered in a survey of a phenotypically normal unselected population. Whether such variants do indeed reflect different amino acid substitutions awaits sequence analyses such as those that have been applied to hemoglobin.

j. Inherited disorders of control mechanisms

As was pointed out in Chapter 1, one becomes aware of injury when an enzymatic activity is affected. This may be due to alterations in the structure of the enzyme (reflecting a genetic lesion in a structural gene), but it may also be due to the amount of the enzyme, or to various necessary non-enzymatic com-

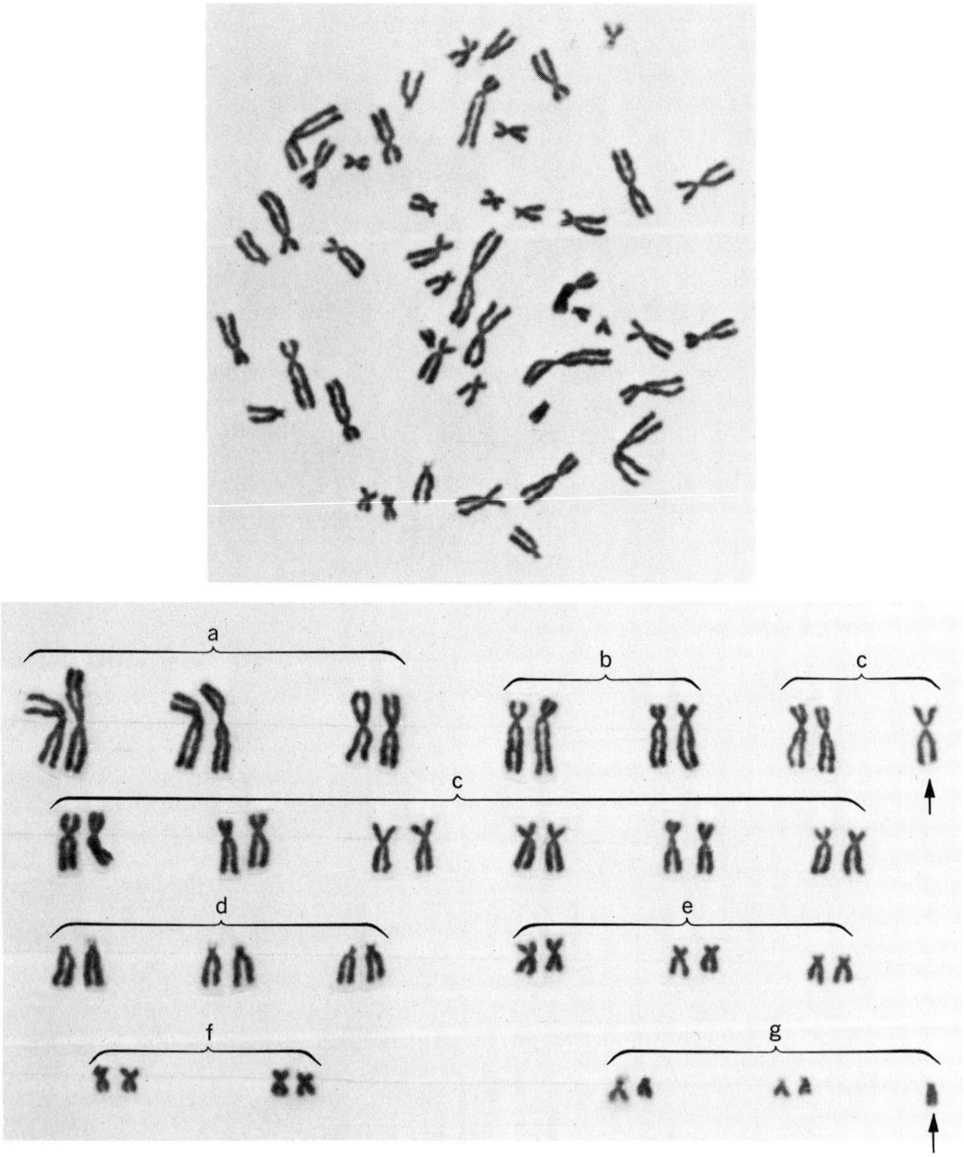

Normal Male

Figure 7-2. Normal male and female karyotypes. Karyotypic analysis involves the examination of a large number of such metaphase spreads obtained from cultured blood or amniotic cells or fibroblasts. One or more representative cells are photographed and the photographed chromosomes are arranged, in pairs, according to the accepted system of classification. Any deviations from normal number, size, and morphology are noted.

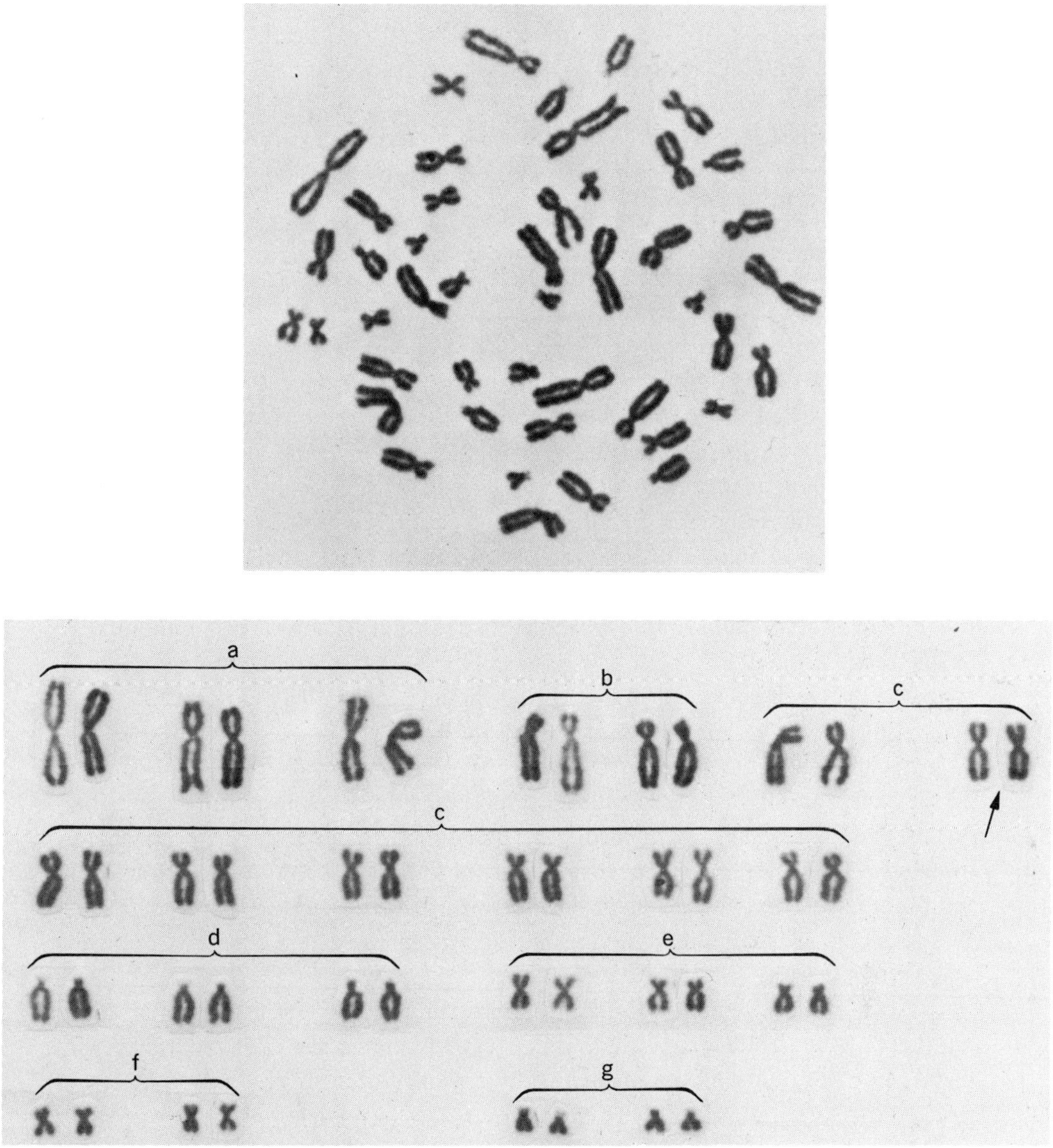

Normal Female

In the male karyotype the X chromosome is in group C (arrow) and the Y chromosome in group G (arrow). In the female karyotype the X chromosomes are in group C (arrow). Courtesy of Dr. Arthur Robinson.

ponents of a reaction. The control mechanisms that have been so expertly investigated and described in microbial organisms may have identical or at least analogous counterparts in animal cells (Dreyfus, 1969). Thus, loss of enzyme activity might be due to a lesion in an operator or promoter segment of the genome or in a gene that codes for a particular inducer or repressor. Genetically determined defects could act at the level of protein synthesis (translation), in the transport and packaging of proteins, or in the attachment of important carbohydrate or lipid moieties within cytoplasmic organelles. Still another possibility lies at the level of the biologic activity itself, with deficient activity due to the lack of a specific activator or co-factor.

A role for controlling factors in determining genetic heterogeneity is implied in several inherited disorders of metabolism. One of these, beta thalassemia, is characterized by severe anemia and growth retardation, terminating in death during childhood or adolescence (Weatherall, 1967). Erythrocyte precursor cells from these patients have a greatly reduced ability to synthesize normal adult hemoglobin, specifically the beta-chain component. The small amount of beta chain that is synthesized is of normal amino acid sequence. Thus, unlike the other hemoglobinopathies, the genetically determined defect is a quantitative rather than a qualitative one. The implication is that the genetic lesion lies in some factor which controls the synthesis of beta chains (Clegg *et al.,* 1968), perhaps at the level of translation.

In the case of hereditary orotic aciduria, it will be recalled that two enzymes are deficient, and that these enzymes act as sequential steps in pyrimidine metabolism. This phenomenon seems similar to mutations of operator genes in microorganisms. More direct evidence for a genetic lesion of a controller factor lies in the observation that the deficient enzymes can be "turned on" when cells from these patients are maintained *in vitro* and grown under certain conditions (Pinsky and Krooth, 1967).

Acute intermittent porphyria, a disease transmitted as an autosomal dominant disorder, may illustrate still another type of genetic lesion of control mechanisms. In this condition, characterized by episodes of neurologic dysfunction, a marked excess (up to 60-fold) of the enzyme delta aminolevulinic acid synthetase (ALA synthetase) is regularly found. The reaction catalyzed by this enzyme is normally a rate-limiting one in the synthesis of porphyrins from succinate; an excess of the enzyme thus leads to an excess of porphyrin intermediates, especially delta aminolevulinic acid and porphobilinogen. This phenomenon seems most likely to involve a constitutive mutation of the operator gene, resulting in lack of ability to repress the structural gene for ALA synthetase: synthesis of the enzyme thus is uncontrolled (Tschudy, 1969).

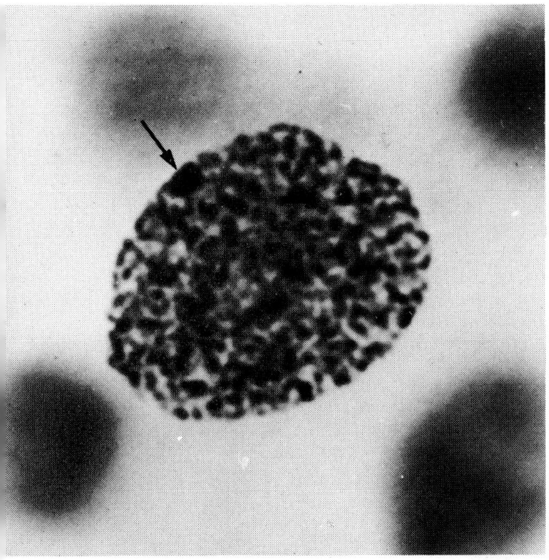

Figure 7-3. Barr Bodies

	Number of Barr bodies	Number of X chromosomes
upper left	1	2
middle	2	3
lower right	3	4

(Courtesy of Dr. Arthur Robinson)

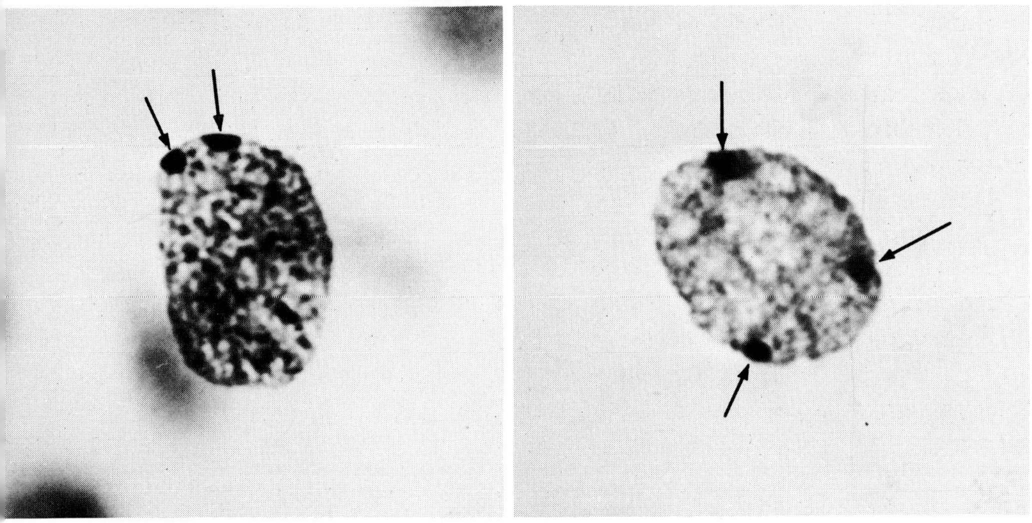

c

3. Chromosomal abnormalities

In recent years advances in cytogenetic techniques have allowed the partial characterization of the human somatic cell set of chromosomes. Large numbers of mitotic preparations derived from unselected populations have been examined by light microscopy, and from this has arisen a generally accepted description of the normal human karyotype, based upon chromosome number, size, and morphology (Chicago Conference, 1966). Using these criteria, the human somatic-

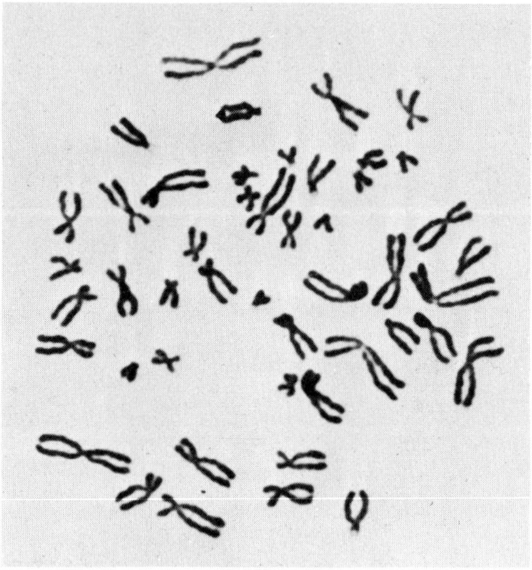

Down's Syndrome

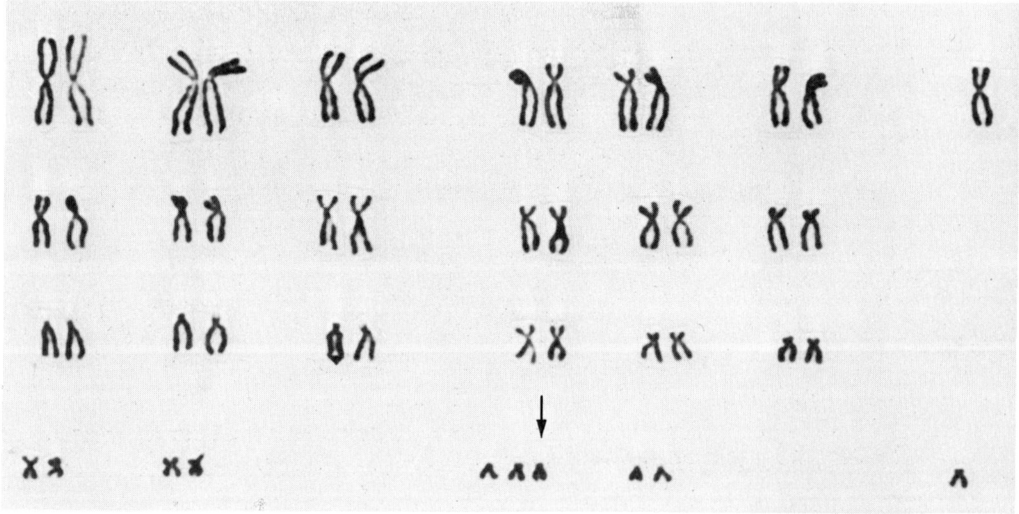

Figure 7-4. Down's syndrome. This patient's karyotype shows 47 chromosomes. There is an additional G group chromosome (arrow). Such a patient would be expected to show the phenotypic features of Down's syndrome. (Courtesy of Dr. Arthur Robinson)

cell complement of twenty-two pairs of autosomes and two sex chromosomes has been divided into seven groups designated A, B, C, D, E, F, and G. Group A includes the three large pairs of autosomes, and Group G the two smallest pairs plus the Y chromosome in the male. Within some groups individual homologous pairs can be distinguished, and within group A, for example, each pair is designated as 1, 2, or 3. Within other groups, such as Group C, such a distinction is not possible (Fig. 7-2).

All human cells contain a single genetically active X chromosome. If one or more additional X chromosomes are present, they are genetically inactive. By light microscopy, such genetically inactive X chromosomes are represented by discrete foci of heterochromatin adjacent to the nuclear membrane (Barr bodies). The number of Barr bodies is one less than the total number of X chromosomes contained within a given cell. Analysis of human material for Barr bodies provides a rapid and easy method for determining an individual's complement of X chromosomes and for establishing sexual genotype (Fig. 7-3).

The application of karyotypic analysis has resulted in an extensive literature describing many human chromosomal variations involving both autosomes and sex chromosomes (Redding and Hirschhorn, 1968; Carr, 1969a; Jacobs, 1969). Many of these variations appear to occur during gametogenesis or early development, and others are transmitted through succeeding generations. Some are associated with no apparent phenotypic abnormalities, while others consistently give rise to significant disease, usually in the form of developmental aberrations of particular organs and other anatomic structures. Some chromosomal abnormalities are characterized by fairly specific constellations of congenital abnormalities in the form of syndromes. The chromosomal abnormalities seen in cancer cells were discussed in Chapter 6.

Chromosomal abnormalities account for a significant proportion of human disease. Karyotypic analyses of fetuses that have died spontaneously *in utero* have shown abnormalities in about 20 per cent (Carr, 1969c). In newborns with obvious congenital malformations the incidence of chromosomal abnormalities is 4 per cent (Stewart *et al.,* 1969), and in phenotypically normal newborns it is about 0.5 per cent (Walzer *et al.,* 1969). Such abnormalities are said to account for 20,000 new cases of mental retardation each year in the United States (Carr, 1969b).

a. Additions

The most frequently observed human chromosomal variant is the presence of an extra chromosome (trisomy), and the first disease to be associated with a chromosomal abnormality was Down's syndrome (Fig. 7-4). Nearly all patients with this syndrome have an extra G group chromosome (trisomy G). The birth defects comprising this clinical syndrome were described long before the chromosomal defect; it includes a characteristic so-called Mongoloid facies, mental retardation, congenital heart disease, and a variety of other less constant developmental anomalies.

Trisomies involving other autosomes are almost exclusively limited to severely malformed aborted fetuses. Trisomy D and trisomy E are occasionally seen in live births, but these infants usually have severe congenital malformations and die early in life.

Additions of sex chromosomes are seen more frequently than the autosomal trisomies. When a Y chromosome is present, the person is a gonadal male regardless of the number of X chromosomes; in the absence of a Y, phenotypic development follows the female pattern. In either situation, however, there is usually retarded sexual development and sterility, and there may be mental retardation and other phenotypic abnormalities as well. In patients with Klinefelter's syndrome (XXY), for example, the testes remain anatomically and functionally immature after the age of puberty, and the secondary sex characteristics of the adult male fail to develop. The XYY genotype, on the other hand, has been associated with an increased incidence of tall stature and sociopathic behavior, and has received much publicity in the past year or two, particularly in connection with sexual crimes. A recent study indicates that this chromosomal abnormality occurs much more frequently than was thought, without clinical manifestations, and thus casts doubt on its sociopathic role.

b. Deletions

The deletion of an entire autosome is a rare phenomenon associated with severe malformations and intrauterine death. A few cases of monosomy G have been reported in infants. More frequently seen, though still rare, are partial autosomal deletions. Of these, the most common is deletion of the short arm of a B group chromosome, which results in the *cri-du-chat* syndrome. Infants with this disease are characterized by mental and growth retardation, microcephaly, abnormal facies, various other congenital malformations, and a typical plaintive cry that resembles the mewing of a cat. Other partial autosomal deletions have been associated with all sorts of phenotypic abnormalities.

The presence of a single X chromosome (XO, Turner's syndrome) is associated with phenotypic "femaleness," but with immature ovaries, infertility, and a variety of other findings including short stature, webbed neck, and mental retardation (Fig. 7-5). The YO genotype has not been observed.

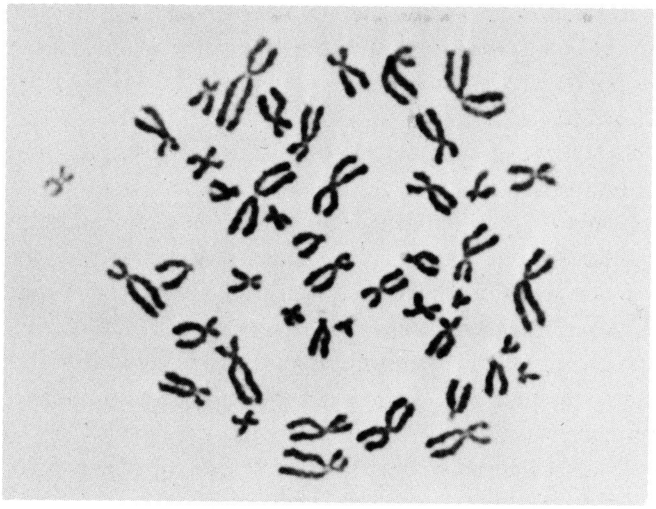

Turner's Syndrome

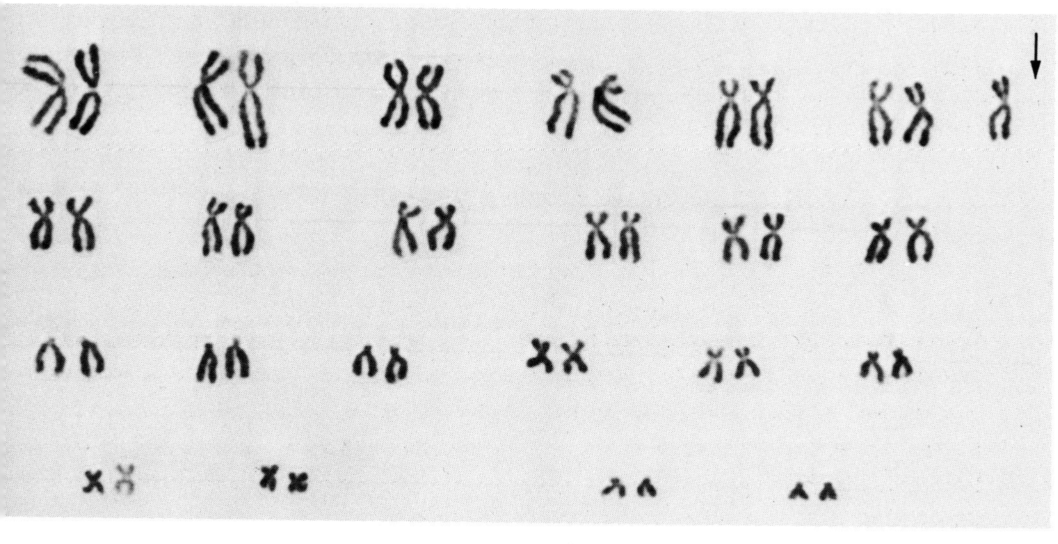

Figure 7-5. Turner's syndrome. This karyotype shows only 45 chromosomes, and although such patients are phenotypic females, there is only one X chromosome (arrow). As expected, cells from such patients show no Barr bodies. (Courtesy of Dr. Arthur Robinson)

c. Rearrangements

Many chromosomal abnormalities appear to result from chromosome or chromatid breaks and subsequent fusions that occur during meiosis and mitosis. Broken fragments may rejoin to form an intact chromosome, or one in which there is an internal rearrangement in the sequence of genetic material. A fragment may be irretrievably lost, or it may unite with another broken chromosome (translocation) (Fig. 7-6). Fragments may be exchanged between homologous or non-homologous chromosomes. Obviously, the variety of genomic rearrangements that can result is enormous. Many of the morphologic aberrations that have been described in autosomes and sex chromosomes are presumed to be due to the consequences of such chromosomal breakage and fusion.

When an exchange of fragments between non-homologous chromosomes is not accompanied by significant loss of genetic material, the resulting translocation is said to be balanced and the host is usually phenotypically normal. The host's offspring, however, are subject to genetically unbalanced situations. For example, one form of translocation that has been frequently described results in the formation of a hybrid chromosome consisting of a large segment of chromosome #15 to which a large fragment of a G group chromosome has been attached. This results in no significant loss of genetic material in the host, who is phenotypically normal. A certain percentage of the host's gametes, however, will contain both this hybrid chromosome and an intact G group chromosome homologous to the G group fragment contained in the hybrid. Fertilization results in a zygote which has a triple dose of this G group chromosome, effectively trisomy G. These patients show the phenotypic manifestations of Down's syndrome and account for about 5 per cent of the cases of this disorder.

d. Minor abnormalities

Included in this heterogeneous group are individuals who show variation in the size or shape of particular chromosomes, or abnormalities of secondary constrictions or satellites. They are termed *minor* because they are usually unassociated with any phenotypic abnormality; many are inherited in Mendelian form.

e. Pathogenesis of phenotypic abnormalities

Gene dosage and the site of genomic lesions are important in determining the phenotypic features of the chromosomal abnormalities.

Gene dosage. Birth defects due to chromosomal abnormalities are almost always due to the addition or deletion of a portion of the genome, regardless of whether the alteration is a trisomy or a monosomy, a partial deletion or an un-

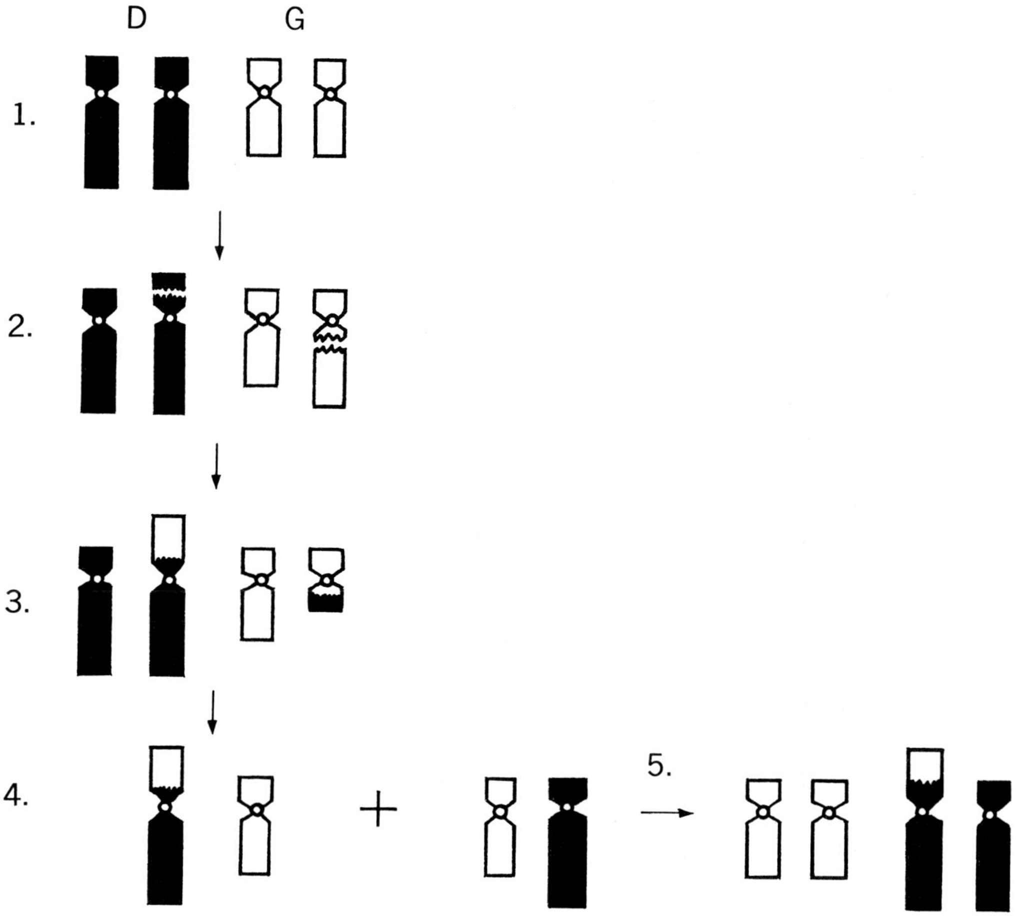

Figure 7-6. Translocation

1. Normal diploid cell containing 2 homologous pairs of D and G chromosomes.

2. Fragmentation of one member of each pair.

3. Balanced translocation. Fragments have been exchanged between D and G chromosomes.

4. Meiotic reduction division. Three patterns of segregation are possible. In this one, the gamete contains an intact G chromosome plus a D chromosome to which has been added a large segment of G chromosome.

5. Fertilization adds still another homologous G chromosome; the resultant zygote contains essentially three homologous G chromosomes—trisomy G.

This is one form of translocation; the treating and joining of chromosomes can result in a variety of other forms of genetic rearrangement and translocation.

balanced translocation. Any deviation from the diploid state apparently results in genetic imbalance sufficient to preclude normal development. How such deviations give rise to the various congenital malformations is unknown.

Site of the genomic lesion. A chromosomal addition or deletion of sufficient size to be detected by light microscopy must affect a very large number of genes; hence, the phenotypic heterogeneity of these abnormalities. Such massive chromosomal lesions, when they occur in most autosomes, are incompatible with fetal survival. Many theoretically possible autosomal additions or deletions have not been found, even in fetuses; if they occur, they must cause death very early in development and may account for a large number of unrecognized, unsuccessful pregnancies.

The relatively mild effects associated with additions of the X chromosome are consistent with the Lyon hypothesis: i.e., no matter how many X chromosomes a cell might contain, only one is expressed. Nevertheless, at least a portion of the second X must be expressed at least some time during development; the genotype XO is phenotypically abnormal, and some effects, however mild, are seen with additions of X chromosomes.

f. Pathogenesis of chromosomal abnormalities

Two major mechanisms have been implicated in the pathogenesis of inborn chromosomal errors: non-disjunction and chromosomal breakage. Non-disjunction refers to the failure of the members of a particular pair of chromosomes (or chromatids) to segregate independently during meiosis or mitosis (Fig. 7-7). In meiotic non-disjunction, the resulting gametes contain either both members or neither member of a homologous pair, and the resultant zygote is either trisomic or monosomic. The incidence of trisomy has been statistically correlated with advanced maternal age and presumably with aging of the ovum. In any human ovum the process of meiosis is interrupted for a period of many years before fertitilization, and this hiatus is even greater in ova of women conceiving late in reproductive life. The passage of time increases the risk of injury and may allow for the accumulation of injuries which, in turn, facilitate aberrant cell division in the form of non-disjunction.

Non-disjunction has been observed in mitotic cells as well and its occasional occurrence in zygotic mitosis cannot be ruled out. That it also occurs early in embryonic development is confirmed by numerous instances of individuals exhibiting various combinations of monosomic, disomic, and/or trisomic cells. Individual mosaics for trisomy G have shown all, some, or none of the phenotypic features of Down's syndrome (Kohn *et al.*, 1970).

Chromosomal breakage is a widespread biologic phenomenon, and the re-

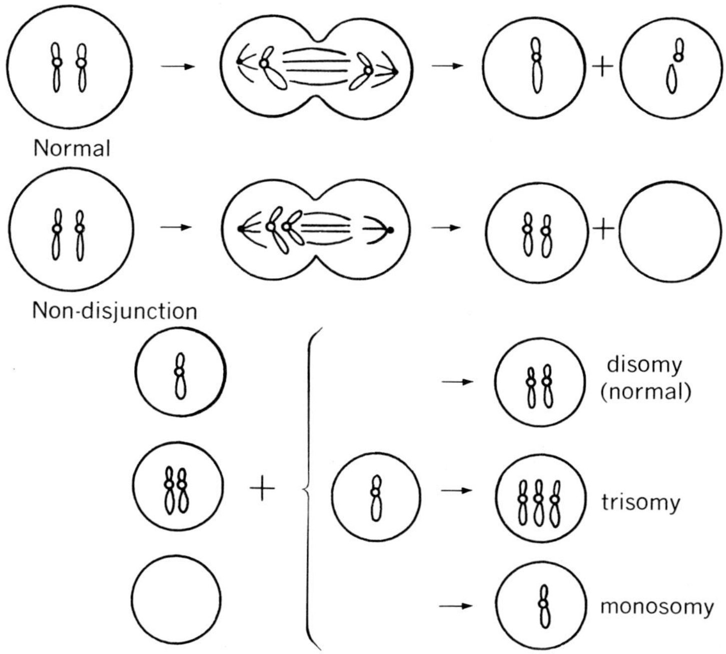

Figure 7-7. Non-disjunction during meiosis of developing gametes. This can occur also during mitosis.

sulting re-combinations of genetic information are important in the evolutionary process. Although most breaks probably heal spontaneously and are without consequence, they can, as we have seen, result in chromosomal rearrangements with deleterious effects upon the host or his offspring. Mosaics may occur in this situation too, again apparently representing errors occurring during mitosis in the early embryo.

Cells derived from patients with two inherited diseases, Bloom's syndrome and Fanconi's anemia, show a remarkable propensity for the development of chromosomal breakage and all sorts of aberrant and rearranged chromosomes (German, 1969). Although these diseases are quite different in their clinical manifestations, they have another feature in common: both often lead to the development of leukemia or malignant neoplasms relatively early in life.

g. Etiology

Experimentally, various agents have been shown to cause chromosomal abnormalities in normal mammalian cells (Nowell, 1969); these agents include ionizing radiation, viruses, chemicals, and immunologic injury. Some of these agents are likely to have a role in the pathogenesis of inborn human chromosomal abnormalities, but evidence for such relations is as yet indirect and far from conclusive.

Irradiation of the gonads of experimental animals has been shown to cause inborn chromosomal abnormalities in their offspring. An increased incidence of trisomy in the children of women who have had diagnostic abdominal irradiation before pregnancy suggests an analogous mechanism in humans (Uchida *et al.*, 1968). Suggestive, too, is a study that shows an increased occurrence of various chromosomal aberrations in cells derived from persons who had been exposed *in utero* to radiation from atomic explosives (Bloom *et al.*, 1968).

Many viruses have been shown to be potent inducers of chromosomal lesions experimentally and, as in the case of neoplasia, a viral etiology for human inborn chromosomal abnormalities has been suggested (Nichols, 1966). It is certainly possible that clinical or subclinical maternal infection could give rise to aberrant meiosis in the ovum or aberrant mitosis in the zygote or early embryo. Reports of seasonally related space-time clusters or "outbreaks" of inborn chromosomal abnormalities are consistent with such a hypothesis (Day, 1966). Epidemiologic data have been interpreted as demonstrating a relation between "epidemics" of infectious hepatitis and the increased incidence of Down's syndrome in infants born nine months after such epidemics (Stroller, 1969).

Although a wide spectrum of biologic and non-biologic chemicals have been shown to cause a wide variety of chromosomal abnormalities in mammalian cells, there is as yet no direct evidence that any chemical is responsible for inborn human chromosomal aberrations. Altered maternal immune mechanisms have also been suggested as a factor in the etiology of chromosomal aberrations; it has been reported, for example, that mothers of Down's syndrome patients have an increased incidence of thyroid auto-antibodies (Fialkow, 1966).

The obvious difficulty in establishing an etiological role for these and other suggested agents of inborn chromosomal abnormalities reflects the difficulties inherent to the study of early normal and abnormal mammalian and human development. Unless such an etiologic relation is overwhelmingly clear, interpretations of retrospective and even prospective studies are fraught with danger. Some of these difficulties may be circumvented by the study of early mammalian development *in vitro*. Mammalian ova, zygotes, and very early embryos have been successfully maintained in culture and, in one instance, a specific agent (the antibiotic, Streptonigrin) has been shown to enter the immature mouse ovum and cause chromosomal abnormalities during meiosis (Jagiello, 1967). The successful application of such techniques to human material (Edwards *et al.*, 1969) will undoubtedly be exploited along these lines.

4. Challenge of the future

The past two decades have witnessed a steady progression in our understanding of basic biological mechanisms in terms of cellular, subcellular, and molecular structure and function. The use of ever more refined methods of morphologic, genetic, biochemical, and physical-chemical analysis continues to define the nature and arrangement of genetic information, the mechanisms by which this information is replicated and expressed, and the system of controls that affect and effect these phenomena. Much of this knowledge is derived from the study of the microbial systems.

The application of the spectacular successes of microbial biology to human genetics presents an exciting prospect to the human biologist. The difficulties of such an endeavor are obvious, but some of them may be circumvented by the use of cell culture (Priest, 1968; Mellman and Kohn, 1970). Lines of "fibroblast-like" cells derived from human biopsies can be maintained *in vitro*. These cells retain the chromosomal and biochemical properties of the host's fibroblasts, and they can be manipulated under controlled conditions in ways similar to bacterial cultures.

The study of microbial molecular biology has been facilitated by the inspired exploitation of naturally occurring and experimentally induced genetic markers or mutations. As we have seen, there are abundant examples of such genetic markers in the human population in the form of protein polymorphism, inborn disorders of metabolism, and chromosomal abnormalities. Many of these markers are carried over to cells in culture, where they can be used to elucidate normal, variant, and pathologic genetically determined biologic functions.

Thus far, the major effort in cell culture has been applied to the demonstration of specific metabolic or chromosomal aberrations. Cultured fibroblasts obtained from patients with Niemann-Pick disease are deficient in sphingomyelinase, and cells obtained from patients with Trisomy G contain an extra G group chromosome. Cells from patients with Lesch-Nyhan syndrome have been used to elucidate the specific enzymatic defect characteristic of that disease. Cells from patients with certain of the inherited disorders of metabolism stain metachromatically with toluidine blue. This characteristic is seen also to a lesser degree in cells derived from heterozygotes, and is used in the identification of such phenotypically normal carriers. The prenatal diagnosis of inherited disorders of metabolism and chromosomal abnormalities is accomplished by the demonstration of these defects in cultured amniotic cells (Nadler, 1969).

The use of genetic markers will eventually achieve the goal of mapping the human genome, possibly through the use of selective cell hybridization or the experimental induction of specific chromosomal deletions and recombinations (Renwick, 1969).

The prevention and therapy of the diseases associated with genetically determined inborn variation are major goals of biomedical science. Prevention of the disease states themselves is limited, as yet, to genetic counseling of prospective parents and therapeutic abortion of demonstrably affected fetuses. In a few of the metabolic disorders, early diagnosis and treatment can prevent some of the significant clinical manifestations. Deletion of phenylalanine from the diet of infants with phenylketonuria significantly retards the development of mental retardation, and supplementation of the diet of patients with hereditary orotic aciduria corrects the anemia associated with this disease. Few of the metabolic disorders and none of the chromosomal abnormalities are at present amenable to therapy, and most are progressive and invariably fatal.

A number of possible approaches to prevention and therapy warrant investigation (Lowe, 1969; Scriver, 1969a). The enzyme (and other protein) deficiencies, for example, may be treated by administration of the deficient enzyme, as in the treatment of diabetics with insulin. For a variety of reasons, this most obvious and direct approach has not been feasible. Many of the enzymes in question have been only partially purified, are not readily available, and are rapidly degraded *in vivo*. Some of these difficulties may be avoided by using new techniques of *in vitro* protein synthesis to produce polypeptides with the desired enzymatic activity and with increased biologic lifespans. Another possibility involves the administration of enzymes in a "protected" state. Catalase molecules, for example, have been enclosed within semipermeable microcapsules consisting of a synthetic polymer. The capsule protects the enzyme from degradation but allows the entry of small molecules such as the substrates of catalase. This technique has been successfully applied to the treatment of a genetically determined deficiency of catalase in mice (Chang and Poznansky, 1968); it has not been used in human acatalasemia.

In the enzyme deficiencies due to abnormalities of control mechanisms, one might hope to be able to bypass the defective controller and "turn on" the deficient enzyme activity. An example of this possibility has been previously discussed in the case of hereditary orotic aciduria, in which production of the deficient enzymes can be induced in cell culture.

Ultimately, one hopes to replace an absent or defective segment of the genome in a process analogous to bacterial transformation. Small segments of intact template will be inoculated into deficient cells in culture, and the cultured cells returned to the host. The introduction of small segments of genetic material may be accomplished by using innocuous "carrier" viruses. Another possibility is the *in vitro* mating of enzymatically sufficient and deficient cells, and the selection of sufficient progeny for administration. The problems involved in such feats of genetic engineering are obviously quite formidable.

The chromosomal abnormalities are acquired during gametogenesis or during mitosis in the zygote or its immediate derivatives, and many of their manifestations are already present very early in development. Their eradication rests upon an increased understanding of such processes as chromosomal replication, breakage, repair, and segregation, and upon the identification and elimination of etiologic factors which cause disarrangements in these processes.

C. Non-Genetic Biologic Variations: Teratology

Thus far, inborn human variation has been discussed in terms of genetically determined alterations. A great deal of human variation, however, is the consequence of alterations at other levels of biologic activity. These account for a large percentage of birth defects. In these instances, the presence of genetic damage is tentatively excluded by the failure to demonstrate chromosomal abnormalities or inheritance of the variant trait. It must be emphasized, however, that the absence of such findings does not completely preclude the participation of genetic phenomena; genetic damage may play a role that is simply undetectable at present.

The emergence of the newborn is the culmination of an exquisitely timed series of integrated anatomic and biochemical events. Although this process occurs within a relatively well protected environment, even this environment is not free of hazards (Ferreira, 1969). Alterations of the environment may occur at any time between formation of the gamete and birth. Their effects are most obvious when they produce injury or death. Injuries occurring during fertilization, implantation, or early embryogenesis probably account for a large number of unsuccessful pregnancies. Since they occur so early in development, they are usually unrecognized and their true incidence is unknown. Lethal injuries occurring later in pregnancy are recognized as spontaneous abortions and as many as 25 per cent of all detectable pregnancies terminate in this way. Sub-lethal injury may occur in the fetus or newborn because of hypoxia, malnutrition, hormonal, vitamin, or electrolyte imbalance, and so on, and can result in a variety of more or less well defined anatomic and physiologic abnormalities.

Teratology refers to the study of congenital malformations: anatomic abnormalities resulting from aberrant morphogenesis of specific tissues, organs, and organ systems. As we have seen, teratologic malformations are a frequent manifestation of inherited and acquired genetic lesions; frequently, however, environmental alterations and injury occurring during critical periods of development are responsible. Specific tissues and organs are particularly susceptible during periods of accelerated growth or when they are undergoing the alterations and rearrangements implicit in the formation of new anatomic structures. The heart and its attendant great vessels undergo profound changes during the fourth and fifth weeks of gestation; sub-lethal injury occurring at this time can result in a wide variety of congenital cardiac and vascular malformations.

In addition to timing, the nature of the environmental alteration is of obvious importance in determining the type and extent of fetal injury. Some agents may act only on specific targets, while others may be unselective in their ability to cause injury. A particular agent that is target-selective may produce no injury if it appears at a time when the target is not susceptible. Conversely, an unselective agent that is present over a long period of gestational time may give rise to a variety of congenital malformations involving multiple organs.

The catalogue of congenital malformations in man is enormous and includes almost every structure in the body. Some malformations are incompatible with prenatal life and others with postnatal survival. Some are compatible with life but cause severe disability, and still others are of no apparent consequence and may be incidental findings at autopsy in nonagenarians. Congenital malformations may occur singly or in random association, and sometimes they are found in characteristic patterns within individuals.

The true incidence of congenital malformations is unknown, and reports vary with the source of material (abortuses, newborns, adults), means of investigation (clinical, autopsy, death certificate), and location of the study (geography, hospital population, socio-economic groups). One meaningful statistic is that 2-3 per cent of all liveborn babies have malformations that are clinically recognizable at birth and are of some medical significance (Warkany and Kalter, 1961). Additional defects become manifest later in life, and by one year of age this figure has risen to 5 per cent. The incidence in abortuses and stillborns is much higher. The frequency with which congenital malformations occur in the general population is indicated by their discovery in nearly half of a large series of unselected autopsies; of these about 50 per cent were considered to be of clinical significance (Sotelo-Avila and Shanklin, 1967).

An extensive list of environmental alterations and specific agents or teratogens has been implicated in the etiology of non-genetically determined congenital malformations. Many have been shown to cause malformations in experimental animals, and some of these serve as experimental models for similar or identical malformations in humans. In addition, there are several examples of human malformation in which a clear-cut etiologic relation has been established; of these, perhaps the best studied is the rubella syndrome (Cooper, 1968).

1. Intrauterine infection

A relation between maternal rubella and the occurrence of congenital malformations was first recognized in 1941 by Gregg, an Australian ophthalmologist; this relation has been subsequently confirmed by extensive epidemiologic analyses, by serologic studies, and more recently, by isolation of the virus from the tissues of affected fetuses and newborns. The clinical syndrome includes cataracts, congenital heart disease, and a variety of other malformations. The fetus of a mother who is infected during the first trimester runs a high risk of being diseased. The consequences may range from spontaneous abortion of a severely malformed fetus to birth of an infant with little impairment. It has been estimated that the rubella epidemic that occurred in the United States in 1964 resulted in as many as 30,000 malformed babies.

When pregnant experimental animals are inoculated with rubella virus, the results are fetal infection and the production of malformations similar to those that occur in humans. This virus does not appear to be particularly cytopathic, either *in vivo* or in tissue culture; it does, however, appear to cause significant retardation of cell growth (Plotkin and Vaheri, 1967). Such growth retardation, occurring during critical periods of development, presumably accounts for at least part of the spectrum of congenital malformations. Rubella also gives rise to chronic infection and can exert its effects over long periods of time; it has been recovered from children years after the initial intrauterine infection.

The demonstration that maternal infection with rubella can be transmitted to the fetus and can cause congenital malformations has led to intensive searches for other examples (Elizan and Fabiyi, 1970; Sever and White, 1968). Herpes virus and cytomegalovirus, as well as toxoplasma, have been shown to cause human congenital malformations; other infectious agents have been implicated as well. The potential role of maternal infection in causing fetal disease is becoming increasingly apparent. Perhaps 5 per cent of all pregnancies are complicated by one or more clinical infections in the mother (in addition to the common cold), and this figure is amplified to an unknown extent by inapparent subclinical or chronic infection. Furthermore, organisms that are ordinarily non-pathogenic for adults can have a significant effect upon the fetus. Recent serologic studies suggest that fetal infection is a far more common phenomenon than has been suspected.

2. Chemical and environmental teratogens

A broad spectrum of exogenous chemicals has been shown to cause congenital malformations in animals and occasionally in man (Smithells, 1966). Thousands of cases of severe malformation have been ascribed to the administration of the sedative thalidomide to pregnant women in Europe. Anomalies of the limbs were particularly prominent in these cases, and the occurrence of these anomalies has been correlated with administration of the drug during a particular two week period in gestation (Nowack, 1965). During this period, limb morphogenesis is particularly active and apparently susceptible to injury.

Other experimental teratogenic agents include various antibiotics and anti-metabolites, anti-thyroid drugs, and corticosteroids; for some of these, a role in human malformation has been demonstrated. Even the ubiquitous acetylsalicylic acid (aspirin) can, under certain conditions, produce malformations in mice and rats, but teratogenic effects in humans have not been demonstrated. Possible teratogenic effects of LSD and other psychoactive drugs are being intensively investigated.

Other exogenous agents may play a significant role in the etiology of fetal diseases and malformation; these include food additives and preservatives, cigarette smoke, herbicides and pesticides, industrial waste products, and other environmental pollutants. In the Minimata Bay area of Japan, a correlation has been demonstrated between a congenital neurologic disorder and the ingestion, by pregnant women, of seafood from the bay. This seafood was heavily contaminated by neurotoxic industrial waste products, methyl mercury compounds (Matsumoto *et al.,* 1965). Another exogenous agent, radiation, is usually discussed in terms of chromosomal damage; yet its injurious effects are extragenomic as well. It may prove to be a significant cause of non-genetic fetal disease (Brill and Forgotson, 1964).

3. Maternal factors

The fetus depends upon an intact maternal metabolism, and changes in maternal health can have profound effects upon the developing fetus. Toxemia of pregnancy, maternal diabetes, malnutrition, and cardiac and renal disease increase the likelihood of fetal death, prematurity, growth retardation, and malformation. The fetal-placental-maternal hormonal relation is a delicate and highly integrated one in which a single alteration can be expected to affect the fetus in a variety of ways (Solomon and Friesen, 1968). Any factor–exogenous, maternal, or placental–that reduces oxygen or nutrient supply or the elimination of wastes, or upsets delicate metabolic balances, will also affect the fetus (Gruenwald, 1968). Morphologic alterations in the placenta are known to take part in the pathogenesis of fetal disease. It has become increasingly apparent that this organ plays an active role in fetal homeostasis, such as in the active transport of specific molecules and the synthesis of hormones and other important compounds. Disorders of specific placental functions will become apparent as mechanisms of normal function are elucidated.

Fetus and trophoblast have an immunologic status similar to that of a homograft, since they contain paternally determined antigens, some of which are foreign to the mother (Lanman, 1965). Although the fetal homograft is protected by the anatomic separation of the fetal-maternal circulations, this separation is not absolute, and cells have been shown to cross this barrier in either direction. While immunologic rejection of the fetus has not been observed, it must be considered as a possibility in the etiology of fetal wastage and malformation.

4. Conclusion

Genetic and non-genetic influences may so damage human development that the biologic variation produced is responsible for much disease, disability, and death. On the other hand, very minor variations can be identified which seem to have no effect on the ability of the host to function in his milieu.

Somewhere between these two extremes may lie a spectrum of inborn human variation whose existence is unproven, whose nature is unknown, and whose effects upon the host are undetermined. It may be genetically and/or non-genetically determined. Its effects may be indirect, subtle, or delayed. Its expression may depend upon a unique concert of other inborn as well as postnatal environmental factors, without which the variant may never have an opportunity for expression. Such a hidden interplay between genetic and environmental factors is illustrated by experiments in which the administration of cortisol to pregnant mice results in cleft-palate in the offspring. This effect, however, is seen only in certain inbred strains of mice and not in others (Smithberg, 1967).

Individual propensities for the development of certain diseases later in life may be a function of inborn variation; such variation might provide the correct setting for the action of various extrinsic agents in the etiology of such diseases as cancer, atherosclerosis, emphysema, hypertension, and mental illness. Environmentally conditioned inborn variation may, in addition, play a role in determining individual uniqueness with regard to various biologic, psychologic, and social functions—aging, intelligence, specific aptitudes, talents, and so on. Provocative hints of such remote relations are beginning to appear (Brozek, 1966). The documentation of additional examples of inborn variation and of their significance in postnatal as well as prenatal life will undoubtedly be forthcoming.

References

Apgar, V., and Stickle, G. (1968), Birth defects: their significance as a public health problem, J. Am. Med. Assoc., *204*:371.

Bearn, A. G., and Parker, W. C. (1965), Genetics and evolution in three human serum proteins, *in* New Directions in Human Genetics. Birth Defects: Original Article series, *1*:57.

Bloom, A. D., *et al.* (1968), Cytogenetics of the *in utero* exposed of Hiroshima and Nagasaki, Lancet, *2*:10.

Brady, R. O. (1966), The sphingolipidoses, New Eng. J. Med., *275*:312.

Brent, R. L. (1966), Immunologic aspects of developmental biology, Adv. Teratol., *1*:82.

Brill, A. B., and Forgotson, E. H. (1964), Radiation and congenital malformations, Am. J. Ob. Gyn., *90*:1149.

Brozek, J. (1966), The biology of human variation, Ann. N. Y. Acad. Sci., *134*:497.

Carpenter, G. G., Auerbach, V. H., and DiGeorge, A. M. (1968), Phenylalaninemia, Ped. Clin. N. Am. *15*:313.

Carr, D. H. (1969a), Chromosomal abnormalities in clinical medicine, Prog. Med. Gen., *6*:1.

Carr, D. H. (1969b), Chromosomal errors and development, Am. J. Ob. Gyn., *104*: 327.

Carr, D. H. (1969c), Lethal chromosome errors, *in* Comparative Mammalian Cytogenetics, K. Benirschke, Ed., Springer-Verlag, New York.

Chang, T. M. S., and Poznansky, M. J. (1968), Semipermeable microcapsules containing catalase for enzyme replacement in acatalasemic mice, Nature, *218*:243.

Chicago Conference (1966), Standardization in Human Cytogenetics, Birth Defects: Original Article series, Vol. II, No. 2.

Childs, B., and Der Kaloustian, V. M. (1968), Genetic heterogeneity, New Eng. J. Med., *279*:1205, 1267.

Childs, B. (1970), Sir Archibald Garrod's conception of chemical individuality: a modern appreciation, New Eng. J. Med., *282*:71.

Clegg, J. B., *et al.* (1968), Hemoglobin synthesis in betathalassemia, Nature, *220*:664.

Cooper, L. Z. (1968), Rubella: a preventable cause of birth defects, Birth Defects: Original Article series, Vol. IV, No. 7, p. 23.

Day, R. W. (1966), The epidemiology of chromosome aberrations, Am. J. Hun. Gen., *18*:70.

Dreyfus, J. C. (1969), The application of bacterial genetics to the study of human genetic abnormalities, Prog. Med. Gen., *6*:169.

Edwards, R. G., Bavister, B. D., and Steptoe, P. C. (1969), Early stages of fertilization *in vitro* of human oocytes matured *in vitro,* Nature, *221*:632.

Elizan, T. S., and Fabiyi, A. (1970), Congenital and neonatal anomalies linked with viral infections in experimental animals, Am. J. Ob. Gyn., *106*:147.

Ferriera, A. J. (1969), Perinatal Environment, Charles C Thomas Co., Springfield, Ill.

Fialkow, P. J. (1966), Autoimmunity and chromosomal aberrations, Am. J. Hum. Gen., *18*:93.

Franklin, E. C. (1967), Genetic polymorphism of gamma globulins in man, Am. J. Med., *43*:1.

German, J. (1969), Chromosomal breakage syndromes, Birth Defects: Original Article series, Vol. 5, No. 5, p. 117.

Gruenwald, P. (1968), Deprivation of the human fetus: forms, causes, significance, *in* Diagnosis and Treatment of Fetal Disorders, K. Adamsons, Ed., Springer-Verlag, New York.

Harris, H. (1966), Genes and enzymes in man, Cancer Res., *26*:2054.

Harris, H. (1969), Enzyme and protein polymorphism in human populations, Brit. Med. Bul., *25*:5.

Hers, H. G., and Van Hoof, F. (1970), The genetic pathology of lysosomes, *in* Progress in Liver Disease, Vol. III, H. Popper and F. Schaffner, Eds., Grune and Stratton, New York.

Hsia, D. Y. Y. (1967), Clinical variants of galactosemia, Metabol., *16*:419.

Jacobs, P. A. (1969), Structural abnormalities of the sex chromosomes, Brit. Med. Bul., *25*:94.

Jagiello, G. (1967), Streptonigrin: effect on the first meiotic metaphase of the mouse egg, Science, *157*:453.

Kelley, W. N., *et al.* (1969), Hypoxanthine-guanine phosphoribosyl transferase deficiency in gout, Ann. Int. Med., *157*:453.

Kohn, G., *et al.* (1970), Mosaic mongolism, J. Ped., *76*:874.

LaDu, B. N., Jr. (1969), Pharmacogenetics, Med. Clin. N. Am., *53*:839.

LaDu, B. N., Jr. (1967), Genetic variation in metabolic disorders, *in* Amino Acid Metabolism and Genetic Variation, W. L. Nyhan, Ed., McGraw-Hill, New York.

Lanman, J. T. (1965), Transplantation immunity in mammalian pregnancy; Mechanisms of fetal protection against immunologic rejection, J. Ped., *66*:525.

Lowe, C. U. (1969), Modification of human metabolism, Am. J. Dis. Child., *118*: 817.

Mathai, C. K., and Beutler, E. (1966), Electrophoretic variation of galactose-1-phosphate uridyltransferase, Science, *154*:1179.

Matsumoto, H., Koya, G., and Takeuchi, T. (1965), Fetal Minimata disease, J. Neuropath. Exp. Neurol., *24*:563.

Mellman, W. J., and Kohn, G. (1970), Human cell cultures–their use in the investigation and diagnosis of disease, Med. Clin. N. Am., *54*:701.

Migeon, B. R., *et al.* (1968), X-linked hypoxanthine-guanine phosphoribosyl transferase deficiency: heterozygote has two clonal populations, Science, *160*:425.

Murayama, M. (1967), Structure of sickle cell hemoglobin and molecular mechanism of the sickling phenomena, Clin. Chem., *13*:578.

Nadler, H. L. (1969), Prenatal detection of genetic defects, J. Ped., *74*:132.

Nichols, W. W. (1966), The role of viruses in the etiology of chromosomal abnormalities, Am. J. Hum. Gen., *18*:81.

Nowack, E. (1965), The sensitive phase of thalidomide embryopathy, Humangenetik, *1*:516.

Nowell, P. C. (1969), The biological significance of induced human chromosomal abnormalities, Fed. Proc., *28*:1796.

Oski, F. A., *et al.* (1969), Congenital hemolytic anemia with high-sodium, low-potassium red cells, New Eng. J. Med., *280*:909.

Pauling, L. (1964), Molecular evolution and disease, Bul. N. Y. Acad. Sci., *40*:1.

Pinsky, L., and Krooth, R. S. (1967), Studies on the control of pyrimidine biosynthesis in human diploid cell strain, Proc. Natl. Acad. Sci., *47*:925, 1267.

Plotkin, S. A., and Vaheri, A. (1967), Human fibroblasts infected with rubella virus produce a growth inhibitor, Science, *156*:659.

Price, J. (1967), Human polymorphism, J. Med. Gen., *4*:44.

Priest, J. H. (1968), Human cell culture: an important tool for the diagnosis and understanding of disease, J. Ped., *72*:415.

Proceedings of the Seminars on the Lesch-Nyhan Syndrome (1968), Fed. Proc., *27*: 1021.

Ranney, H. M. (1960), Clinically important variants of human hemoglobin, New Eng. J. Med., *282*:144.

Redding, A., and Hirschhorn, K. (1968), Guide to Human Chromosome Defects, Birth Defects: Orginal Article series, Vol. IV, No. 4.

Renwick, A. (1969), Progress in mapping human autosomes, Brit. Med. Bul., *25*:65.

Scriver, C. R. (1969a), Treatment of inherited diseases: realized and potential, Med. Clin. N. Am., *53*:941.

Scriver, C. R. (1969b), The human biochemical genetics of amino acid transport, Ped., *44*:348.

Sever, J., and White, L. R. (1968), Intrauterine viral infections, Ann. Rev. Med., *18*:471.

Smith, L. M., Jr., Huguley, C. M., Jr., Bain, J. A. (1966), Hereditary orotic aciduria, *in* The Metabolic Basis of Inherited Disease, J. B. Stanbury, Ed., Blakiston Co., New York.

Smithberg, M. (1967), Teratogenesis in inbred strains of mice, Adv. Teratol., *2*:258.

Smithells, R. W. (1966), Drugs and human malformations, Adv. Teratol., *1*:251.

Solomon, S., and Friesen, M. G. (1968), Endocrine relations between mother and fetus, Ann. Rev. Med., *19*:399.

Sotelo-Avila, C., and Shanklin, D. R. (1967), Congenital malformations in an autopsy population, Arch. Path., *84*:272.

Stewart, A. L., *et al.* (1969), A chromosome study of unselected live-born children with congenital anomalies, J. Ped., *74*:449.

Stoller, A. (1969), Virus-chromosome interaction as a possible cause of cases of Down's syndrome and other congenital anomalies, Adv. Teratol., *3*:113.

Tschudy, D. P. (1969), Porphyrin metabolism and the porphyrias, *in* Diseases of Metabolism, P. K. Bondy, Ed., W. B. Saunders Co., Philadelphia.

Uchida, I. A., Holunga, R., and Lawler, C. (1968), Maternal radiation and chromosome aberrations, Lancet, *2*:1045.

Walzer, S., Breau, G., and Gerald, P. S. (1969), A chromosome survey of 2,400 normal newborn infants, J. Ped., *74*:438.

Warkany, J., and Kalter, H. (1961), Congenital malformations, New Eng. J. Med., *265*:993.

Weatherall, D. J. (1967), The thalassemias, Prog. Med. Gen., *5*:8.

Wyngarden, J. B. (1970), Genetic control of enzyme activity in higher organisms, Biochem. Gen., *4*:105.

INDEX